D1583640

Health Policy Reform

Global Health versus Private Profit

Health Policy Reform

Global Health versus Private Profit

John Lister

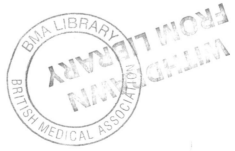

LIBRI
PUBLISHING

First published in 2013 by Libri Publishing

ISBN 978 1 907471 78 0

A CIP catalogue record for this book is available from The British Library

Design by Carnegie Publishing

Cover design by Helen Taylor

Printed in the UK by Ashford Colour Press

Libri Publishing
Brunel House
Volunteer Way
Faringdon
Oxfordshire
SN7 7YR

Tel: +44 (0)845 873 3837

www.libripublishing.co.uk

Contents

PRAISE FOR *HEALTH POLICY REFORM – GLOBAL HEALTH VERSUS PRIVATE PROFIT*

"As the global health discourse embraces the idea of universal health coverage, the political economy of health care remains largely camouflaged in 'zombie' ideas with deep roots in a neoliberal orthodoxy. Ironically strengthened, rather than weakened, by the global financial crisis, the poverty of these ideas is laid bare in Lister's masterful, detailed and highly readable account. Re-asserting the importance of a Marxist analysis to health reforms of the past three decades, his book makes an important contribution to informed health-policy debates and should be essential reading for progressive health reformers worldwide."
Ronald Labonté, Canada Research Chair, Globalization and Health Equity, and Professor, Faculty of Medicine, Institute of Population Health, Ottawa

"John Lister's latest book is also his most ambitious – the summation of half a lifetime's research and teaching on health and health policy by a committed scholar–activist. He pulls no punches and ideologues of the market will hate it. But they will have to raise their game if they want to criticise it in terms of evidence and logic. Lister's knowledge of the literature, lucid reasoning and clean prose are a class act. A major achievement which everyone interested in health needs to read."
Colin Leys, Emeritus Professor of Political Studies, Queen's University, Canada, joint author of *The Plot Against the NHS*

"John Lister's book is a must-read for anyone passionate about universal health care [who wants] to understand its greatest obstacle and where we must focus our fight."
Anna Marriott, Health Policy Advisor, Oxfam GB

"The Soviet model of communism collapsed in the late 1980s because it became clear that the governments concerned were being run for the benefit of a tiny elite, the *nomenklatura*. Two decades later, it has become equally clear that the neoliberal model of capitalism is doing the same, with wealth being concentrated in the hands of a few while the living conditions of 99 per cent of the population are being steadily degraded. Yet not content with riches beyond belief, this new global elite is mounting a sustained attack on what remains of the welfare state, with health care as one of their prime targets. In this penetrating, highly readable and extremely well-researched book, John Lister takes on the narrative being peddled by this elite and their cheerleaders and shows that there is an alternative, but it is up to us to seize it."
Professor Martin McKee CBE, Professor of European Public Health, London School of Hygiene and Tropical Medicine

"Now is a critical time for public health care and health systems across the world: bank bail outs and loan agreements are being used to front market-driven reforms in public services in what is rapidly becoming a race to the bottom. John Lister's book gives us valuable insights into the forces arrayed against universal health care and how capitalism is consuming our basic rights and entitlements. It's up to us to organise to take them back."
Allyson Pollock, Professor of Public Health Research and Policy at Queen Mary, University of London

"This is a welcome update of John Lister's 2005 book: and an encyclopaedic, thoroughly referenced update it is! The use of extensive direct quotes puts important issues in the words of real protagonists in our field. A critique of the 'missing' Millennium Development Goals addresses the serious omission of health care for the elderly ('customers' nobody wants) and the attitudes of the market towards mental health and towards disability ('the hidden giants'). It goes without saying that John Lister gives us a crucial, elegant and comprehensive update on many issues as we begin to discuss what next after the MDGs."
Claudio Schuftan, People's Health Movement, Ho Chi Minh City

"John Lister's excellent book explains how worldwide disintegration of public healthcare services into competing commercial units has passed into law, and how organised professionals, carers and users are now starting to organise resistance. It is essential reading for all students and practitioners of health and social care who want to understand the context within which they are now being condemned to work, and start changing it."
Julian Tudor Hart, author of *The Political Economy of Health Care: A Clinical Perspective*

"John Lister has written a really important book. In meticulous detail and with enormous care, it combines a comprehensive critique of the failings of the neoliberal approach to the provision of UK health care with a careful exploration of the links between poverty, inequality and health. The book combines a comprehensive overview with a series of high-resolution, high-definition case studies to explore illustrative examples in meticulous detail and without using doctrinaire paradigms. In all, this book is as ambitious, as all-encompassing and as undoctrinaire as to qualify as a sort of Doyal's *Political Economy of Health* for the 21st century."
Professor John S Yudkin MD FRCP, Emeritus Professor of Medicine and former Director, International Health and Medical Education Centre, University College London

Acknowledgements

As I have outlined in the Preface, a large number of people have played a part in enabling me to complete this book, so this is for them: I apologise to any who feel overlooked. And while they have inspired the strengths of the book, the weaknesses, as ever, are my responsibility alone.

Huge thanks of course once again to my publishers Libri and their whole team who have again done sterling work, and in particular to main man Paul Jervis and tireless copy-editor Matt Skipper for their efforts and encouragement, and Matt's vital eye for detail.

I also want to thank Coventry University for the support which enabled me to attend a number of international conferences, and the Faculty of Health and Life Sciences and the School of Art and Design which helped me to organise a successful IAHPE conference in the University in 2009.

Internationally, I want to mention Natalie Mehra and her fantastic trade-union colleagues and supporters in the Ontario Health Coalition, friends and colleagues working with Alexis Benos in the Aristotle University in Thessaloniki, and the brave Spanish anti-privatisation campaigners in CAS Madrid, all of whom have extended practical support and hospitality, welcomed me on visits and helped shape up my experience and deepen my knowledge.

At home, where the fight has had to go on against the neoliberal health policies of a Labour government and now a Conservative-led coalition, I am hugely grateful for the continuing support from colleagues and campaigners from Keep Our NHS Public including Wendy Savage, Jacky Davis, Louise Irvine, Peter Fisher, Ron Singer, Julian Tudor Hart and Allyson Pollock. Union activists from UNISON, Unite, BMA and others have loyally stood firm to support my own organisation, London Health Emergency, to keep it running and me still employed and annoying people after almost 30 years. I also want to thank a very select group of union officials whom I won't name, to spare any embarrassment on their behalf, but whose support has been invaluable.

And thanks, too, to all the many dedicated campaigners, academics and activists I have been lucky enough to work with, all of whom work to keep the spirit of criticism and the principles of universal health care and social solidarity alive.

But above all, I have been hugely privileged to have had such support from close family and friends for the work that I am sure they feel has consumed an unreasonable amount of my time and energy over the years. I could not have completed this book without the efforts and support every step of the way from my wife Sue (Professor Sue Lister, whose tremendous work on quality and service improvement has also helped inspire my work), my son Kevin and his lovely, patient family.

This volume is dedicated to Kevin's two daughters, Kaitlin and Abbie: both they and their mum Elaine owe their lives to timely intervention at crucial moments by the National Health Service. They epitomise for me the need to preserve the values and the model of the NHS – as a universal health care system, free of charge at point of use – and the need to extend these principles for their generation around the world, and for later generations too.

The fight goes on until we win!

John Lister, Oxford, April 2013

Preface

This book is the outcome of a long-held ambition to rewrite and improve upon the first edition (*Health Policy Reform: Driving the Wrong Way*, 2005). Although I was proud of it, pleased with the content and delighted to get a platform to raise the issues to a new and wider public, the book always felt to me much too much like the PhD thesis which was its central element.

My ambition to do better was fuelled and driven by the experiences I have been lucky enough to have in discussing these issues with a widening circle of friends, colleagues and campaigners: the book opened new doors for me. As a journalist who had previously worked almost exclusively on issues relating to the National Health Service in the UK, and largely in England, the new debates, conferences and projects with colleagues around the world brought a dramatic expansion of my knowledge and understanding.

The invitation from two Canadian academics, Ron Labonté and Ted Schrecker, to join the Global Knowledge Network they were organising, to feed into the ongoing WHO Commission on Social Determinants of Health[1], brought me into contact with a whole group of academics, many of whom were also active in the People's Health Movement – including David Sanders and Claudio Schuftan. These people and the work of the Network enabled me not only to update and deepen my awareness of the WHO, but also challenged me to come to terms with the concepts of Public Health and engage more seriously with the goals of Alma Ata, including Primary Health Care. The positive impact of that is visible in this volume.

Ongoing work with Alexis Benos and colleagues from the International Association of Health Policy (Europe) (IAHPE) helped deepen my understanding of the ways in which health 'reform' processes were rolling out in different parts of Europe.

At the IAHPE conference I organised in Coventry University in 2009, we were lucky enough to get Anna Marriott from Oxfam to present her paper 'Blind Optimism' on the role of the private sector in health care in developing countries. This led to me further updating my analysis of the World Bank – and learning more about Oxfam and other NGOs, some of which have developed an increasingly serious critique of neoliberal policies and their impact on the poorest peoples.

A journey to Istanbul to celebrate the Turkish translation of the book challenged

---

1   This working party was originally going to be given the more explanatory title of the Social Inequalities Working Party, but the name was changed to the clumsier, vaguer alternative as a result of US pressure.

me to explore the contradictions of the Turkish health reforms. Working visits to Ontario, Finland, Spain and Greece, and further conferences in Canada, South Africa, Greece, Turkey, Sweden and Brazil, have all helped to keep me learning and underlined the need to rework the first book to do justice to these friends, campaigners and colleagues who had helped and inspired me on my way.

This book was planned some time ago: but work on it had to be put on hold as the British coalition government embarked upon a major new offensive, with legislation to break up the National Health Service and reduce it to a pool of taxpayers' money to purchase care from a fragmented 'market' of competing providers. Despite the problems explaining the complexity of the proposals and the desperate lack of press and media coverage, especially in the early months, we fought a growing rear-guard action against the White Paper and the Health & Social Care Bill, from the summer of 2010 to the spring of 2012. In the latter stages of the fight, more professional organisations and health unions joined in, the Labour Party belatedly began to take a limited interest and, in the final few months while the Bill was in the House of Lords, we even managed to get some headline coverage, although BBC reporting remained consistently poor. Despite our efforts, it was all too little and too late to stop the Bill, which became law in April 2012, and is due to be fully implemented from April 2013. Only when we had definitely lost that fight could I find time to devote myself to the work on this wider project.

The main body of the book was written between May and October 2012, and even as it was completed a new phase of dialogue over Universal Health Care was beginning to take rather ambiguous shape. There were positive and impressive declarations on this from the WHO and international institutions, and apparently ambitious initiatives by governments, including the Indian government – although subsequent events in India have called into question the extent of genuine commitment, and the outcome of the process remains largely undecided.

There will never be a point at which all is settled and a complete and final analysis can be made of an almost infinitely complex world picture: but the final chapter on alternatives tries to give the most up-to-date assessment of where we are and what could be done. I have steered clear of 'maximal', completely idealistic solutions (socialist revolution etc.) which make up in simplicity what they lack in plausibility and connection to the real world we have to live in. In my own opinion, the key is not to map out ever-more-elaborate visions of the ultimate solution, but to identify tangible means to get there, building on what we have, working through policies which help to develop consciousness and awareness as people embrace them and put them into practice.

In the work of finishing and preparing the text, a number of 2013 documents have been added to the mix, where this was appropriate and possible without substantial rewriting. As a journalist by trade, I have always craved the most up-to-date sources for any story and have done my best to bring this approach to the work on this book.

The rewriting, expansion and updating has led to the first part of the book becoming book-length in its own right, leaving no space for the more detailed country studies, 40 of which formed the final chapters of the first edition. But the timescale for the work did not allow the type of analysis I wished to develop for this section either: so the plan is now that these will be a separate volume, hopefully in the form of an on-line e-book, to be completed in 2014. This will also allow a limited updating to follow up on the debates and developments on Universal Health Care.

All this offers an opportunity to widen still further the base for the research for this second volume: I would love to be able to include the widest range of the most up-to-date material and, where possible, interview material. So my invitation to international readers of this book is that if you agree with the approach and the analysis you see here, and would like to see your country and information on developments which concern you reflected in the analysis in volume 2, please contact me, j.lister@coventry.ac.uk, preferably in English, and we can work together on it.

This volume concludes, as its title suggests, that 'global health is in conflict with private profit' and points out that most people are clear which they would prefer to prevail. It is intended to encourage all those working for political and popular action to challenge the status quo. We are many: the neoliberals are few. Their control and their world view blocks global progress on every front.

The facts and the arguments are on our side: but good ideas must be turned into political action to change the world. That's why this book offers not only evidence to academics and professionals but also fuel to boost and encourage campaigners. It's a book I hope will not sit gathering dust on library shelves but be brandished – even used as a weapon – by those fighting for change. A reinforced hardback edition may yet be needed to ensure we win!

John R Lister
Oxford, March 2013

Chapter one

Introduction

For many present it must really have felt, at least briefly, as if another world of health care was really possible. In September 1978 the Alma Ata Declaration and its objective of ensuring 'Health for All' by 2000 were endorsed by an overwhelming vote of the WHO's World Health Assembly, comprising 3,000 delegates from 134 governments and 67 international organisations (de Rivero 2003, Irwin and Scali 2005). But sadly, this marked both the high-water mark and the beginning of the end for the 'post-war political consensus' that had brought the extension of welfarist policies to most Western European countries, and even seen some of these same principles briefly extended to the newly independent countries of former colonial empires.

Thirty years later there was little evidence of that consensus when the WHO attempted to revive the spirit and values of Alma Ata amid a chaotic process of 'reforms', austerity, privatisation and marketisation of health care. Indeed, many of the countries that had functioning welfare states including access to health care in 1978 have in recent years been scaling down and undermining these systems (Lister 2011b, McKee et al. 2012, McKee and Stuckler 2011) while, ironically, some of the emerging economies, especially in Asia (India, China, Indonesia, Philippines), are moving in the opposite direction and beginning to put some rudimentary forms of social protection and affordable health-care provision in place (*Economist* 2012).

Meanwhile, for the low-income developing countries stuck at much lower levels of economic development and plagued by a heavy burden of disease – and increasingly, by the additional problem of chronic, noncommunicable disease – the picture is very different. The global solidarity of Alma Ata has been replaced by a refusal of donors to support the extension of free health care even in the most desperate of emergency situations; an insistence on retaining user fees for treatment and drugs; and proposals by donors and aid agencies to impose rationing of antiretroviral drugs – all in the name of 'sustainability', eking out the pathetically limited resources and pretending this amounts to a health-care system (Ooms 2006). A more recent World Bank report on the fiscal dimensions of HIV/AIDS repeats a very similar position (Baker 2012). For all the talk about 'universal health care' which is now coming from the WHO, 'Health for All' remains a very distant dream indeed in these poorest countries, and the debates over policy seem to have hardly advanced at all.

East and West

The values of Alma Ata in 1978 were not by any means limited only to countries which held on to the capitalist system or to those which enjoyed democratic government. Eleven years before the fall of the Berlin Wall, the rhetoric of social solidarity and universal entitlement also rang out loudly, if not sincerely, in the internal and external propaganda from the bureaucratic 'socialist' regimes of Eastern Europe and the Soviet Union. Free health care provided by the state had proved to be a useful tool to help legitimise the totalitarian bureaucratic regimes installed within the new Soviet 'buffer zone' in the aftermath of the Second World War – especially in the aftermath of decades of authoritarian governments and inadequate health cover which preceded the war (Wohlforth and Westoby 1978).

In Asia, the Chinese and newly independent Vietnamese regimes also projected egalitarian values in 1978, especially with the memories of the recent health benefits of Mao's 'barefoot doctors' in rural China (Horn 1969, Weiyuan 2008). After the 1959 Cuban revolution, Che Guevara's insistence on the need for an independent medical school resulted in a new generation of doctors, many of whom were then dispatched overseas to deliver health care in developing countries. They helped spread the message of the health gains to be achieved (despite the relentless US blockade) from a new model of health care – one combining public health, primary care and high-tech medicine – even in what had been, up to that point, a small, profoundly unequal and economically vulnerable developing country (Brouwer 2011).

Even the fascist regimes that had just fallen, in Portugal with the 1974 revolution and in Spain with the death of Franco, had cynically maintained and extended the social health insurance systems that they had taken over, recognising the need to buttress the state by providing some form of collective safety net to provide health care for those who would otherwise have none (Lister 2008a). In Chile, the brutal Pinochet dictatorship which had taken power with CIA support five years earlier, while basing its policies on the harsh notions of the Chicago school of free-market economics and ruthlessly privatising and slashing back Chile's public sector, did not privatise the public health-care system: preferential treatment and incentives were given to the private sector, but the public hospitals (although with drastically reduced resources) were retained as a lower-tier service for those too poor to afford the private schemes (Lister 2005).

The outlier: the US rejects collective provision

By 1978, therefore, almost every country with control over its own destiny and policies had established some form of collective provision to finance or provide health care – with one notable and massive exception. The US health-care system, for a combination of social, economic and political reasons, had emerged as a 'medical–industrial complex' – too large and powerful even then for any federal administration to restructure or reform fundamentally (Relman 1980). It has remained as an outlier ever since. The continued travails of the Obama administration – in its limited attempts to reduce the massive numbers of uninsured and in its vain quest to make health insurance affordable and attainable to low-income families – have again demonstrated the pre-eminence of the health insurers and health providers. They have enormous resources to dedicate to the funding of political lobbying. This is one among many political, cultural and ideological obstacles to be surmounted if radical health-care reforms are ever to be implemented or soaring health spending contained in the 'land of the free' where health care is widely unaffordable and health bills are the major cause of personal bankruptcy (Garrett 2012).

It is hardly surprising that the three principles at the centre of the Alma Ata policies were not only anathema to the Americans but everywhere flew in the face of the prejudices of the ideological right wing. The Alma Ata declaration was a simple and clear statement of an alternative approach based on:

- Health as 'a fundamental human right'. 'Health' itself had already been defined by the WHO as 'a state of complete physical, mental and social well-being, and not merely the absence of disease or infirmity'. This has subsequently been criticised as over ambitious and/or idealistic, but it has the strength of clearly locating health and health care in a public health context. It embraces the health concerns of all ages and issues beyond physical health, rather than adopting a narrower, less-effective curative focus or 'medical model'.

- Universalism: the ambition to include the whole population within a protective network of health care and health services, available on the basis of clinical need rather than the ability to pay. This led inevitably to WHO opposition to user fees and charges, which everywhere have the effect of excluding the poor.

- Primary health care: this was defined as 'essential health care based on practical, scientifically sound and socially acceptable methods and technology made universally accessible to individuals and families in the community through their full participation and at a cost that the community and country can afford.' To be effective, local, flexible and responsive primary care – incorporating physicians, nurses, midwives and other health professionals and support staff – should be combined with the availability of accessible hospital and secondary care services for those who need them. Primary health care also requires systematic promotion and enhancement of public health, through preventive measures, education, immunisation, and provision of clean water, nutrition and sanitation.

(Lister 2007)

The apparent, if fragile, consensus around these values in 1978 was already being undermined by an economic crisis that had been growing, deepened by the 'oil shock' of 1973–4. It was soon challenged by political developments which changed the dominant ideological paradigm of the capitalist countries.

The next year, 1979, brought the election of Margaret Thatcher in the United Kingdom; then Ronald Reagan was elected US President in 1980. The economics of monetarism and the politics of deregulation and privatisation, which these key figures advocated, foreshadowed a revitalisation of the brutal ideology elaborated by Friedrich von Hayek and Milton Friedman, which was soon dubbed 'neoliberalism' (discussed in more detail in Chapter 2 below). This powerful political and ideological shift resulted in a 'Washington Consensus' in which the leading global financial institutions, the Washington-based International Monetary Fund (IMF) and the World Bank, more openly embraced the political and ideological agenda of the US Administration (Williamson 1990, 2000). By contrast, the Geneva-based and more inherently 'democratic' WHO, with its Assembly of member states, was increasingly marginalised and starved of resources from the early 1980s (Godlee 1994a, b, c).

As a result, despite all the high hopes, the progressive values and aspirations of the Alma Ata declaration had few lasting echoes in the years that followed. One notable exception was in Canada, where a fundamental reform of health care had begun in the mid-1970s (almost 30 years after the big wave of welfarist reforms in Europe). This was against the grain even then, as many capitalist governments moved towards austerity. In 1984 the Canadian government completed the legislative framework for its Medicare system, which broke definitively from the previous US-style system based on private insurance and instead established a tax-funded 'single payer' system, giving universal cover: health care was to be provided by private, but non-profit, providers. Profit and private medicine were squeezed out of the mainstream Canadian system and the rapid year-by-year increases in spending, which Canada had until then shared in common with its US neighbour, were brought under control. From 1984, each year saw a growing divergence between soaring costs in the US and the more controlled share of GDP allocated to health spending in Canada (OECD Health Data 2012).

Social action to improve health

There was also another important dimension to the principles behind the Alma Ata declaration: the commitment not simply to establish systems that can deliver health care and health services to those who have become ill, but also to take *social action* to improve living conditions, thereby improving health and limiting or preventing the development of ill health amongst whole populations. This is based on a clear materialist understanding that population health is determined to a large extent by social conditions – housing; access to clean water and sanitation; living standards and basic income sufficient to ensure adequate nutritional intake; education; and equitable access to health resources when needed, including immunisation against preventable disease.

Action on these 'social determinants of health' requires involvement in areas well beyond the conventional remit of health ministries, hospitals and health professionals. Like the original 'public health' movement, much of which had its roots not in modern medicine but in nineteenth-century local government, action on social determinants seeks to secure improvements in health for whole populations (Irwin and Scali 2005). It also requires a commitment to progressive and equitable policies by governments over the long term rather than the offering of short-term 'quick fix' or 'early win' solutions.

This principle has also proved controversial and support for it has fluctuated in the last 35 years, along with levels of commitment to the implementation of policies flowing from it. In the mid-1980s, the WHO followed up on Alma Ata with conferences and discussions on ways to act on social determinants of health, culminating in the 1986 Ottawa Charter for Health Promotion. This identified eight key factors which between them determine health: peace, shelter, education, food, income, a stable ecosystem, sustainable resources, social justice, and equity (Irwin and Scali 2005).

However, it proved much more difficult to live up to these principles and deliver the necessary action in the political climate that emerged during the 1980s and consolidated in the 1990s. A 25-year balance sheet on the eight key factors shows that advances have really only been made on income – and this in an uneven way, heavily distorted by the very large-scale changes and growth of the Chinese economy (Yuwei 2010) and by the desperately low level of daily income which is used as a benchmark for 'middle income' compared to 'low income' on a global scale.[1]

Market forces

On most other issues, movement has been in the opposite direction. The World Bank, the ideological centre of the Washington consensus, became increasingly involved in financing health initiatives from 1980 and, from 1983 onwards, began discussions on alternative approaches that could bring some of the market mechanisms and disciplines favoured by the Bank into the financing and organisation of health care (Lister and Labonté 2009). In 1985, the year in which the US administration first withheld its contributions to the WHO – after conflicts over WHO campaigns against the promotion of manufactured baby milk, against smoking tobacco, and over family planning initiatives which worked with organisations that provided abortion – the Bank's David de Ferranti produced an initial paper on 'paying for health services in developing countries'. Two years later, the year after the Ottawa Charter was adopted, the Bank itself published its own very different 'Agenda for Reform' along similar lines, outlining the case for the imposition of user fees in even the poorest countries, and other measures to limit demand and government intervention in a potential health-care market (De Ferranti 1985, World Bank 1987).

The Bank was in a strong position to press for its policies to be adopted: many governments in developing countries faced financial problems and required financial support to implement any health programmes at all – and the Bank, echoing the Structural Adjustment Programs of the IMF, began to require health systems to be structured along lines it proposed as a condition of guarantees and loans. In many countries these political proposals were happily received and implemented by authoritarian governments, most of which in any case looked to Washington, London and Paris for their political allegiance rather than to developing popular support through radical or progressive policies at home.

By 1993, just 15 years after Alma Ata, the WHO had been almost completely sidelined as a global leader on health policy as a result of US economic sanctions. Despite its occasional progressive-sounding rhetorical flourishes, with regular talk of equity and targeting resources at the poor, the Bank's approach as the new dominant global voice on health care completely contradicted the Alma Ata principles of health

---

1 'Income group: Economies are divided according to 2011 GNI per capita, calculated using the World Bank Atlas method. The groups are: low income, $1,025 or less [$2.8 per day or less]; lower middle income, $1,026–$4,035 [$2.8–$11.05 per day]; upper middle income, $4,036–$12,475 [$11.05–$34.2 per day]; and high income, $12,476 or more' (World Bank 2012b).

as a human right, universalism and primary care. Its discussion had matured into a full-scale *World Development Report*, rather inappropriately titled *Investing in Health*. This landmark report consolidated the previous policy proposals, but went further in suggesting that the poorest countries should abandon any hope of developing comprehensive or universal health-care systems, instead focusing on delivering a 'minimum package' of health measures, largely confined to public health, immunisation and maternal and child health measures, and costing an estimated $12 per head per year. Everything else should be left to private sector (World Bank 1993).

Unaffordable minimum

However, the proposal for the policy was not linked to any proposals to ensure that many of the poorest countries, most of which were spending far less than $12 per head, were able to afford even this most minimal of minimum packages – indeed, WHO figures show that at least 19 countries were still falling below this average spend per head (14 of them in Africa) even by 2000. The estimated cost of providing even a minimum package of health provision has risen to an overall average of $38 per head per year ($34 in low-income countries, CMH 2002: 157): however, the most recent WHO figures suggest 24 countries are still currently below even this minimum level of spending, 18 of them in Africa (WHO 2012c).

There were other major political upheavals taking place at the same time. In 1989 the Berlin Wall was brought down by popular action and many of the totalitarian so-called 'socialist' bureaucracies of Central and Eastern Europe fell in rapid succession: soon afterwards the Soviet Union itself began to splinter and the once all-powerful political leadership of the Communist Party apparatus (as reshaped into a counter-revolutionary police state by Stalin) was weakened, then marginalised. Most Stalinist rhetoric was revealed to the world as empty bluster and, in particular, its 'egalitarianism', imposed everywhere only from the top down by a vicious secret police apparatus, was shown to countless millions at home and abroad to be a flimsy façade concealing the privileges of a vast and corrupt nomenklatura. This in turn helped lend a spurious credibility to the claims of the US and to those seeking to privatise the East European economies to be somehow 'liberating' a captive people and allowing them the 'freedoms' of a competitive market system. Socialism, and with it Marxism, was widely seen as having been discredited by those who had spuriously claimed to uphold it.

These changes in government and apparatus were followed by a growing process of privatisation and restructuring which also had a profound impact on health-care systems. The empty promises, hidden inequalities, chronic under-investment in health care, corruption and appallingly low standards of health systems in self-styled 'socialist' regimes have been supplanted by the equally fraudulent, corrupt and exploitative systems and illusory promises of benefits in newly emerging 'markets' and privatised systems.

In 1992, the rich nations' club, the Organisation for Economic Cooperation and Development (OECD), began its efforts to monitor, compare and spread market models in health care, promoting barely tested models of 'reform' (OECD 1992).

By 1997, the World Bank's Health Nutrition and Population directorate had developed beyond *Investing in Health* to set out a more comprehensive strategy aimed at creating embryonic health-care markets in even the poorest countries (World Bank Group 1997).

The WHO's retreat from universalism

The following year, the new ideological climate was reflected when a new director general of the WHO took over, former Norwegian premier Gro Harlem Brundtland, steering the organisation firmly away from its Alma Ata principles and recruiting senior staff from the World Bank. The resultant *World Health Report 2000* (henceforth *WHR 2000*[2]) simultaneously embraced Bank principles and explicitly rejected some of the WHO's own core values, notably the commitment to universalism (which was replaced by a new oxymoronic notion of 'selective universalism') and the preference for public-sector provision and funding of services. This report unleashed an angry debate. The new, controversial WHO policy criticised the Alma Ata declaration's failure to embrace the private sector and instead embarked on the quest for 'Global Public Private Partnerships' with pharmaceutical corporations and with the Bank (Lee et al. 2009).

As this retreat was taking place, a little-noticed but significant report by the European Health Management Association examined the available evidence for reforms that had already attempted to apply market methods to health care. The EHMA concluded that the policies do not work either to improve efficiency or to reduce costs (EHMA 2000). This underlines a crucial aspect of the drive for neoliberal and market-style 'reforms': their implementation has continued despite the absence of any substantial evidence that they either work or even partly deliver their claimed objectives. Even the most committed managers don't believe in them.

In the same year, it became inescapably obvious that the attempt to deliver 'Health for All by 2000' had not succeeded. The WHO had already shifted ground to some extent, arguing for the vaguer and more distant prospect of 'Health for All in the 21st Century' (WHO 1998), but even this position proved untenable in the harsh ideological climate. The debate over why this failure had occurred continued, alongside the development of a completely different approach from the Bank and others who had clearly never shared the initial aspirations and were more concerned to see the extension of free-market values – in which health care is seen as a commodity to be bought and sold rather than a human right, universal or otherwise. The wider aspiration to 'Health for All' was replaced by the narrower, more target-based 'Millennium Development Goals', adopted by the UN in 2000 – with the timetable set another fifteen years into the future. In fact, the resources to make it achievable were not agreed in outline until the G8 meeting of 2005 (UN Millennium Project 2005).

In place of the health focus of Alma Ata, only three of the eight Millennium

---

2   This is an abbreviation of the title; *WHR 2000* is listed in the bibliography under WHO 2000.

Development Goals related to health, and even these related only to a part of the population. The targets were reducing child mortality rates, improving maternal health and combating HIV/AIDS, malaria and other diseases. While it is possible to see the entire package of MDGs as a commitment to work on the social determinants of health (Irwin and Scali 2005), it is also clear that the three specific health-related MDGs fall far short of the much-broader aspirations to improving health for all as spelled out in the Alma Ata declaration. And, like the World Bank's 1993 proposals for a minimum package of health-related policies, there was no initial commitment to raising the funds necessary to implement the MDGs.

The new health donors

The change of direction also brought an increased privatisation of health aid for developing countries: the Bill & Melinda Gates Foundation was formed and a steadily growing share of the resources available to implement immunisation and other programs began to come from newly formed donor bodies including the Global Fund to Fight AIDS, Tuberculosis and Malaria, and George W. Bush's Presidential Emergency Plan for AIDS Relief (PEPFAR).

With the very partial exception of PEPFAR, which at first clearly reflected the ideological prejudices of its bigoted Republican initiator, George W. Bush, and sought very firmly to steer the use of funds and spell out which social policies were acceptable and which were not, these huge funds are notable for the absence of any specific governmental control. Like PEPFAR, they all lacked any real democratic accountability, most of all to the people in the recipient countries, who have no voice on the policies implemented on their behalf. They are run from the top and have mostly developed top-down 'vertical programs' based almost exclusively on medical models and paying only limited if any reference to public health principles or the longer-term development of sustainable health-care systems in the recipient countries. Indeed, there are concerns that some programs serve to attract local health professionals to better-paid and more satisfying work, leaving the country with even weaker health provision than before (Muraskin 2004, Vujicic et al. 2011).

In other words, while embracing an overtly benevolent approach to the peoples of the poorest countries, these donor organisations – themselves to a large extent recycling vast surpluses from highly profitable businesses and economies which exploit cheap raw materials and labour from the developing world – have epitomised and entrenched, rather than questioned, the underlying ideology of neoliberalism and capitalism.

In 2004, the Bank was forced into a partial retreat from its 1993 approach, as pressure from campaigners secured the declaration that the Bank had 'no blanket policy' of imposing user fees for health care. This came only after dozens of countries, most notably in Sub-Saharan Africa, had been obliged by Bank pressure to impose fees for even the most basic health services. Yet the evidence was unequivocal and damning: the policy which the Bank had promoted for more than a decade had generated little if anything in the way of resources for health care, but was shown to have one clear effect: sharply reducing demand and access to treatment especially amongst the poorest, while doing nothing to reduce health needs (Oxfam 2006, Human Rights Watch 2006, Save the Children 2005).

The Bank's retreat was partial and temporary: in 2007, its explicitly pro-privatisation wing, the International Finance Corporation (IFC), published a major report 'The Business of Health in Africa', researched for it by McKinsey. This proclaimed the merits of expanding the private sector in even the poorest countries and the prospects for profitable markets for health care (IFC 2007b). The IFC committed itself to raising a total of $1 billion for the promotion of private-health-care initiatives in Africa and two similarly named private equity funds were launched – with little impact (see Chapter 4 below).

After the crash

The following year came the collapse of Lehman Brothers and the dramatic crash of the banking sector in the US and much of Europe, heralding a fresh drive to austerity and an even more vigorous retreat from the ideals of universalism and solidarity in health and welfare.

The OECD redoubled its efforts to promote market-based 'reforms' despite an embarrassing failure to identify any significant evidence that the reforms already implemented had delivered any improvements in efficiency or reduction in costs (OECD 2009, 2012c). And in Britain, the right-wing coalition government elected in 2010 embarked on a massive, trailblazing plan to reform the 62-year-old, £100-billion-per-year National Health Service, changing it from an overwhelmingly publicly funded and delivered service into a fund of taxpayers' money to purchase services from a range of private non-profit and for-profit providers (Lister 2012a, Pollock and Price 2011, Leys and Player 2011).

Behind the British reforms and many similar reform packages in the high-income countries lies an ideological commitment to the use of markets and competition as ways to deliver and improve health care, despite the continuing lack of evidence that this is a viable approach.

The process towards greater privatisation of provision and greater competition has been effectively a one-way process only, with no obvious means by which the new policies can be reversed, even when proven ineffective, or more collective, planned and progressive systems reintroduced. Increasingly restrictive competition laws are being policed globally by the WTO, in Europe by the EU and at national level by governments, which in many cases also have their own political agenda for extending competition and privatisation. These restrictive laws are available to be exploited by private companies, large and small, seeking to carve out a growing share of what have until relatively recently been public or social insurance budgets for health care, which in many cases has previously been delivered by public or non-profit providers (Leys and Player 2011).

Moreover, the ideology of reliance on markets and competition is being pushed by the large-scale multinational corporations which draw large profits from health-care budgets, whether these flow from individual out-of-pocket payments, insurance companies or from governments and collective health-care provision. The same large-scale corporations, headed by the drug companies, have acted as the major obstacles to President Obama's limited attempts to reform the chaotic and costly American health-care system. Their vast lobbying power – reinforced by the individualist and anti-collective zeal of the so-called 'tea party' Republican movement in the US – has held up the implementation of the reform legislation and raised questions as to how far even the laws that have been passed can be implemented.[3]

For these private companies, issues of cost efficiency in the use of public and collective health funds are very much secondary to their continued ability to secure large and growing profits for their shareholders and extravagant salaries for their leading executives. Their benchmark is not value for the tax dollar so much as the percentage of tax dollars that are recycled back into the private sector by spending on private provision – and (in the case of the insurance companies) how little of that money can be spent on delivering services for patients[4] and how much retained for shareholder dividends and executive salaries.

Upholding and reinforcing these values, another lucrative product of US capitalism is the vigorous trade in consultancy services, delivering research and other services for the World Bank and for governments around the world. US-based companies like McKinsey, Abt Associates and John Snow Associates, along with consultancy services from UnitedHealth, the largest US health insurer, have become profitable global brands, exporting the dubious nostrums and assumptions of free markets and the US health-care system whilst preaching a parsimony in other countries that contrasts with the colossal levels of waste, fraud, overhead costs and inefficiency in the US system (Kelley 2009).

The scavengers of capitalism

To cap it all, there has been a global rise in 'private equity' capital – comprising venture capital firms, growth capital and buyout firms. Private equity companies produce nothing and commit to nothing: in general, they are not even using their own money for their acquisitions but borrowing at relatively high rates of interest, intending to make even higher returns on their short-term investments. They use the selective investment power of vast accumulated wealth to speculate with industries and services, buying up with borrowed ('leveraged') funds, asset-stripping and reconfiguring to maximise short-term returns. They have also developed successful strategies for exiting investments when growth rates fall back after 3–7 years, 'harvesting' further profits by selling the company on. Their targets have

---

3   By contrast, American health-insurance companies that in 1996 set out to create new markets for their policies in Latin America and in Europe (after having largely exhausted the potential subscriber base of middle America and the larger employers in the US) have been happy to do a deal with President Obama in which private health insurance remains at the very centre of even the reformed system. There is freedom to raise insurance premiums without question by as much as 9 per cent per year – well in excess of the likely increases in income for all but the wealthiest American families (Waitzkin and Iriart 2004).

4   Interestingly, this spending is described as 'medical loss'.

increasingly included health care, where companies have seen the possibility of returns as high as 20 per cent or more (Robbins et al. 2008). The role and scale of private equity has increased especially rapidly in the US (where the flow of capital into the health-care industry doubled in the year 2010–11 (Bain & Co. 2012)) but has also become much more significant in the UK, where PE has a stake in, or owns, many of the key players in providing private-sector health care.

The impact of all these key players on health-care systems goes well beyond the huge sums of money involved and the resulting strain on financial resources. The model they seek to build upon runs counter to the values and fundamental approach of primary health care and social determinants of health:

- The pharmaceutical companies and all of their vast lobbying power are clearly committed to a medical, curative approach, and the use of high-tech measures to treat diseases after the effect, rather than preventative or public-health approaches. The rest of the private sector is also committed to this same approach which is the easy route to profits.

- The large-scale private donors that fund many interventions in developing countries in general sign up to the same approach; indeed, many of their partnerships and vertical programs work hand in hand with the pharma corporations.

- Private hospital chains – and the private insurance companies that widen their potential market – are also based on a curative, medical model. They add to this a focus on uncomplicated surgery rather than more risky or complex treatment and an exclusive approach which limits access for the very poor (and very sick), who cannot afford the fees or premium payments and, in many cases, cannot access the buildings themselves, which tend to be located in more prosperous urban areas.

- Meanwhile the private financiers seeking to build large new hospitals and facilities through 'Public Private Partnerships' are also promoting a model which fundamentally contradicts the values of Alma Ata, by focusing heavy investment in highly centralised and expensive hospital facilities. This drains resources from potential investment and funding of more local and accessible community and primary-health-care services, mental health and chronic care. The recently opened PPP/PFI-funded hospital in Sub-Saharan Africa, the new Queen Mamohato Memorial Hospital in Lesotho's capital Maseru, is set to consume upwards of 30 per cent of the country's limited health budget, despite having a catchment covering just 16 per cent of the population. Profits from the scheme, not least from the private hospital co-located on the new hospital site, will largely go to the principal operator, the South African multinational hospital company Netcare (Lister 2011a).

- And private equity, like a carrion crow, stands by to seize upon openings for profitable investment, giving fresh and speedy impetus towards more intensive commodification of health care – with not the slightest commitment to improving health outcomes or balancing the availability of services with levels of social need.

The squeeze on spending

While the ideological foundations of collective health care have been actively under-mined from these directions, the financial foundations have also been weakened by the impact of the banking crisis and the resultant economic slump and widespread austerity policies. National health services in the Spanish state and Portugal, Greece and Ireland have faced very substantial cutbacks in government resources as a result of their countries' membership of the Eurozone, along with additional pressures as growing unemployment results in tens of thousands of workers losing their work-place-funded health insurance. Countries in Eastern and Central Europe have also faced severe economic pressures and sought to impose cutbacks and cash-cutting 'reforms' (McKee et al. 2012).

But regressive reforms have not been restricted to countries in dire financial straits. One of the few countries to have bucked the trend towards slump, Turkey, is putting into place a new system which, on one level, extends a limited health insurance to wider sections of the population (Tatar and Kanavos 2006), but with cover limited and patients required to 'top up' their entitlement with out-of-pocket spending ('extra billing' of up to 30 per cent of the amount covered by the insur-ance). This policy is strongly favoured by private insurers, who will expect many middle-income families that can afford to do so to take out insurance against the risk of substantial top-up costs (OECD 2008). Romania and Bulgaria, with their publicly funded health systems crumbling from chronic lack of investment, haemorrhaging doctors and health professionals by the thousand to better-paid posts in the US or elsewhere in the EU, and plagued by low morale and corruption involving massive bribes to be paid to access 'free' treatment, have been looking towards similar poli-cies. However, public resistance to this and other regressive reforms has impeded the progress of the Bulgarian government and been a major factor in the downfall of at least two Romanian governments since 2011 (Tsolova 2012, Ilie 2012).

Elsewhere, the decline and collapse of former Semashko-style systems in Eastern and Central Europe has also been followed by the legacy of rock-bottom levels of spending and the problem of what to do with their extensive networks of large hospi-tals. These are neither economic to operate in the existing framework nor attractive as going concerns for private health care. Low average wages, low government spending and an accumulation of social problems resulting in long-term health needs mean that the systems are far from ideal for any full-scale market in health care. Salaries averaging well below €1,000 per month mean that the large majority of people of working age are unable to afford the market price of any treatment they may need or to deliver regular premium payments high enough to guarantee profits to insurers. Pensioners and young children are even less financially viable for potential private insurers. These health systems were first assembled by what is now a failed political and economic system; but they are now classic examples of market failure by another, older economic system to deliver comprehensive and universal health care. Only the wealthiest can feel immune from these problems and, in the main, these can only escape by accessing private care in other countries.

Markets where nobody wants to compete

Similar contradictions beset the development of health-care systems in the poorest developing countries. Despite the World Bank's injunctions to keep government involvement to a minimum and to provide only the most basic 'essential package' of health services (World Bank 1993), the private sector has shown little if any interest in filling the resulting gap. They are reluctant to target a 'market' in which a huge proportion of the population lacks the ability to pay even a portion of the market cost of the treatment and services they require. Instead, they have opted to focus a limited effort on targeting the emerging middle class and wealthy minority in up-and-coming developing countries (IFC 2007b). Research has confirmed that the least-useful allies for governments in developing health-care systems are for-profit private health providers. These are less likely to coordinate with public services; prone to inducing demand, giving more costly treatment and prescribing more drugs in order to keep their profits high; more focused on those with high incomes; and less likely to stick around when donor funds stop flowing (Forsberg et al. 2011). Moreover, the rhetorical endorsement by the Bank and IFC of the notion of health insurance (whether at 'micro' or state level) in low-income countries has been less than convincing, especially in the light of experience that shows the schemes that have been introduced have been partial in their cover and their reach, in some cases to the extent of hardly offering insurance at all (Akazili 2012, Marriott 2011).

The other big issue for the Bank has been its policy on user fees, which seems to be in some disarray. Despite its formal change of policy in 2004 (moving to 'no blanket policy' on user fees), the Bank has not explicitly sided with those arguing for access to health care to be free; nor has it been proactive in urging countries to lift the fees that have already been put in place. For some that have done so, such as Zambia and Uganda, the desperate shortage of public funds has created fresh problems as pent-up demand puts services under strain (Gilson and McIntyre 2005). The Bank now seems to have endorsed and funded one scheme offering free access to maternity care (Marriott 2011).

Evidence for a different model

By contrast, fresh evidence has emerged that systems based on public ownership and control are a more effective means of delivering the objectives of universalism, equity and cost-effective treatment than any of the standard policy proposals embraced by the World Bank. The ambitious Equitap project ('Equity in Asia-Pacific Health Systems') was a collaborative research project of 17 institutional partners from the UK, Europe and Asia, which spent three years jointly assessing equity in the health systems of 16 Asian nations. Principally funded by an EU INCO-DEV research grant, it also received additional funding support from DFID, the World Bank, the WHO, the UN (UNDP), the Rockefeller and Ford Foundations, and the governments of Hong Kong SAR and Taiwan. The authors state that 'The work of the Equitap study represents the most comprehensive and systematic assessment to date of the available empirical evidence of health system equity performance in Asia'

(Rannan-Eliya and Somanathan 2005b).

The project concluded that universal, free or extremely low-priced services are more effective at achieving equity and widening access than two-tier systems with specific services 'targeting' the poorest and, moreover, that user fees could be reduced or eliminated by governments spending as little as 2 per cent of GDP on a universal health system that would give most benefit to the poor. Other major studies have also reviewed the literature and experience on public services in developing countries and underlined the importance of well-organised and properly resourced universal public services, pointing to the gaps and failings that are common occurrences when profit-driven private services are involved in the delivery of services intended to benefit poor people (Emmett 2006). Unger and colleagues press the case for integration of health care in place of failed 'disintegrated' medical models based on disease control, commodification and privatisation of health care (Unger et al. 2006).

Further examples of initiatives and projects which can be regarded as successful can be found in WHO (Spinaci et al. 2006) and World Bank studies. Significantly, none of these successful models revolves centrally around the neoliberal/market-driven policy menu: most involve only non-profit NGOs, if they require any private-sector input at all.

In an extensive book of articles studying the impact in Asia, Africa, Latin America and the Caribbean of the standard reform menu from the standpoint of sexual and reproductive health, De Pinho rejects the idea of a 'global blueprint' and argues that, to be successful, reforms have to be 'context-specific' rather than centrally driven by agencies and donors. She calls for more research to identify some of the information required to ensure services – especially those for sexual and reproductive health – are correctly focused (Ravindran and de Pinho 2005).

Publicly funded private sector

The stakes are high: not only are health and health care crucial political issues for elected governments around the world, they are also a focus of eager attention from a powerful private sector that seeks to carve out more profit from a larger share of the global total of almost $5 trillion annually spent on health – much of which still remains (at least in most of the wealthier OECD countries) dominated by public-sector and not-for-profit organisations. This is because the 'inverse care law' dictates that, in most instances, the communities and individuals most subject to ill health and in need of health care are those least able to pay a market price for it.

Ironically, the contradictions of health care under capitalism mean that the expansion of the private sector still hinges not on the creation and functioning of a free market, but on prising open and plundering the coffers of social insurance and public-sector health budgets in the wealthiest countries. Slicing more from collective budgets and transforming non-profits into for-profit businesses are key to the private sector's efforts to move beyond simply redividing the estimated $500–550 billion global total of profits (Bain & Co. 2012).

Nowhere in the world can the private sector on its own sustain a comprehensive or universal health-care system or even a competitive market in health (Hart 2010: 36): it needs a combination of public subsidy to train staff with either the scope to cherry pick the most financially lucrative patients, or public provision for the most demanding cases that will never be profitable to treat. The pattern throughout the world still confirms that the private for-profit sector in particular is averse to risk and, for this reason, unwilling to deliver full-scale emergency services or open-ended services for the chronically sick and elderly – unless a substantial premium payment is attached to guarantee a profit stream.

The five-fold crisis for health care

Thirty-five years after Alma Ata, health-care systems around the world are now confronting a five-fold crisis, driven by the convulsive crisis of the capitalist system:

- A crisis of health needs driven by climate and ecological change, described by authoritative research as 'the biggest global health threat of the 21st century' (Costello et al. 2009);

- A rapidly rising, costly burden of noncommunicable disease (Anderson 2009);

- A crisis of financial resources – health-care systems in many high-income countries face cuts whilst those elsewhere continue to suffer a desperate lack of funds;

- A crisis of human resources (WHO 2006a); and

- A crisis of fragmented, 'disintegrated' systems, riven by competition and conflicting interests, in which rational planning and efficient use of resources, or any coordinated international effort to resolve the problems listed above, are effectively blocked (Unger et al. 2006).

Each of these issues could be a full-scale book in its own right. Whilst the final four points are addressed in varying degrees of detail in the chapters that follow, it is worth looking a little more closely here at the one which has been the least discussed. This is in many ways the most insidious threat to health and health-care systems across the planet: climate change and the degradation of the environment by a rapacious and chaotic capitalist system.

Awareness of the health implications of climate change has been growing since the 1980s and has been driven by the establishment of the Intergovernmental Panel on Climate Change in 1988. The IPCC has been at the forefront of mapping the acceleration of man-made climate change through rising emissions of greenhouse gases coupled with deforestation, which has stripped the planet of the natural means to trap carbon from the atmosphere. The changing climate poses threats to health through various direct and indirect channels, including changing patterns of disease, growing problems of water and food insecurity, and extreme climatic events that endanger human settlements and force mass migration from low-lying coastal areas and river basins (Costello et al. 2009).

Broader but related environmental damage also threatening health comes from: air pollution in cities and rural areas; fouled drinking water; the deterioration of the ozone layer, which threatens to bring increases in a variety of health problems; soil exhaustion and resulting desertification; the over-fishing of seas and oceans and the damage caused by vast trawling operations to coral reefs and the seabed; the huge and unmanageable accumulation of waste, including highly radioactive nuclear wastes; and food contamination (Löwy 2006).

Poor bear the brunt

The damage done to the climate and environment will have its most brutal impact on the poor, the elderly, the very young and the vulnerable. It is unfolding in a profoundly unequal world in which 10 million children already die each year; 200 million children under five are not developing to their potential; 800 million people go to bed each night hungry; and more than 20 per cent of the earth's population (1.5 billion people) lack access to clean drinking water (Costello et al. 2009: 1,694).

Responding to the growing threat, in 2003 the WHO set out the main health risks of climate change and calculated that, comparing 2000 with 1990, 150,000 additional deaths and 5.5 million 'disability-adjusted life years' could be attributed to just four aspects of climate change[5] (WHO 2003: 18). Left out in this estimate are: the more complicated possible impacts of changes in air pollution; altered transmission of other infectious diseases; effects on food production from changed environment for plant pests and diseases; drought and famine; population displacement as a result of crop failure or natural disasters; destruction of health infrastructure through natural disasters; conflict and war over natural resources; and the direct impact of heat and cold. The WHO warns that:

> Human populations vary in their susceptibility, depending on factors such as population density, economic development, local environmental conditions, pre-existing health status and health care availability.
>
> (WHO 2003: 31)

It's clear from this that the most vulnerable are the poorest people in the poorest countries – the countries which are the lowest producers of greenhouse gases and the least able to effect any change in the environmentally unsustainable activity of the wealthiest and heaviest-polluting countries.

The *Lancet*-UCL project on climate change, spelling out the scale of the challenge, also points to the need for technological development to boost food output while maintaining the integrity of ecosystems and developing less-polluting methods of farming (agriculture is responsible for an estimated 22 per cent of greenhouse gases). Technological solutions are also needed to improve the treatment, recycling and desalination of water; to create low-carbon building materials and energy-efficient buildings; and to produce alternative supplies of non-polluting energy (Costello et al. 2009: 1,695). But the project also notes that the private sector is an unreliable partner in developing green technologies, especially for low-income countries, and warns that this gap will need to be filled by public funding.

---

5   Food- and water-borne disease (as measured by diarrhoea episodes), vector-borne disease (malaria cases), weather-related natural disasters (floods and landslides) and malnutrition.

Malnutrition and capitalism

Together with low birth weight and suboptimal breastfeeding, malnutrition is estimated to cause the deaths of 3.5 million mothers and young children every year, and to cause stunting in a third of children under five in developing countries. While there are technical 'fixes' that address vector control,[6] the threat of millions more people suffering malnutrition is a far more complex question, exposing the harsh contradictions of capitalism:

> In the case of malnutrition due to food shortages, public health and medical approaches can provide, at best, only temporary relief, and a sustainable solution can only be found in measures that match food supply to need and ensure economic entitlements in the most vulnerable groups.
>
> (Costello et al. 2009: 1,702)

While a complete change in the political and economic system is required to tackle the underlying problems of inequalities, poverty and deprivation in the poorest countries, the urgency of reducing carbon emissions and stemming the reckless plundering of the planet's resources for the profit of a super-rich minority is obvious. Yet the capitalist system makes it almost impossible to coordinate a serious effort to change course. Seventeen annual international conferences have taken place within the Convention on Climate Change, yet carbon emissions continue to rise – and are now 50 per cent higher than they were 20 years ago. The June 2012 UN 'Earth Summit' in Rio de Janeiro was larger and cost more than the first such conference in 1992 – and achieved nothing. As satellite pictures revealed even more dramatic melting of the Arctic icecap, government leaders from the UK, Germany and USA were among the 60 leaders that did not turn up from the 190 countries involved, sending second-string functionaries to take their place. Capitalist eyes have remained firmly averted from the necessity to cut emissions, being focused instead on the possibilities for further profitable exploitation through the so-called 'green economy'. This was the main proposal of the Earth Summit organisers – rebranding capitalism, maintaining a firm private-sector grip, and seeking new ways to extend private-sector ownership of natural assets (Conway 2012).

The *Lancet*-UCL researchers conclude their detailed 40-page report by arguing that:

> The most urgent need is to empower poor countries, and local government and local communities everywhere, to understand climate implications and to take action.
>
> (Costello et al. 2009: 1,728)

Yet there is no sign of the poor being empowered at any level. The system grinds on indifferent to the lives and deaths of the poorest, focussing on maintaining and

---

6 For example, mosquito nets, new vaccines, and improved health systems offering swifter diagnosis and treatment.

increasing the profits of the super-rich. In the absence of any concerted action, the deepening environmental crisis will be an added pressure on health services and a driver of social and economic crises in the developing countries, while it also undermines the viability of human life on the planet as a whole.

The right reforms for health

More recent events and findings tend to underline and expand upon the analysis presented in my earlier book, *Health Policy Reform*.[7] This new book is intended as a further contribution to the ongoing debate on which type of health-care reforms can achieve progressive change to benefit those most in need of health care – the poor, the elderly and those suffering from mental illness – something which, despite copious rhetoric, never seems to have been established as a priority in health provision.

More debate, more solutions, more case studies need to be worked through; but the fundamental problem to be addressed is that the market-style policies that are the subject of this critique are driven neither by economics nor by the quest for efficiency. In many cases, they are more costly and more bureaucratic than either the systems they replace or progressive alternatives. They are being driven by the quest for profit and by ideological commitment – in defiance of the evidence and experience of front-line health workers around the world.

For that reason, I make no apology for addressing neoliberal ideology, challenging the assumptions that it builds upon and insisting that more rational, helpful, efficient and economically sound alternatives can and do exist – and offer the only real way forward.

7   Middlesex University Press, 2005

Chapter two

A framework for analysing changes

For those who like to keep their analysis simple and superficial, the paradoxes of health care under capitalism present some serious problems. In a way, the contradiction between the interests of global health and private profit can be summed up in a curious phrase used by the American health insurers to describe every dollar and cent spent on delivering health-care services to their customers: this is described with chilling bluntness as 'medical loss' (Hall and McCue 2012).

Here we have summed up the counterposition of, on the one hand, the material interests, wishes and needs of the *consumers* of health care; and on the other, the competing material interests, wishes and needs of those entrusted with providing care as required. The former pay high and handsome for insurance, either directly as individuals or indirectly, through collective employer-provided cover or through taxation towards Medicare and Medicaid, which many believe entitles them to the best health-care system in the world; whereas the latter provide services in exchange for a generous margin of profit and extravagant expenses which together make up the very substantial 'overhead' costs of health insurance.

So complete is this counterposition that, as Michael Moore's film *Sicko* so clearly documents, major US insurers (and no doubt others, if perhaps on a smaller scale) spend large sums of money and extensive management and administrative effort seeking to ensure that, wherever possible, high-cost claims are not paid and that, in fact, health insurance does not take on the risk of catastrophic cost, but dumps this back in the laps of those needing treatment. Hence the enormous costs of health care remain a major cause of personal bankruptcy in the US, with many of these unfortunate people having falsely believed themselves to be 'insured'.

We also have the naiveté of the customer who is tacitly willing to accept the deduction of a large proportion of the money they pay into the system and the cynicism of the insurer who regards the whole fund as essentially belonging by right to them and their shareholders – and who regards any spending at all on the intended purpose as a 'loss', 'waste' to be minimised. This also illustrates the inequality in power relations and resources between the major insurers, who play the most pivotal role in the massive $2.7-trillion-a-year US health system, and those who are supposed to benefit from this system. Both insurer and insured are notionally 'stakeholders' – but in the kind of relationship which Canadian academic Ted Schrecker has shrewdly compared to the interaction in a garden between cats, on the one hand, and small rodents and birds: 'All are 'stakeholders' in such interactions, but their stakes are quite different' (Schrecker 2011b).

Health care brings other conflicts and contradictions which highlight the real essence of the relationships between consumer and provider: for example, the fact that the cherished neoliberal principle of competition between rival providers (which is allegedly the magic fountain from which efficiency, quality, cost-effectiveness and almost all good things are supposed to flow (OECD 2012c)) can only operate in health care with the aid of very substantial public subsidies. Raised through taxation, these are necessary to ensure that at least some of the services are affordable to the poor. US pharmaceutical corporations depend on price fixing to protect their profits against lower-priced equivalent products from abroad.

In a similar contradiction, the full benefits of new scientific advances, technological and pharmaceutical research cannot be brought to bear on many of the world's most destructive and costly diseases, which blight hundreds of millions of lives, because the drug companies and suppliers who might wish to market any resulting treatment are convinced that the global poor and their governments (who would be their principal customers) simply won't be able to afford them.

Or to take a fourth and final example: the level of actual regulation and control over the quality and safety of private-sector provision has remained so feeble that analysts actually argue that, in some sectors, public-sector provision of services is required in order to 'crowd out' poor-quality but low-cost private-sector providers – whose patchy and deficient care could, for example, result in the emergence of new, drug-resistant strains of HIV and thus reverse years of global effort to contain this health problem (Over 2009: 20–1). Far from being the dynamic driver of quality and efficiency, the private sector is admitted to have become dilatory and dangerous, scooping up profits at the expense of quality and elementary public safety, and insufficiently accountable to anyone – including governments.

System of conflict, crises and contradiction

However, as Bob Evans has so eloquently pointed out (Evans 1997), few if any of these contradictions present themselves obviously to the consumer/customer/patient in their relationship with corporate health care and the system as it appears to them day by day. This study will argue that to draw out and examine such contradictions, a consistent method of approach is required which can embrace the concept of capitalism as a system of conflict, crises and contradiction, split apart the complex whole and analyse its component parts. So, unlike many existing comparative studies of the reform process,[1] this study employs a Marxist framework, seeking to develop an approach based on a political, economic and historical analysis which is therefore able to offer a coherent explanation of events, economic forces, policies and ideologies, while also embracing complexities, contradictions and tensions. A Marxist approach

---

1   These include Flood (2000), Freeman (2000), Moran (1999), Preker and Harding (2003), Ranade (1998), Saltman and Figueras (1997), Saltman et al. (1998), Saltman et al. (2002), Schieber (1997), Scott (2001) and Tuohy (1999).

offers the possibility of a consistent and critical analysis of the context and content of particular policies; and where necessary, will use this to assess the motivation and the material (class) interests which are being served.

This flexible, dialectical approach is of course very different from wooden and dogmatic 'Marxist' assertions that seek to reduce every policy and event to an issue of 'class versus class' or to dismiss health-care systems as purely mechanisms invented by capitalists to control and facilitate reproduction of the working class. Such approaches are boring and laborious to read, lacking both subtlety and credibility in a period where defence of affordable and accessible health care – or fighting for such services in countries where they are not already available – is an active concern of working people and the poor.

In contrast to Marxism, however, the contending analytical methodologies offer a choice between a variety of relatively static, apolitical and ahistorical approaches. This study is primarily one of health-care policy reforms rather than philosophy and methodology, so no attempt is made here to engage in an in-depth explanation or critique of the multiplicity of possible alternative approaches.[2]

The strength of the Marxist method, as exemplified in Lesley Doyal's landmark study *The Political Economy of Health* (1979), is that it recognises that history is made by a complex interaction of individuals, interest groups and social classes – 'all the many wills' that combine to make history, though not in a manner of their own making or choosing (Marx 1852). The underlying roots of ideology, politics, culture – and the health of individuals and communities – are seen to lie in the material conditions of societies divided along class lines.

Marxism (in common with the 'Marxism-light' approach of political economy) recognises that the provision of health care has to be understood as an issue of both political and economic significance (Armstrong et al. 2001). As a political phenomenon, the provision of health care is both a device to secure the legitimacy of ruling regimes and (as understood by Bismarck and by authoritarian and fascist regimes since) a potential way of binding sections of workers to the state: but at the same time, it is also a material benefit to the working people who receive it, a concession to their strength and a focus for their demands.

Historical context

As a tool for analysing the development of the health reform agenda, Marxism also sets the development of social and political phenomena in a historical context and recognises that ideas and policies change and evolve over time, rather than emerging ready-made in the minds of individuals. Marxism does not reject the need for progressive reforms nor dismiss the possibility of achieving significant improvements

---

2 It is not the purpose of this study to engage in a detailed examination of, or polemic with, the various academic Marxists, neo-Marxists, post-Marxists and critical theorists, in the hands of many of whom, in the period since the rise of Stalin and especially since the post-war period, 'Marxism' has evolved in a very different direction, back towards the levels of abstraction and contemplative disengagement which Marx himself rejected in 1845 (Pierson 1998, Therborn 1996).

for working people even within the framework of capitalism: but Marxists do not automatically conclude that all reforms are socially progressive and neither do they see reforms as an end in themselves.[3]

Rather than assuming that in every case 'Reform means positive change' (Berman and Bossert 2000), a Marxist analysis of 'reforms' to the health-care system within a capitalist framework will explore and evaluate the inevitable limitations, contradictions and unresolved political aspirations that will arise from even ostensibly progressive measures implemented by capitalist governments – such as the Turkish government's reforms to give all citizens universal access to a standardised benefits package. This is achieved through social health insurance which not only makes room for the inclusion of private hospitals as services providers, but also promises to result in many middle-class people taking out complementary private health insurance cover (OECD 2008).

A number of the global bodies whose policies have helped drive reforms in health care and which are central to this study – notably the World Bank, the International Monetary Fund (IMF), the Organisation for Economic Cooperation and Development (OECD) and USAID – are themselves 'the financial agencies of international capital' (Alcock and Craig 2001: 4), institutions founded with the specific and declared objective of sustaining and developing capitalism (and, in the case of USAID, supporting US foreign policy). This makes it especially relevant to subject their proposals and their involvement in health-care policy to a Marxist critique.

Marxism is also very pertinent because health care is not only a vast complex of organisations that deliver varying health treatments to countless millions: it is also perhaps the world's biggest single industry, turning over around £5 trillion per year on the latest WHO statistics and employing around 60 million staff worldwide (WHO 2006a). Even within the larger health-care industry, sub-sections – such as many of the major pharmaceutical corporations – enjoy budgets and turnover larger than many governments of smaller and low-income countries, and exert far more political influence than most elected politicians.

The politics of reformism

However, the predominant line of criticism and opposition to market-style reforms and neoliberal-influenced policy reflects not a Marxist but a reformist perspective, which sees it as possible to resolve or at least ameliorate the gross inequalities which

---

3   *The Communist Manifesto* notes the success of British workers in forcing the legislation of the Ten Hours Bill and stresses (Section IV) that 'The Communists fight for the attainment of the immediate aims for the enforcement of the momentary interests of the working class, but in the movement of the present they also represent and take care of the future of that movement' (Marx and Engels 1970). The Communist International, in the *Theses* of its Third and Fourth Congresses, developed tactics and a programme which required the new communist parties to be involved in every 'individual and partial' demand of the workers (Adler 1980). Trotsky's 1938 *Transitional Programme* also insisted that 'The Fourth International does not discard the programme of the old "minimal" demands to the degree to which these have preserved at least part of their vital forcefulness. Indefatigably it defends the democratic rights and social conquests of the workers.' (Breitman and Stanton 1977: 113–14)

persist within global capitalism through a series of policy reforms that will also leave the underlying system (and its class divisions) intact. Many of the policies of the World Health Organization derive from precisely this reformist approach, which helps to explain events such as the 2011 Rio Summit, in which heads of state and technical experts adopted a series of largely empty and rhetorical declarations pledging action on Social Determinants of Health. This flies in the face of the very different policies being carried out in practice by governments and global bodies, especially in the aftermath of the 2008 banking crisis[4] (Kirigia et al. 2011).

A Marxist standpoint offers the possibility of identifying the socially progressive aspirations of such policies, while also demonstrating the recurring contrast between progressive rhetoric and less progressive reality – the ideal and the real. Most of the literature and documents on which this (and almost any) study must be based also assume that the capitalist market – especially if it could be regulated in some way – offers a suitable model for the development and reform of health-care services. Many studies and policy proposals reflect the prevailing 'health-care reform agenda' which, as Drache and Sullivan (1999: 1–2) point out:

> has been dominated by economists and policy-makers narrowly focused on deficit reduction and spending controls. ... All advanced economies now admit some role for markets in their financing and delivery systems.

This study aims to critique and challenge this approach, and to strengthen the case for a consistent alternative.

The underlying contradiction of health care under capitalism

Health is by no means simply a product of health care and medical intervention: it is arguable that most of the gains in increased life expectancy and improvements in health have resulted not from health care or medical treatment at all, but from improved living standards, housing, access to clean water and sanitation, education and basic public health measures. Health is above all a social construct and, as such, inevitably reflects class differences in living standards and conditions. This means that effective action to improve health and address illness must combine interventions that go to the roots and causes of ill health – the Social Determinants of Health – with steps to ensure that the poor, rural populations and the lowest-income urban communities, men and women alike, can access suitable health-care services when needed, without facing obstacles of affordability, distance or discrimination (WHO 2012a).

---

4 Kirigia and colleagues (2011) surveyed African governments on the known and expected impact of the global financial crisis: of those that responded, more than a third had been notified by the Ministry of Finance that the budget for health would be cut; almost one in six had been notified by partners of their intention to cut health funding; nearly two-thirds indicated that the prices of medicines had increased recently; more than three-quarters had seen prices of basic food stuffs increase; and almost half said levels of unemployment had increased since the onset of the global financial crisis.

Of course, this ignores the fact that some men (the poor, ethnic minorities and those who are other than heterosexual) and all women already face various forms of discrimination at various levels, most notably in the arena of health care. Women's needs as consumers of health care are often neglected, while women also form the overwhelming majority of the health-care workforce. In an unpaid capacity, too, and often with little if any support from any other agency, women shoulder most responsibility in the provision of informal care for family members, young and old. Within the health workforce, the hierarchical structure often means that the senior management positions and strategic roles are held by men (Langer and Catino 2006). The health needs of women include maternal mortality, reproductive and sexual health, cervical and breast cancer, while heart disease in women is a neglected killer that often goes undetected. Living longer on average than men, older women are often also dependent upon health- and social-care systems and are the most at risk where these are inadequately funded, subjected to fees (since many women face problems accessing family budgets) or cut back (Nanda 2002). Many working women are still on incomes lower than their male counterparts, resulting in lower pensions for older women and pushing more into poverty (Lethbridge 2011). So while health reforms are clearly not specifically designed to impact most heavily on women, those that are not specifically designed to meet women's needs will fail properly to address key social determinants of health.

Analysis of the health-system reforms has to begin from a grasp of what is a fundamental underlying contradiction: each of the structural and managerial reforms that will be examined is an attempt to remedy the continuing – possibly inevitable – failure of the profit-driven capitalist system to deliver a universal, comprehensive and affordable supply of health-care goods and services to a global 'market' which is driven by health needs rather than consumer 'wants' and which is dominated numerically by people too poor to pay a profitable rate for them (Drache and Sullivan 1999).

While reformist approaches seek ways to reduce inequalities in health, the results of these reforms are always limited by the fact that capitalism itself is a system that both thrives on and generates inequality – in status, income and living conditions. This inequality is reinforced through political mechanisms which are themselves controlled or heavily influenced by the wealthiest minority: in Britain, for example, BBC journalist Robert Peston pointed out in 2008 that:

> The new super-rich have the means through the financing of political parties, the funding of think-tanks and the ownership of the media to shape Government policies or to deter reform of a status quo that suits them.
>
> (Peston 2008)

The low wages and high rates of exploitation of the majority are key to the profits of the wealthy and the sky-high salaries of the senior managers who run the system on their behalf. While entrepreneurs are lavishly rewarded for taking 'risks' with the capital they have already accumulated, workers are much less lavishly compensated for risky work such as mining, construction, work in polluted environments and so on – or for the accidents and disability they may suffer as a result. And to ensure that there are always enough applicants for any job, there is a 'reserve army' of unemployed on minimal, subsistence-level income, which also helps to discipline those in work and hold down salaries and aspirations. Where the home-grown workforce rejects especially arduous or low-paid work, ways will be found to use migrant workers, legal or illegal. All this helps ensure that even while incomes and living standards for many have improved in cash terms since the Second World War, levels of inequality have continued to increase (Ortiz and Cummins 2011, Mathiason 2012).

Another way of looking at this same contradiction is that, while most health care is required by poor people, whose average levels of chronic ill health are far higher than those of the wealthy, most political and economic power in deciding whether or not appropriate services should be made available lies in the hands of the rich.[5]

Perhaps the simplest embodiment of this contradiction between 'need' and demand is the dilemma facing the pharmaceutical companies over the development of a vaccine to prevent further infection in people already suffering from the AIDS virus. Owen Dyer (a *Financial Times* correspondent) aptly summed this up in 2003:

> The economics of such a vaccine would be difficult. Dr Berkley points out that the target market would be in poor countries. There would be little demand in the wealthy markets where vaccine developers might hope to recoup investment.
>
> (Dyer 2003)

Economic overview

A major global industry

Health care is one of the world's biggest industries, potentially affecting every individual on the planet at some time in their lives. Policy decisions affecting health-care systems therefore affect not only service users but also potentially the jobs, pay and conditions of the staff employed as professionals, and the large numbers – often on very low comparative rates of pay – providing support services.

Health-related industries, notably those manufacturing pharmaceuticals and modern diagnostic equipment, along with US private health insurers and health maintenance organisations, are among the world's biggest companies, with turnover in tens of billions of dollars. They generate huge returns for shareholders: for over 30 years from 1960 to 1991, the US pharmaceutical industry was first or second in the Fortune 500 league table of post-tax profitability (Mossialos and Mrazek 2002).

This level of commercial investment places additional pressures on health-care systems: for example, one of the hardest factors to control in health services anywhere in the world has been the upward pressure in pharmaceutical spending – and the profit margins jealously guarded by the multinational corporations which dominate this market. But the requirement to maintain and increase large profits flows from the very nature of capitalism itself – to justify the huge levels of capital investment.

---

5   This in turn may be seen as an alternative and updated variation on the 'inverse care law' identified by Julian Tudor Hart more than 40 years ago, according to which the provision of accessible health care is inversely proportional to the level of need (Hart 1971).

The sheer scale of the multinational drug corporations now acts to maintain their monopoly position, making it almost impossible for any new competitors to enter the market.

Health care as a special type of commodity

Capitalism is a system driven by the accumulation of capital, through the production and exchange of commodities. Commodities, as Marx analysed in *Capital*, embody two contradictory values: their use value, without which they would not be saleable in the marketplace; and their exchange value, defined by the hours of necessary labour time for their production (Marx 1867).

Marx begins his critique of the whole system with the analysis of the commodity, seeing in it a microcosm of the social and economic relations within society. An analysis of the health-care episode can in similar fashion offer a basis on which to appraise the predominant values and social relations in a given society.

Health care shares with other commodities the combination of 'use value' (in this case additional healthy life, which for the patient remains the key factor). But since it is the product of human labour, embodying necessary hours of work (and in many cases access to modern, capital-intensive 'means of production'), it also embodies potential 'exchange value'.

Like other industries under capitalism, health care has moved from small-scale and often primitive 'petty' production (the early predominance of the individual practitioner) to larger-scale socialised production (the development of large and complex modern hospitals and health-care systems, which rely on the combined efforts of a wide variety of professionals, technicians and support staff). Costs long ago grew beyond the point where any but the wealthiest individuals could afford to pay medical bills without some form of insurance, at least against catastrophic costs: as a result, health insurance itself, as an intermediary industry, has emerged as a major player and a source of profit.

As a system, capitalism has consistently demonstrated its tendency to develop and revolutionise the productive forces, and with them science and technology (Hoggett 1994); but it has not done so evenly. The underlying quest to accumulate surplus value dictates which techniques and which areas of production receive the greatest level of investment.

In health care, since the emergence of scientific medicine, the most profitable areas have been hospital-based and pharmaceutical-based treatments: and on a global scale, the greatest investment has focused on the health issues affecting the wealthiest countries, those with the greatest ability to pay.

The limits of markets

Markets as a means for the exchange of commodities and the realisation of surplus value are the natural state of capitalism. Goods and services are primarily produced *not* for their use value, to match social need, but for their *exchange value*, to generate profit. In a classical market, producers compete to maximise profits while mini-mising the costs of production: the logical conclusion of successful competition is to win maximum market share and to force competitors out of business (Malin et al. 2002).

Perversely, therefore, the outcome of the ultimate in competition can be its very opposite – *monopoly*, control of a market by a few large-scale producers. While competition can be seen as a means to force producers to hold down costs and prices, monopoly gives producers the opportunity to maintain *high* prices and to exclude new entrants to the market. As the Russian Bolshevik leader Lenin argued in 1916 in his keynote analysis *Imperialism: the Highest Stage of Capitalism*, the exten-sion of the capitalist market and major corporations onto the global level opened up the possibility of *worldwide* monopolies, delivering 'super-profits' to the ruling rich minority at the expense of poverty and exploitation in developing (many of them then colonial) countries (Lenin 1917).

The inherent drive to monopoly within the competitive dynamic is possibly even more obvious today than it was in 1916, but appears to be little discussed by advo-cates of the market system. Instead, neoliberals, and the classical economists harking back to Adam Smith, emphasise the role of each individual being free to maximise their own income and happiness, guided only by the 'invisible hand' of the market: 'a competitive system is an elaborate mechanism for unconscious coordination through a system of prices and markets' (Samuelson 1967, cited in Malin et al. 2002: 67). Preferring this 'unconscious' mechanism to conscious attempts at planning provi-sion to meet need, neoliberals seek a minimal role for the state, which they see as distorting the market through attempts to intervene, regulate and control. They take strongest exception to measures such as public funding and provision of health care, which effectively 'decommodifies' and removes a large section of this industry from the market.

As a counter to planned, collectively funded and publicly provided health systems, market-style systems have been seen one-sidedly by their proponents as a means of increasing efficiency in health care and reducing the costs of treatment by stimulating competition – whether this is between financing bodies (insurance funds or health maintenance organisations (HMOs) which purchase care on the behalf of the patient/consumer) or between health-care providers (hospitals and other facili-ties) working under contract for the purchaser. Yet there is at least a tacit recognition that a full-scale free-for-all in an unregulated competitive market could not deliver satisfactory results. Hence competition between rival funds is commonly termed 'managed competition' and the wider system is described as 'managed care' (Flood 2000).

The European Health Management Association investigated the proposition that market mechanisms increase productivity – and found little evidence to support it. But they also investigated other propositions: that market mechanisms *increase* costs, that they separate public health policy from other reforms, and that they *reduce* the autonomy of professionals. They found evidence from various countries in Europe to support each of these views, while noting that market systems are in general incom-patible with greater equity in access to health care (EHMA 2000).

The EHMA study also clearly demonstrates that it is not necessary to embrace a Marxist analysis to conclude that unbridled market mechanisms are incompatible with the efficient or equitable provision of health care. Empirical evidence, consistently collected, can lead to the same conclusion: this helps to explain why so few neoliberal policies for health care are based on clear evidence of effectiveness. That markets are the wrong solution is the overwhelming consensus view of academics, economists and governments; it is disputed only by the most fundamentalist of neoliberal theorists[6] (Glennerster and Midgley 1991). Even the much-constrained 'managed' competition and 'planned markets', proposed as a means to utilise what is seen as a progressive dynamic of competition to improve publicly funded services (Saltman and von Otter 1992), have proved controversial, being unpopular with many governments and offering little evidence of success.

Market failure in health care

The various sources of 'market failure' in health care have been frequently rehearsed and debated by a wide range of authors from very different standpoints, so this study will examine the argument only briefly. World Bank studies summed up by Dunlop and Martins (1996: 196) concurred long ago that market mechanisms for the financing of health care:

> will not ensure either equity or economic efficiency, because of the characteristics of the health care market on both the supply and demand side, which suggest the presence of market failure conditions.

What, then, are these characteristics? According to Dunlop and Martins (1996: 190), the supply side (i.e. health-care providers) is characterised by imperfect competition and monopolistic practices, among other reasons because:

a.   Too many economic units are large enough to exert an influence on the prices of goods and services.

b.   There are too few providers to allow competitive pressures to drive down prices, creating effective monopoly positions.

c.   It is prohibitively expensive for new providers to enter the market and difficult for existing providers to pull out.

d.   There is insufficient standardisation of quality.

e.   There is unequal knowledge on the part of both consumer (patient) and supplier (provider).

On the demand side, the characteristics which undermine the workings of a free

---

6   Among the many varied authors embracing the consensus view that a free-market mechanism is inappropriate for health-care systems, while not necessarily sharing a common analysis of which systems are appropriate, are: Saltman and von Otter (1992), Walt (1994), Mohan (1995), Dunlop and Martins (1996), Laurell and Arellano (1996), Enthoven (1997), Appleby (1998), Figueras et al. (1998), Drache and Sullivan (1999), Buse and Walt (2000b), Deber (2000a), Freeman (2000), Ferge (2001), Leys (2001), Scott (2001), Malin et al. (2002) and Koivusalo (2003).

market are seen as including:

- Unequal knowledge (dependence on the professional expertise of doctors and nursing staff), which opens up the possibility of supplier-induced demand – or of patients failing to receive adequate care.

- The prevalence in advanced economies of 'third party' payment systems (public or private insurance or tax-funded systems), which means that neither the doctor nor the patient has any incentive to minimise the cost of care.

- The often uneven and uncertain demand for health care: previously healthy individuals may suddenly suffer catastrophic and costly accidents or illness, raising the need for risk-pooling.

- The lower likelihood of a patient suffering pain or life-threatening illness 'choosing' not to have treatment than a customer for other, more optional, goods and services. Indeed, patients requiring costly treatment commonly make far-reaching and, on one level, irrational decisions to sell assets, liquidate savings or run up unpayable debts in the hope that the costly treatment they are buying will give them additional months or years of life.

- The potential for exclusion of patients – especially those with chronic conditions or from low-income groups – from insurance cover through 'adverse selection'; while conversely, young, fit and prosperous adults of working age and low risk of illness may be 'cherry-picked' by insurance companies, thus reducing the risk pooling and increasing the cost to individuals.

- The vulnerability of insurance systems to 'moral hazard' (excessive use of services once the cost for the individual patient is covered by insurance).[7]

An additional problem arising from a market mechanism for the financing and delivery of health care is that it may well not provide for 'externalities' – the provision of immunisation or other public health measures which necessarily extend even to those lacking insurance cover: such a service will benefit the population as a whole by reducing the risk of communicable disease, but financing and delivering such a service effectively requires state intervention.

Free markets, politics and social forces

Whether or not there is an attempt to realise the exchange value, by trading health care as a conventional commodity (or service, like hair-dressing) for sale in the market-place, is determined by a combination of social, political and economic factors – all of which are *external* to the health-care episode itself. Drache and

---

7   'Moral hazard', although referred to as an established fact by some health economists (Dunlop and Martins 1996), might more realistically be seen as a largely imaginary creation of health economists, under which patients might in theory be tempted to avail themselves of additional unnecessary treatment if it were available to them free of charge. However, as Deber (2000) points out, even where health care *is* available free, demand for it is far from infinite: people demanding it are restricted to those suffering the appropriate condition: 'I doubt if many readers... would gladly accept free chemotherapy or free open-heart surgery, unless they "needed" it.'

Sullivan offer three possible approaches:

- That health care should be regarded as a service like any other, to be bought and sold in the market

- Or as a 'public good that only states can effectively provide'

- Or, alternatively, as something 'closer to what Adam Smith described as a non-market "necessary" for the support of life, that no society can afford to be without'.

(Drache and Sullivan 1999: 5)

Which of these variants applies (or which combination of variants) will depend in each case upon a complex balance of forces, including the politics and electoral or other social base of the government in the country concerned, and the extent to which key decision makers face democratic political or social pressure from different social classes.

The post-war development of welfare-state provision in many European countries brought an extension of publicly funded services or universal social insurance which effectively 'decommodified' health care and other benefits.[8] The extent to which welfare services have been decommodified is one measure used by Esping-Andersen to categorise and compare different types of welfare state (Esping-Andersen 1990), while critics of latter-day social democracy under Tony Blair and then Gordon Brown in Britain warned of the 'recommodification of the residual public sector, to promote the role of market forces' (Leys 2001; see also Jessop 2003).

The commercial trading of health care as a commodity serves above all the interests of those who are in a position to profit personally from such trade, and who feel themselves sufficiently wealthy and/or powerful to be able to withstand the costs of any treatment they or their families may themselves require. By contrast, it may be argued – not least because the 'exchange value' of health-care treatment, drawing as it does on the skills and training of specialist and professional staff, means that it can command a price higher than most working people could afford to pay – that the commodification of health care is against the interests of the working class and the rural poor.

Hart argues that the limitations to the expanded production of health care arise not from the boundaries of knowledge, which continue to widen, but the 'ruling assumptions about the nature of the medical care economy':

The minds of politicians with their hands on state power recognise only one possible kind of economy and one possible mode of production, capitalist production for the market, expanding not to meet human needs but to maximise profit.

(Hart 2003)

---

8   After years in which it was largely unchallenged, many health-care professionals and consumers have come to see the post-war 'social-democratic' consensus of socially funded health-care provision as a moral principle, and would tend to agree with Vienonen et al. (1999) that 'Markets are amoral'. Yet the failure of health care in the free market is not a *moral* problem: as has been discussed above, economic factors and the social relations of production under capitalism make health care an exceptional commodity.

When is a market not a market?

Many of the health-system reforms that have emerged since the 1990s claim to make use of the dynamics of market forces such as competition, 'quasi-markets' and market-style measures – not, it is claimed, primarily to maximise profit, but to improve the efficiency of public health-care services. Various contradictory phrases have been coined to sum up this new, supposedly benign application of a system which is inherently unplanned and ill-equipped to secure equity in access to services.

Responding to market-style reforms in Sweden, Finland and the UK, Saltman and Von Otter (1992) argue the case for 'a hybrid territory between politics and markets'. However, the notion of 'planned markets' (in which patient choice between providers becomes the driving force of 'public competition') is as inherently oxymoronic as the fashionable notion of 'managed competition' promoted by Flood (2000) but derided by Marmor (2001, 2002).

Saltman and Von Otter seek to distinguish between 'planned markets' and 'regulated markets', and propose a system of 'public competition' which:

> partially uncouples health sector management from political control on matters of economic productivity, but retains public responsibility for normative outcomes...
>
> (1992: 152)

However, the notion of exploiting market-style incentives to remodel publicly funded services while not embracing the classical operating objectives of genuine markets (personal gain, corporate profit) is even more problematic in the context of other government objectives – such as reining in state spending and reducing taxation. Saltman and Von Otter[9] argue that under the new paradigm:

> the patient's decision about where to obtain care becomes the decisive factor for steering system-wide resource flows...
>
> (1992: 153).

The contradiction is that – partly because it is NOT a genuine free market, in which all potential providers would have free access to additional borrowing for capital investment – this new regime cannot ensure the availability of sufficient resources to enable the public-sector providers to meet the wishes of patients, even though it appears to prioritise the patient's choice. Full and unfettered availability of services to allow any patient to choose any provider would require a surplus of capacity among public-sector health-care providers – thus diminishing efficient use of resources, increasing unit costs and creating new pressure to increase global budgets to facilitate expansion. Meanwhile, there is always the underlying threat that, if the public sector cannot deliver the capacity and resources to meet levels of expressed demand, the private sector can be expected to take advantage of the opportunity to pick up additional work, thus draining precious resources from public-sector budgets.

---

9   Foreshadowing the 'Patient Choice' and 'financial flow' policies ushered in by Britain's New Labour government in 2003.

Elsewhere, apparently oblivious to the contradictions inherent in the concept, Saltman has upheld the view that 'the idea of a planned market is a straightforward one' (Saltman 1996). Differentiating between three variants of 'planned markets', to be based on price, on quality or on market share, he argues that:

> A central element of these planned market models is that only system-level expenditures are capped. In both the price-based and the quality-based approach a particular provider doesn't have a fixed prospective global budget...
>
> (Ibid.: 9)

The tension between a globally fixed budget and competition between providers, in which 'each provider competes for a bigger share of a fixed pie' (ibid.: 10), is that if any providers make gains, others will lose out in revenue terms, while the system overall cannot expand to offer the additional capacity required to offer genuine free choice or to remedy problems of quality or inadequate capacity in individual providers. With no overall increase in resources, providers seeking to increase their 'efficiency', to reduce prices, or cope with reduced budgets will have no choice but to cut jobs or squeeze increased effort from their workforce – with a consequent risk to the quality and safety of care.

Costs of market reforms

Perhaps an even bigger problem is ignored by the Saltman formula: the *cost* of implementing market-style reforms, in terms of increased complexity in administration and accountancy. The British market-style reforms, which introduced a new system of pricing, billing and annual contract negotiations between a large number of purchasers and providers, dramatically increased the previously very low administrative costs of the National Health Service, requiring thousands of additional managerial and clerical staff (Paton 2000). The decision of the New Labour government to retain the purchaser–provider split meant a further substantial (59 per cent) increase in numbers of senior managers in the six years from 1997[10] (DoH 2004b). The complex 'payment by results' system of reimbursement – allowing private-sector competition to draw on NHS funds – is also expensive to implement and the British market-style reforms seem to have more than doubled the overhead costs of administrating the NHS (Leys and Player 2011).

Behind this ostensibly 'straightforward' suggestion of applying competition to publicly funded health services, therefore, is a fundamental shift from planning, solidarity and cooperation to division, conflict, competition and fragmentation. Any efficiency savings achieved in the delivery of front-line health services can be undermined by increased costs of more complex bureaucracy, and by the alienation of staff and less coherent treatment of patients in larger, impersonal units (Boyle at al. 2004).

---

10 Management numbers in proportion to front-line nursing and administrative staff also increased, with almost 25 per cent fewer admin and clerical staff, and 50 per cent fewer qualified nurses per manager in 2003 than in 1995 (DoH 2004b). The numbers peaked in 2009 as a financial squeeze began to take effect.

And while the maintenance of 'global' cash limits to purchasers and providers may appear to squeeze better value out of public services, it can result in the longer term in a shortfall in investment which leads to a growing reliance on private-sector provision. In other words, 'planned' markets carry with them all of the contradictions of 'unplanned' markets.

This study explores the extent to which changes stem from, lead to or tacitly reinforce and legitimise defective market-based models. It argues that the dynamic of the policies means that they will result in a less egalitarian, less efficient and eventually more expensive system – as shown by the evidence so far – one that will hold back rather than assist improvements in the health and health care of millions.

Marx was clear in his analysis that capitalism came on to the historical scene as a revolutionary, dynamic force, driving forward technical progress, developing and expanding the means of production well beyond the confines of preceding feudal systems. This is also true in health care, which, since the emergence of modern medicine in the early twentieth century, has opened up huge new possibilities to diagnose and treat diseases and to control long-term conditions that were previously fatal.

But Marx also warned that, just as competition eventually turns into its opposite, the progressive role of capitalism would also find its limits, in which the grip of the bourgeoisie and its drive for profits would become a limit, a fetter, on the further development of the means of production. Lenin took this analysis further with the concept of imperialism as the highest point of monopoly capitalism, blocking further progressive development. There are clear signs that the possibilities of medical technique and technology have now run well past the point where they can be sold profitably to the larger multi-million strong market of poorest people who need them most: the possibilities of treating AIDS and HIV, and of preventing malaria and other diseases are limited by the fact that the patents are held by massive multinational corporations, and the quest for profit forces prices unaffordably high for those on impossibly low incomes.

Moreover, the way the system is structured, towards profit streams for the large corporations with heavy investments, limits the options for actions which focus primarily on prevention and social determinants of health, that must compete for resources with systems focused on curative medicine.

The limits of 'globalisation' as an explanation for reforms

As a commonplace term of abuse and criticism aimed at transnational capitalist corporations, 'globalisation' came of age in the Seattle protests against the World Trade Organization in 1999, by which time the phenomenon of global expansion of transnational corporations and their systematised exploitation of the world's resources and labour markets was already well developed. At the same time, an 'anti-capitalist' movement was born, embracing a wide spectrum of interests and political views, ranging from traditional trade unions seeking to protect jobs against competition from low-wage economies overseas, to anarchists and socialists questioning the very fundamentals of the capitalist world economy (Sabado 2009).

As a political current, anti-capitalism has remained diffuse, divided and weak despite the numbers it has attracted on occasion to mass protests: but the issue of challenging world capitalism and its logic has remained as a background to the fury at the costs and consequences of the banks' crash in 2008 and afterwards, and the subsequent waves of austerity budgets seeking to pass the buck for these problems on to working people and the poor. Yeates (2001: 4) argues that:

> Globalisation is a highly contested term, the frequent use of which has tended to obscure a lack of consensus with regard to what it entails, explanations of how it operates and the directions in which it is heading.

The lack of consensus is even more marked when it comes to deciding what to do about it: in some ways it is a soft option to blame 'globalisation' in abstract for political and economic policies which may flow more from individual governments, or from the policies and ideological prescriptions of global bodies and institutions, than from globalisation itself or the new world order it has ushered in.

However bad it may be, it is impossible from within the limits of any one country (even the US) to fight 'globalisation' as such: the fight has to begin with targets that are within reach and can be identified. Global capitalism is not an abstraction: it works through agencies and has material connections against which people can act politically.

The dynamics of the various aspects of globalisation drive in different ways towards changes in health systems. For instance:

- The scale and speed of cross-border movement of goods, services and finance capital leaves many national economies and their governments potentially vulnerable to short-term movements of capital. This might therefore be seen as a driving force towards more frugal and cost-effective health systems that could keep levels of taxation low in order to attract and retain inward investment. Yet there is relatively little evidence to demonstrate this effect (Gough 2000). More recently, the austerity policies vigorously promoted by governments across Europe and elsewhere in the aftermath of the 2007–8 banking crash are routinely justified by references to the demands of external 'markets' and 'investors': the cuts in public spending and health care are thus blamed on absent and theoretical capitalists rather than the real, living domestic capitalists whose profits are enhanced by low taxation while working people carry the costs of bailing out global bankers.

- Most governments appear to be committed to working towards further 'globalisation' – economic integration, backed by policies of labour-market flexibility, low taxes and tariffs, privatisation and minimal regulation. But the consensus is stronger in theory than in practice. And in health care, while there have been sustained and continuing attempts to apply market-style reforms to health systems in developing countries, until recently very few of the wealthier OECD countries have opted to do the same. Indeed, with the notable exception of the unique ongoing and unresolved situation in the US,[11] most OECD countries have retained welfare-state protection and social solidarity on health and some (Mexico, Turkey) have even begun (at least partially) to extend it.[12] Some early moves towards more extreme market reforms in the 1990s were halted and reversed in the light of negative experience (New Zealand). Since 2000, within the OECD, the United Kingdom (primarily in England) and Portugal have been well out in front in their commitment to the implementation of market-style reforms in health systems, regardless of their cost, their political unpopularity and the lack of any evidence that they deliver the promised improvements; while Australia and Ireland have been exceptional in persisting with their expensive option of encouraging greater use of private medical insurance.

- The establishment of binding rules, through the WTO and other bilateral and regional treaties (including EU competition law), which have begun to constrain the policy flexibilities of governments to expand publicly provided services and – particularly regarding extended patient rights – access to new medicines, vaccines and potentially life-enhancing science.

Yeates, citing Petrella (1996), elaborates seven types of globalisation, relating to

- Finances and ownership
- Markets and strategies
- Technology and knowledge
- Modes of life, consumption patterns and culture
- Regulator capabilities
- Globalisation as the political unification of the world
- Globalisation of perception and consciousness.

(Yeates 2001: 5)

However, while the first three of these variants of globalisation as analysed by Yeates can clearly be seen to play a role in the developing pressure on health-care systems, none of them can be seen as the ultimate driver of the reform process within health-care systems. The notion of globalisation as a driver of health-sector reform[13] has generated a substantial literature but little agreement from the various authors, either on the basic definition of 'globalisation', the extent to which it can be seen to influence specific policies and changes, or on whether that influence can be seen as for

---

11 The US health-care system is by far the most expensive in the world, consuming over 16 per cent of GDP (almost $2 trillion) in 2005 (Tanne 2007), spending upwards of $400 billion on administration (Woolhandler et al. 2003) and wasting up to $700 billion a year (Kelley 2009) while leaving 45–50 million Americans without full insurance cover (Cohen and Martinez 2006). Much of this spending flows from, or is subsidised by, the government at federal and state level: US government spending as a share of GDP was equivalent to the UK in 2003, leaving the bulk of additional spending to the private sector and out-of-pocket payments (Hsiao and Heller 2007).

12 However, a number of countries have seen an erosion of entitlements to social security, pensions and benefits for people with physical disabilities.

13 As Palier and Sykes (2001) point out, so many accounts have been developed since the mid-1990s that it is not feasible here to cite all of the available references on globalisation, let alone to explore them in this study.

better or for worse, or a combination of the two (Labonté et al. 2004: 1–12). Palier and Sykes (2001: 2) argue that globalisation is a 'buzz-word' used to suggest 'a whole range of phenomena'.

Globalisation and governments

As Yeates argues, reference to 'globalisation' has been used to help explain changes in very different areas of enquiry: political science, economics, geography, sociology and social policy among them (2001: 15). Yeates is also careful to distinguish between two concepts: 'strong' globalisation, an irresistible economic force compelling governments into action, which she criticises as economistic, deterministic and reductionist; and a more nuanced version which incorporates issues of political agency and social conflict.

Palier and Sykes draw a similar distinction between 'apocalyptic' versions and versions in which globalisation is 'as much a political and ideological phenomenon as an economic one' (2001: 5). These authors argue that there is a two-way process of pressure and legitimisation, in which the ideological globalisation perspective of bodies such as the World Bank, OECD and European Commission 'provides welfare reformers with a certain repertoire of reforms' (often neoliberal), while 'the threat of globalisation provides governments with ideological justification for their welfare state changes' (2001: 11).

Globalisation of capitalism therefore *does* have an impact on health systems, although in general the policies for change come only indirectly from the global economy. More often, they come through the ideology and policy prescriptions – the 'hidden politics' – of the Washington Consensus (Deacon 2001) and related approaches and assumptions ('Third Way', 'New Public Management'). These look to market mechanisms, competition, choice and the supposed 'efficiencies' of the private sector rather than to the previous consensus of 'social-democratic' social solidarity, focused on proactive planning and allocation of resources to meet health needs and achieve goals of equity, universalism, access and inclusion.

Yeates (2001: 28) argues that the 'globalization of the social policy process' is centred on 'general agreements reached by participants in international fora, such as the UN or G7 summits'. Yet, while these bodies can in theory be seen as gatherings of equals, almost all health-system reforms appear to have been transmitted from the wealthier countries to the poorest. This does not take place through voluntary engagement, partnership or agreement, but through the pressure and even through the intervention of less egalitarian global organisations – notably the World Bank and the IMF. While the basic menu of reforms – the 'one size fits all' derided by Stiglitz (2002) and other critics – may be similar everywhere, the policies *adopted* are not by any means identical. Until recently, few governments with any room for choice have opted to push through systematic market-style reforms in health care.

Historical and political overview

The material and political roots of reform

The reforms examined here are relatively recent and represent a new stage in the evolution of health-care policy. In many cases, they appear to have been inspired by 'globalised faith in market mechanisms' (George and Wilding 2002: 64). However, it is useful to recall that today's reforms are in many cases re-shaping systems which were themselves the product of substantial earlier reforms and which were also a response to material and political circumstances and ideological pressures. These pressures do not work evenly or mechanically. Marx (in *The German Ideology*) argued that:

> The ideas of the ruling class are in every epoch the ruling ideas, i.e. the class which is the ruling material force of society is at the same time its ruling intellectual force.
>
> (Marx and Engels 1970b: 64)

However, if this general statement – which Marx intended to locate the material and class origin of 'ruling ideas', which otherwise might simply be seen as abstractions – were taken too literally, one might assume that market-style policies would have enjoyed continued dominance for as long as the capitalist system remains in place: the problem is in understanding the preceding 40 or 50 years of welfarist consensus. But no political process is that simple. Marx also makes clear that there is always scope for differences of opinion and a degree of disunity within the camp of the ruling rich, just as there is within other social classes.

This is because thought and ideas inevitably reflect the material world, within which constant and complex changes take place, requiring adjustment to both theory and practice. As Kelsey (1995) argued, analysing New Zealand's reforms in the 1980s, governments may be confronted by objective pressures and situations – but these do not lead automatically to any one inevitable conclusion: governments always have choices.

The post-war welfarist consensus

One of the key historic periods of choice came in 1945, when Europe's weakened and bankrupt ruling classes faced a new post-war political reality. They had to devise a new approach that could safeguard stability and rebuild a system that had been shattered and destabilised by war. The emergence of Keynesian economics and a 'welfarist' consensus in much of Europe reflected a new balance of class forces, in which capitalist classes found themselves having to deal with the expectations and demands of a more militant working class (reflected also in the strengthening of social-democratic and communist parties) which they were poorly placed to confront. Only the USA was largely unaffected by the new situation, its economy having been relatively untroubled by the war and its lack of even a social-democratic party of the working class helping to ensure that the post-war wave of trade-union militancy remained largely confined to economic rather than political objectives (Armstrong et al. 1984). As a result, the divergence between US and European politics continued to widen.

The new economics and welfarism were no threat to capitalism, but a means of ensuring its survival. Even the 'socialists' and 'communists'[14] brought into post-war reformist and coalition governments in Western Europe[15] lacked either the courage or the political commitment to press for the socialist solutions they adhered to on paper; instead, they joined with the capitalists, who in turn embraced the Bismarck technique of co-option and purchased a degree of social peace by offering concessions to the working class and the middle classes. The policy was shared by most major political parties: in Britain, for example, where some of the most sweeping changes took place,[16] the post-war Labour government's development of a welfare state as part of a reconstructed capitalism followed a blueprint for social policies drawn up during the war by a Liberal. Moreover, it reflected a broad (if not precise and detailed) consensus with the Conservative Party – even if the precise form of the NHS proved contentious (Doyal 1979, Timmins 1995).

The political consensus around this type of 'post-war settlement' dominated much of Western Europe through the boom years of the 1950s and 1960s, during which time health care and other welfare spending grew substantially (Alcock 2001) and almost every developed country other than the US began to develop some form of collective provision for health care (Lister 2008a). But a generalised recession in 1974–5 ended what had been a prolonged period of economic growth and expansion of welfare-state provision. Since then, most OECD governments have been seeking policies to contain what had been, from the early 1960s, an inexorable rise in health-care spending (OECD 1995a).

As Saltman and von Otter sum up, by the 1980s:

> The logic of neo-classical economics had begun to replace that of classical democratic politics as the core theoretical basis upon which to evaluate all types of social activity. Markets were increasingly seen to embody the virtues that politics, and with it public sector organisation, appeared to lack.
>
> (1992: 6)

---

14 Despite the abolition of the Communist International during the war, communist parties in Western Europe were at this stage still firmly controlled by the Kremlin and followed Stalin's general strategy of 'peaceful coexistence' with capitalism, including the 'Parliamentary Road to Socialism' (Black 1970, Wohlforth and Westoby 1978).

15 While the US cranked up a massive anti-communist witch-hunt and an even longer period of Cold War hysteria.

16 Not least with the nationalisation of the hospital network and establishment of a new National Health Service offering universal access free at point of use, based on need rather than ability to pay (Armstrong et al. 1984, Lister 2008a).

Constrained consensus: market-driven reforms

Health-care spending statistics show that these efforts at containment were generally less than completely successful and, in most of the wealthiest countries, health care has continued to consume an ever-growing share of national wealth and of government spending (Moran 1999: 2–3). However, most observers agree that, in this early period, policies for restructuring and rationalising health services were often drawn up more for financial than health reasons. An OECD study, analysing changes in the 30 years to 1990, argues:

> the combined weight of medical technology *and of financial pressures* contributed to a rationalisation in the supply of [acute] beds.
>
> (OECD 1992: 166)

The same OECD report also noted the extent to which cost-cutting measures in the wealthier countries were driven by the wider pressures of a competitive world market. The signs of an 'overall convergence' in the health-care policies of OECD countries were seen as 'the result of market forces which lessen each country's discretion to go its own way' (OECD 1992: 16). These measures are therefore examined in this study under the general heading of 'market-driven' reforms. However, it is also necessary to explain why they need to be addressed as 'reforms' at all, rather than as economy measures: the issue is one of political presentation.

Most cost-saving measures, involving cutbacks in popular, publicly funded services are inherently politically unpopular, especially when they declare their intentions openly: most Western European-style health-care systems offer near-total coverage of the entire population[17] and are so dependent upon public (government) spending that any attempt to cut or even hold down health spending becomes a highly charged political issue (Chinitz et al. 1998, Armstrong et al. 2001: 2). One consequence of this is that cost-cutting changes are often presented not as straightforward economies but as 'reforms' – 'centralising', 'rationalising' or 'modernising' services.

Although such thin disguises are seldom sufficient to conceal the underlying purpose,[18] these market-driven measures are therefore analysed in this study as a specific category on the wider 'menu' of reform.

---

17 As such, European systems have more in common with each other than any of them does with the US model (Freeman 2000, Kokko et al. 1998).

18 Examples in Britain include the Worcestershire Health Authority's boldly titled 'Investing in Excellence' (1997), which involved the loss of more than a quarter of the county's acute beds including all in Kidderminster Hospital, and West Hertfordshire's 'Choosing the Right Direction' (1998), which again centred on substantial cost-saving rationalisation. In 2012, a new raft of similarly blandly titled plans has been proposed in a bid to drive through a rationalisation of hospital services in various parts of England.

Breaking the consensus: market-style reforms

However, the other main strand of reform has very different political and ideological roots. Far from saving money, many market-style reforms have actually brought a commitment to *increased* state and private spending – not least the sharply increased costs of administering the new 'market-style' system in New Zealand after 1993; the higher costs of private health insurance, encouraged by government tax incentives in Australia (Ham 1999, Drache and Sullivan 1999, Birrell et al. 2003); and of course, the increased administrative costs of market reforms in Britain from 1991 and since 2001 (Lister 2008a, Leys and Player 2011).

The key driving factor in these changes has clearly *not* been financial pressures (Moran 1999, Mossialos et al. 2002). Rather, they flow from the ideological New Right, a political current championed by Hayek and Milton Friedman, which had never disappeared in the US or relented in its opposition to welfare-state provision and Keynesian economics (Harrison et al. 1990). In a context of growing economic crisis from the mid-1970s, this strand of ideology began to influence a new section of right-wing political leaders seeking a break from welfarism, who now felt strong enough to opt for confrontation with the working class, rather than consensus. It led to a new approach based on 'rolling back' the 'nanny state', privatisation, competitive tendering, deregulation, reduced taxation and an emphasis on 'possessive individualism' as an alternative to collectivism and social solidarity (Jones 1994, Malin et al. 2002).

As Jones (1994) argues, such ideas were also able to find a purchase in genuine problems and shortfalls in health and welfare provision. Some of the arguments developed by the New Right as weapons to attack the welfare state as 'bureaucratic', 'inefficient', 'remote' and 'ineffective' were shamelessly taken from criticisms originating on the left, among campaigners pressing for more responsive, local and democratic services, protesting at the perverse incentives of the 'poverty trap' effect and complaining of continued inequalities in health.

In Britain, Margaret Thatcher's rise to the leadership of the Conservative Party in the 1970s coincided with, and reinforced, the gathering ideological challenge to welfarism. In parallel, Thatcher and Ronald Reagan, from the Republican right in the US, each bid for office arguing that 'big government' was strangling enterprise (Clarke et al. 2001). Thatcher's election victory in 1979 brought in a Conservative government which could experiment with some of the policies devised by the New Right.[19] For health care, this began with a combination of market-driven constraints on health spending, coupled in the mid-1980s with two policies which anticipated elements of what was later to be branded as the 'New Public Management':

- Managerialist changes designed to break from the old ethos of NHS administration and consensus, strengthening the hand of management in dealing with senior

---

19 However, the health service remained so hugely popular with the electorate that even Thatcher repeatedly insisted it would be 'safe in our hands'. Her government also resisted continual efforts from the right wing of the Conservative Party to promote more radical, right-wing reforms such as wholesale privatisation, voucher schemes, opt-out schemes – and other devices that would expand private provision at the expense of declining services for the poor and elderly (Caldwell et al. 1998).

medical professionals; and

- The imposition of competitive tendering for most non-clinical hospital support services ('steering, not rowing').

The neoliberal agenda: a 'Washington consensus'

These were the opening shots in a 'New Right' offensive on welfarism, the underlying ideology and assumptions of which combine the neoliberal[20] assertion that the private sector is inevitably more efficient and more responsive as a provider of services with the neo-Conservative emphasis on the traditional role of the family and the individual (Clarke et al. 2001).

On health and other areas of policy, the neoliberals aimed to:

- Reduce the role of the state

- Change the role of the state from provider to purchaser and regulator

- Break up the state monopoly of welfare provision

- Encourage 'consumers' to make choices about the services and service providers they used.

Such structural reforms can run alongside cost-cutting: soaring spending on

---

20 'Neoliberal' is the general description of a set of economic policies related to economic liberalism, the notion of allowing the fullest freedom of the market, originally associated with the writings of Adam Smith. His study *The Wealth of Nations*, published in 1776, has inspired a new generation of 'free market' fundamentalists since the late 1960s, amid the decline of the post-war Keynesian/social-democratic consensus. Among the more prominent and influential neoliberals have been University of Chicago economist Milton Friedman (whose 'Chicago Boys' advised the Pinochet dictatorship in Chile from 1973) and philosopher–economist Friederich von Hayek. Backed by important sections of the US super-rich, their ideas have been promoted by a powerful network of right-wing foundations, institutes and research centres. Neoliberals and neoliberal policies have also been prominent in the work of the IMF, the World Bank and USAID. Von Hayek was a direct influence on British Prime Minister Margaret Thatcher, while neoliberal institutes have long been linked with the US Republican Party: the Heritage Foundation, the principal think tank for Ronald Reagan's administration, has remained an influential force in US politics. The main elements of neoliberalism can be summed up as:
   - The rule of the market, liberating 'free' private enterprise from any restrictions or regulations and de-unionising workers
   - Cutting public expenditure for social services, health and education
   - Deregulation
   - Privatisaton of state-owned enterprises, including utilities supplying power and water as well as health care, schools, railways and roads
   - Eliminating the concept of 'community' and the 'public good', replacing them with individual responsibility.
   (Martinez and Garcia 1997, George 1999, Coburn 2000)
   The influence of neoliberal ideology in the formulation of health-system reforms has been noted by many critics, including Collins and colleagues who point specifically to the links with so-called 'user choice', promotion of the private sector, the introduction of competition, markets, decentralisation and new incentives, limits on the public sector, and changes in the finance of health care including user fees and private health insurance (Collins et al. 1999: 76).

both public and privately funded sectors of health care in the USA in the 1970s had brought a succession of measures aimed at curbing costs.[21] The new Reagan administration from January 1981 lost no time in pressing home cuts in spending and a deregulation of medical care, but followed this with more elaborate measures to hold down spending, introducing the concept of diagnosis related groups of treatments which would receive fixed payments – a model later emulated in England by Tony Blair's New Labour government (Patel and Rushefsky 1999).

The monetarist, free-market policies of the British and US governments of Thatcher and Reagan brought wider acceptance of what became the dominant 'neoliberal' model for politics and economics, the basic package of which was summed up by Williamson (1990) as the 'Washington consensus'. Among the ten basic broad propositions for policy reform at the centre of this 'consensus' were five which relate directly to the subject of this study: fiscal discipline; redirection of public expenditure priorities toward health care, primary education and infrastructure – offering both high economic returns and the potential to improve income distribution; liberalisation of foreign direct investment; privatisation; and deregulation (to abolish barriers to entry to, and exit from, the market) (Williamson 2000: 252–3).

Williamson has since argued that his list stopped short of some of the more extreme neoliberal propositions. Writing for the World Bank's own journal, he insisted that the 'consensus' he described should have been seen not as a policy prescription based on the most hard-line free-market principles, but as a 'lowest common denominator' of the reforms 'Washington' could agree on for Latin America in 1989. He argues that the term 'consensus' was merely intended to sum up the dominant approach of both the US government and the Washington-based institutions shaping the world economy – the World Bank and the IMF – and that by 1990 some of the most radical free-market policies had been toned down or dropped: 'The market fundamentalism of Reagan's first term had already been superseded by the return of rational policymaking' (ibid.: 255).

However, Williamson also concedes that the various Washington policy makers *were* looking to develop global models that would be applied to a very wide range of diverse countries. Interestingly, he admits that in this sense there *was* at that time a form of underlying 'blueprint' for all developing countries, so that 'There probably would not have been a lot of difference if I had undertaken a similar exercise for Africa or Asia' (ibid.: 254–5).

The 1990s saw the 'Washington consensus' widely applied as the basis of policy advice and prescriptions from global bodies to developing countries. And while the primary targets were lower state spending, privatisation and the maximum deregulation of the market, the accompanying neoliberal rejection of notions of social solidarity was summed up by Margaret Thatcher's now infamous insistence

---

21 Including support from the Nixon administration for the launch of the first Health Maintenance Organisations (HMOs) in 1973, and failed attempts by Jimmy Carter's administration to impose limits on hospital costs, thrown out by Congress in 1980 after three years of debate (Patel and Rushefsky 1999).

– echoing von Hayek and a long tradition of laissez-faire advocates of individualism going back to Adam Smith and de Tocqueville – that:

> 'There is no such thing as society. There are individual men and women, and there are families'.
>
> (Timmins 1995: 433)

Pressures to conform

By the 1980s, many governments were already embracing the ideology of the free market in many areas of economic activity: many were seeking to privatise public services and utilities, and to step away from direct ownership and control. This helps explain why, even as European governments struggled to hold down the costs of largely state-funded health services, they became more receptive to ideas drawn from the very different, hugely expensive, but technically very advanced health-care system in the USA. Moran argues that even though the UK had developed a health-care system that was very good at cost containment, the new model for health system reform became the 'stunningly expensive' US, where health care was a 'complete policy fiasco':

> More generally the diffusion of institutional innovation seemed to be from the system that was conspicuously failing at cost containment: it was the United States, not the United Kingdom or Scandinavia, that was state of the art as far as health care reform was concerned. In the international diffusion of health care reforms, apparently nothing succeeded like failure.
>
> (Moran 1999: xi)

In this context, one of the influential figures who won an audience among Western governments was American economist Alain Enthoven. Although his ideas were a costly flop in the defence industry, where he honed his skills in the 1960s (Waitzkin 1994), he was one of the many economists, politicians and academics seeking ways of 'managing' the chaotic and ruinously expensive private market in health care in the USA. His proposals for restricting the costs of private medical insurance through the introduction of 'managed care', offering a restricted range of funded treatments from a restricted range of 'preferred providers', led to an influential paper on the British NHS (Enthoven 1985). This pamphlet, with its proposal for a competitive 'internal market' within the NHS, was acknowledged to be the kernel of the Conservative government's market-style reforms,[22] once the more outlandish New Right notions from back-bench Conservatives had been discarded. The British health-care reforms, in turn, served to encourage other governments to contemplate their own market-style reforms, notably New Zealand, which also looked to Enthoven for inspiration as it implemented its own variant of a 'managed market' system in 1991 (Enthoven 1988).

---

22 Embodied in the White Paper *Working for Patients* and the subsequent NHS and Community Care Act (DoH 1989b, DoH 1990, Ham 1999).

In most cases, such as in Sweden during a brief three-year period of conservative-liberal government in 1991–4, the changes which resulted have been slower and much more partial than those in the UK (Freeman 2000). However, these pioneering health-care reforms triggered a new worldwide interest both in the corporatisation of hospitals (established as NHS trusts in the UK, Crown Health Enterprises in New Zealand) and in the introduction of competition and quasi-markets into publicly funded health services (Preker and Harding 2003). The early 1990s saw further moves towards private-sector involvement in public services, with the development in the UK of the Private Finance Initiative (PFI) as a means to privatise the capital investment programme in publicly funded health care (Sussex 2001, Lister 2008a, IFC 2002).

The limitations of neoliberalism

Although the term 'neoliberal' is widely (and often loosely) used by critics to describe the ideology and reforms proposed or inspired by sections of the New Right, the most radical section of neoliberals embrace policies which very few politicians or publicly accountable health-care planners could be seen to endorse. One example of this extreme view is Aubrey, a doctor writing in the *Medical Sentinel*, who explicitly defends the idea that medicine should properly be seen as 'a commodity produced by profit seeking entrepreneurial physicians, working in a free market, and purchased by their patients' (Aubrey 2001). It's interesting to speculate how this doctor would respond to the fundamentalist anarcho-capitalists who, ten years later, following the logic of neoliberalism, went even further – advocating an end to the registration of doctors and other health professionals, arguing that anyone wanting to practice as a doctor should be allowed do so, with the market deciding who succeeds or fails (Wellings 2012).

Pauly (2000), approvingly introducing a volume of neoliberal essays, states:

> Is health care so different from other goods and services that a dominant role for government is inevitable or desirable? *American Health Care* addresses that important question and answers it with a qualified 'no'.
>
> (Pauly 2000: ix)

Any policy designed to ensure equity in health care, especially if it involves government intervention to regulate private-sector providers in the health-care marketplace, or the raising of progressive taxation to subsidise care for the poor, is likely to incur the wrath of the hard-line defenders of the free market.[23] In American neoliberal publications and on US websites such as those of the Heartland Institute and Independence Institute, doctors, right-wing theorists and academics decry as 'socialism' or even 'fascism' any attempt by government to intervene in the market or to

---

23 'Any limit on technology, any restraint on drug-firm profits, any fee schedule for doctors – all will apparently ruin the quality of US health care. Those willing to challenge that assumption are hard pressed to gain access to the media' (Marmor 1999: 262).

'manage' competition (Aubrey 2001, Dorman 1999). For such ideologically driven proponents of the free market, even such elementary public-health precautions as gun control and the discouragement of tobacco smoking are unreasonable intrusions into the lives of individuals.

Neoliberalism has been well described by Bourdieu (1998) as a 'utopia of endless exploitation'. However, health-care systems, like other aspects of the economy in democratic countries, are shaped and driven not only by economics and ideology, but also by *political* considerations and interests. In democracies, governments have to be elected and policies have to win the backing of an appropriate alliance of forces in order to be implemented: key players include the pharmaceutical industry, other major suppliers of health-care equipment, medical professionals, and of course the main political parties, each with an eye to the practical and electoral consequences of the policies they adopt.

For neoliberals, therefore, there is a serious and insoluble problem: their ideas presume the workings of a free and perfect market, which clearly does not, and cannot, exist. Worse: their ideas are so inherently unpopular among the majority of the population that it is almost impossible for any democratically elected government to implement and test them out (Mills et al. 2001, Collins et al. 1999). Decades of experience in the USA, the most heavily private health-care system in the OECD, with the world's most powerful lobby of neoliberal pressure groups and academics, have left American neoliberals frustrated and bitterly critical of successive governments' failures to carry through their favoured model. This culminated in the extremist Republican 'Tea Party' movement, seemingly on a mission to make their party completely unelectable[24] (Health Policy Consensus Group 2001, Armey 2001, Scandlen 2003, Taranto 2012).

Because of this inherent problem, the pressure from neoliberalism has been channelled into other, more pragmatic 'market-style' policies, centred not so much on establishing the full freedoms of the market, but on attempting to devise or copy (especially from the USA) methods of maximising the role of the private sector while restraining and 'managing' the market, competition and entrepreneurialism, to avoid their worst, most wasteful, excesses (Enthoven 1985, 1997, 2003, Hunter 1998, Saltman and von Otter 1992, Saltman et al. 2002).

Laurell and Arellano (1996) and Deacon (2001) are among those who have detected the confusion and contradiction running through many of the policy documents of the World Bank, which is instinctively aligned with neoliberalism, but which feels obliged in its policies to make reference to 'equity'. Indeed, the Bank's more astute analysts appeared by the end of the 1990s (Johnston and Stout 1997) to have begun to concede pragmatically that the neoliberal model cannot be fully implemented in the area of health care. Even the most eager proponents of private-sector solutions recognise the fact that public provision must play a key role if key

---

24 Their anger is paralleled by the disappointment of those seeking a more socially progressive reform, which also foundered under the Clinton Presidency, having also failed to construct a suitably broad coalition of political support (Marmor 1998). The influence of neoliberalism in the USA is underlined by the fact that even socialist campaigners have in recent years focused on socialising the finance rather than the provision of health care (PNHP 2003a).

areas of health care are to be delivered to those in greatest need: 'It is evident that government intervention is essential to ensure equitable and efficient delivery and financing of health care' (IFC 2002: 16).

Significantly, the Bank (here represented by its sub-division the International Finance Corporation[25]) intends this public-sector intervention to restrict itself to those low-cost peripheral areas of public health, health education, immunisation and preventive services which the private sector is least interested in providing.

Neoliberalism meets social democracy: the 'Third Way'

Doyal (1979) argues that even among those most wedded to the capitalist mode of production there have been different approaches to the question of whether health care should be bought and sold in the same way as any other commodity. Most political parties are committed not to abolishing, but to reforming capitalism. The most influential of these have been 'social-democratic' (sometimes calling themselves 'socialist') parties, which – having decades ago renounced their Marxist origins in the Second International – have become wedded to the notion of purely parliamentary action to secure progressive legislation for reforms benefiting their largely working-class electoral base.

The post-war 'social-democratic consensus' led governments of various political parties in most of the industrialised countries to develop 'welfare state' provision, including health care[26]: other European governments followed suit, developing public health-care systems at a later stage[27] – as did Canada, which broke from a US-style private insurance system to establish Medicare in 1971. These developments took place in the context of generalised economic expansion, partly on the basis of post-war reconstruction and partly driven by an expansion in mass production of consumer goods.

Even the most expensive of the publicly funded schemes have also proved to be relatively cost-effective systems for capitalism, incurring only a fraction of the massive overheads in administration costs which help inflate the costs of US health care. (Some even manage to incorporate a role for private non-profit and even for-profit providers without racking up the stratospheric costs of the US system.) Indeed, while proposals for publicly funded health care have been largely unsuccessful in the US, there has nevertheless been a degree of socialisation of financing of services for

---

25 The IFC's main concern is expanding the role of the private sector (Lethbridge 2002a).

26 Welfare-state systems can be seen as concessions to the strength of the working class, or as a means to ensure the active or passive acquiescence of a strong working class in the continued operation of capitalism (Saltman and von Otter 1992). However, social concessions to co-opt workers are by no means the prerogative of left-wing or social-democratic governments: in the late nineteenth century, the authoritarian Bismarck government in Germany was the first to identify an advantage in binding the otherwise alienated and increasingly organised working class to the capitalist state with a social-insurance system (Freeman 2000).

27 Italy (1978), Portugal (1979), Greece (1983), Spain (1986)

the elderly, children and the very poor through Medicare, Medicaid and state-level funding of public hospitals (although these remain a constant target for spending cuts or new ways to carve out a role for private insurers and providers). These, plus extensive provision of tax breaks for privately financed insurance schemes,[28] have meant that the result has been a situation in which the US population is (more than) 'Paying for National Health Insurance, but not getting it' (Woolhandler and Himmelstein 2002).

The further dilution of social democracy

However, the end of the period of capitalist 'boom' opened a new period of intensified global competition, bringing a rise of neoliberalism and the simultaneous erosion of old-style social-democratic parties and politics. According to Saltman and Von Otter (1992), the reason why the health-policy debate in northern Europe increasingly began to focus on the question of the introduction of competition into publicly operated health services was linked with the demise of 'classical democratic politics' as a result of various factors. These included:

- A decline in the strength and organisation of the working class, leaving governments freer to mould services to the more individualistic, consumerist needs and wishes of the middle class

- The increasing reluctance of younger people to accept standardised services

- The service sector becoming larger than manufacturing in most Western economies – as the biggest service industry, health care thus became a focus for attempts to increase efficiency.

All of these things are obviously true: but like so many plans drawn up from ideological assumptions rather than the real world, this analysis of the forces driving change appears to focus more on the conditions in which a political offensive *might* be waged than on explaining why governments would feel obliged to run the political risks involved in forcing through controversial changes in highly popular public services. The fact that some governments have advanced far further and more rapidly than others on market-style reforms suggests that more deep-seated political and ideological factors are driving the process of change, rather than general and objective trends.

The new conditions helped create a new element which became dominant within social democracy: it has been termed the 'Third Way'. This was the political approach supported from the mid-1990s by such leading politicians as former US President Bill Clinton, British Prime Minister Blair, Brazil's President Lula and German Chancellor Schroeder. Conferences and events to discuss and showcase Third Way politics were for a while sponsored by sections of big business – no doubt attracted by the way in which these 'new' social democrats effectively wound the clock back to before the advent of social democracy. This was done by incorporating

---

28 According to neoliberal critics, the tax-break subsidy for employment-based health insurance in the US is worth an estimated $125 billion a year (Health Policy Consensus Group 2001).

elements of the neoliberal agenda and discarding (for those who had ever held them) many traditional concepts which had previously defined social democracy[29] (Elliott 2003b, Madarasz 2003).

The Third Way claimed to distance itself from class politics and collective 'socialist' objectives, focussing instead on the individual consumer and on 'partnerships' between public and private sectors. But this was an illusory independence because it firmly embraced the main precepts of the 'New Public Management'; and while professing to smooth away inequalities through reforms designed to appear 'radical', in practice – as its own MPs admitted – it widened inequalities, making repeated concessions to the wealthy capitalist elite (Blair 2001b, 2003, Ramesh 2010, Woolf 2006).

While traditional social democracy favoured reforms involving planning and active management of capitalism, Third Way politicians have favoured the free working of the capitalist market system, with a minimum of regulation[30] – summed up in Britain as 'Thatcherism with a Christian Socialist face' (Jessop 2003). The Third Way also differs sharply from traditional social democracy in drawing no distinction between the purchase of services from the private or from the public sector.

In Britain, this led to: the use of private capital to finance 94 per cent of around 100 new hospitals built after 1997 through the Private Finance Initiative[31] and dozens of new health centres through a variant of PFI; a new 'Concordat' with the private sector to treat more NHS-funded patients; the establishment of a new network of private, for-profit Diagnostic and Independent Sector Treatment Centres delivering care to NHS patients; and the establishment of a new 'patient's choice' system that is already beginning to divert more NHS patients to private hospitals, financed from the public-sector budget.[32] In addition, 100 hospitals and mental health services were given autonomous 'foundation trust' status, standing outside the managerial structures and accountability of the NHS. Community health services were separated out, broken up and a process of privatisation to for-profit and non-profit providers began, initially inviting 'any willing provider' to bid for contracts. GP contracts, too, were offered to private corporations and smaller companies of entrepreneurial

---

29 Elliott (2003b) sums up by arguing that 'Third Wayers are free marketers who have learned how to play the chords to Stairway to Heaven'. The conference in the UK was attended by 400 think-tank analysts: it was followed by a summit meeting of leaders from 14 nations, including Germany, Canada, Poland, Hungary, Romania, the Czech Republic, Chile, Argentina, Brazil, New Zealand, South Africa and Ethiopia.

30 Clearly, minimal regulation is not the same as no regulation at all – which despite the enthusiasm of today's neoliberals and their predecessors has not prevailed as a policy with any government since the brief heyday of 'laissez faire' economics in Britain in the early nineteenth century.

31 PFI was aptly described by Conservative chancellor Kenneth Clarke in 1993 as 'Privatising the process of capital investment in our key public services, from design to construction to operation' (Lister 2002: 1).

32 Tony Blair in an article on 'Where the Third Way goes from here' goes even further, suggesting 'We should be far more radical about the role of the state as regulator rather than provider, opening up healthcare for example to a mixed economy under the NHS umbrella, and adopting radical approaches to self-health. We should also... be willing to experiment with new forms of co-payment in the public sector' (Blair 2003).

GPs seeking profit: a whole new 'partnership' was announced with private-sector providers invited by Tony Blair and ministers to join the 'NHS family'. Even the commissioning of services and planning was prepared for privatisation with the formulation of an approved list of 14 companies and consortia, comprising city-slicker management consultants, accountants and so-called 'think tanks' like the servile King's Fund (Leys and Player 2011, Lister 2008a).

Department of Health figures show spending by the NHS on non-NHS providers of services rocketing from £1.1 billion in 1997 to £7.4 billion in 2009 (Davies 2012), with the trajectory continuing upwards and even more rapid increases since the right-wing coalition government took over in 2010. This switch of resources to the private sector runs alongside a freeze on NHS funding and a drive to generate £20 billion in 'efficiency savings' between 2010 and 2014 (Ball and Sawer 2009). This is a more subtle approach than simply 'privatising' care: it enables the private sector to select its chosen areas and services, and to benefit from popular public-sector budgets. Far from offering any variant of socialism, New Labour proved itself the model advocate and architect of a piecemeal privatisation of services, beginning to reverse the historic 'modernisation' that had been achieved with the establishment of the NHS in 1948 (Lister 2008a). As Julian Tudor Hart points out:

> There is no question of total privatisation in the sense that medical care for the mass of people will ever be returned to the market. The new global capitalism is a true and devoted partnership between governments and multinational corporations.
>
> (Hart 2003)

2008 and after: seizing the opportunity of austerity

> 'Never let a serious crisis go to waste. What I mean by that is it's an opportunity to do things you couldn't do before.'
> Rahm Emmanuel, November 2008, cited by WSJ.com (January 2009)

These famous words of President Obama's former Chief of Staff sum up the way in which the aftermath of the 2008 banking crisis has opened the door for policies which previously would have been politically impossible, including massive and disproportionate cuts in public spending and in health budgets, accompanied by far-reaching rationing of services and 'reform' in Europe and elsewhere.

As Campaigner Naomi Klein argued, the crisis brought a brief pause in the neoliberal rhetoric – for long enough to allow for governments to pump in public money to prop up the private financial institutions brought down by irresponsible speculation – before normal hostilities resumed in the form of brutal austerity cuts to pay for the bail-out:

> During boom times, it's profitable to preach laissez faire, because an absentee government allows speculative bubbles to inflate. When those bubbles burst, the

ideology becomes a hindrance, and it goes dormant while big government rides to the rescue. But rest assured: the ideology will come roaring back when the bailouts are done. The massive debts the public is accumulating to bail out the speculators will then become part of a global budget crisis that will be the rationalisation for deep cuts to social programmes, and for a renewed push to privatise what is left of the public sector.

(Klein 2008)

The post-2008 crisis has also opened up opportunities for the scavengers of capitalism, the private-equity companies moving in on flagging non-profit and for-profit health-care providers to squeeze out the last vestiges of profit before moving on. The period 2010–11 marked a new boom in private-equity activity, mainly based in the US and Europe (Bain & Co. 2012). Becker and colleagues surveying the US scene identify no fewer than 13 'hot' areas of investment, while noting that four sectors have become less desirable to private-equity companies. By far the biggest investment has been in hospital systems which are seen as 'too big to fail': billions have been pumped into large financially struggling 'not for profit' US hospital chains, turning them into for-profit systems. But other profitable areas include the market in highly specialist hospital doctors, including anaesthetists and radiologists; ambulatory surgery; health-care information technology; drugs, devices and technology to deal with chronic disease; cancer care; and perhaps most gruesomely of all the prospects for profits from death through investment in the US hospice sector[33] (Becker et al. 2011).

Private equity cleans up

The takeover by private equity has also brought a shift of emphasis, from insurance companies screwing value from hospitals to hospitals becoming more aggressive in their billing of insurance companies (including the public-sector Medicare) (Creswell and Abelson 2012). One of the key exponents of this approach, generating copious profit streams, has been the giant US hospital corporation HCA, which was bought up in 2006 by Bain Capital, the private-equity firm co-founded by the Republicans' 2012 US Presidential hopeful Mitt Romney. The new PE-led HCA has stopped its hospital ERs treating patients with non-urgent conditions unless they pay a co-payment of $150 up front; and they changed their billing codes for hospital emergency rooms, boosting the numbers said to require more care (and therefore incurring higher fees): it increased earnings by almost $100 million in a quarter. Within the hospital, too, PE went on the offensive: staffing levels were squeezed down and hospital doctors were required to focus more on generating profits for the parent company. One California hospital increased income for the most serious classification of treatment almost 20-fold from $48,000 in 2006 to $949,000 in 2010 (Creswell and Abelson 2012). However, the ruthless tactics employed by private equity have led to critics warning that they were creating an unsustainable 'bubble' in US health care (Denning 2012).

---

33 One company has begun to set up 'hospice campuses' combining hospice and home care.

In the UK, private equity is behind the high-profile but not yet profitable Circle Health, which owns a small number of bijou and costly private hospitals and became the first company to take over the management of an NHS hospital (Hinchingbrooke in Cambridgeshire) since a failed experiment in the West Midlands 2003 (Lister 2008b). Circle presents itself as some form of social enterprise or mutual, but 51 per cent of it is owned by a number of private-equity investors. A number of the other large operators in the UK private health market have also been taken over by private equity, as well as Southern Cross, the UK's largest chain of nursing homes, which collapsed suddenly and spectacularly under the stewardship of private equity in 2011 (Shipman 2011).

In India, the rapidly growing health-care industry and medical tourism have attracted a number of private-equity investors: the giant Apollo Hospitals group is now partly owned by Apax Partners; and General Atlantic, Actis and Jardine Rothschild have also been showing an interest (Apax 2012, Kurian et al. 2011), although the market has cooled a little (Anand 2012).

Ideological bias of reforms

The overall political thrust of the reforms in health-care systems in the last 30 years has been politically rightwards, away from notions of social solidarity. The range of alternative policies for welfare backed by global (World Bank and IMF) and supranational (OECD) organisations is limited and 'currently confined to variants of liberalism', while the ideological retreat of traditional social democracy has been faster and more complete than the vanishing of the ice caps. As far back as 2001, Yeates pointed out that there was 'a marked absence of any international institution advancing a social-democratic or redistributive agenda' (Yeates 2001: 29).

Deacon (2001) drew a similar conclusion – that no international organisation, with the possible exception of UNICEF, still embraced an old-style 'Scandinavian-type' redistributive approach to social policy. Even the Scandinavians have been dragged to the right: their social model has been increasingly fractured and public-sector budgets milked by market-style reforms (Martinussem and Magnussen 2009, Vrangbæk 2009). Rightward-moving sections of the one-time political left have found it too easy to refer to 'globalisation' as the root cause of social problems such as unemployment, poverty, austerity and 'structural adjustment programmes', without recognising the extent of complicity and corruption of national governments and political leaders, or coming to grips with the social dimensions of globalisation. Universalism appears to have been sidelined without any real resistance (Deacon et al. 2005). Such political factors can be decisive: Ferge, examining developments in Central and Eastern Europe, raises the key issue of the ideological driving force behind the reform process, identifying priorities – and targets for cuts:

> In the short term, cutbacks in state spending are an economic necessity. This does not fully explain, however, why the welfare system had become the main target of cutbacks, and why the cuts are implemented in a way that affects long-term commitment in all areas of public well-being.
>
> (Ferge 2001: 150)

Arguing that 'politics matter', Yeates (2001: 127) also criticises the excessive weight given to economic forces and the downplaying of political factors by all those who argue a 'strong' role for globalisation as a force 'bulldozing' reluctant governments into policies. She stresses the importance of political counter-pressures which can limit the scope for implementation of market-style reforms – notably social conflict, political opposition and class struggle at a national level – and points out that this has increasingly led to international pressures and campaigns explicitly challenging capitalist globalisation. Pierson, too, argues that 'Few serious commentators on social policy accept the globalisation story in its simplest and most draconian form' (Pierson 1998: 64).

But of course, globalisation has its supporters. The political right and 'Third Way' social democrats have welcomed 'globalisation' as offering new opportunities and advances, while studiously ignoring – and through their policies even intensifying – the negative side-effects of growing inequality and social exclusion on a global level.

Chapter three

The World Health Organization

One of the global organisations which might be expected to uphold a more progressive agenda, addressing some of the genuine social and economic issues involved in the improvement of health on a world scale, is the World Health Organization (WHO). Launched in 1946, with 61 countries signing its constitution and 55 attending its 1948 World Health Assembly, the WHO now has 194 member countries (2012) and is the United Nations' leading specialist agency for health (Vaughan et al. 1996).

The WHO is not an NGO and does not deliver services directly: instead it works with governments and health ministries, in a manner designed to 'avoid charges of imperialism' (Godlee 1994a). Its Secretariat has 4,500 members of staff and the WHO employs 8,000 overall, covering six regional offices as well as the Geneva HQ, and 147 national offices.

The WHO is best known for its projects and public-health campaigns reaching into the poorer countries of Africa and Asia, and for its ambitious – ultimately unattainable – Health for All 2000 project. This was launched in 1977 and promoted alongside UNICEF at the international conference in Alma Ata in 1978. HFA 2000 aimed at improving the health of the world's population by the turn of the century (WHO 1992). Linked to the HFA programme was a new emphasis on primary health care (PHC) as the key to developing an infrastructure of basic health care, public health and preventive measures that could reach the poor and rural areas in developing countries rather than squander the largest share of resources on one or two high-cost, showpiece hospitals in the capital or urban areas.

As a global body credited by the UN in 1979 with coordinating the elimination of smallpox, and which continues a focus on preventing communicable disease in developing countries, the WHO also has the potential to be a significant force in influencing health-care policies, especially among the poorest member states – although in practice, its freedom to act, and even its ability to publish accurate data which may be perceived as embarrassing or damaging to influential member states, can also be constrained (Murray et al. 2004).

Conservative beginnings

During its first 25 years, the WHO was a fairly conservative, specialist, medical-led agency, consciously avoiding political or potential religious controversy that might arise from dabbling in issues such as contraception (Godlee 1994b). However, the rising number of independent member states and the influence of the Non-Aligned Movement countries meant that political control of the World Health Assembly, like that of the UN General Assembly, had visibly slipped from the grasp of the USA and the wealthier developed countries by the late 1970s. While the increasingly representative membership gave the WHO potentially greater authority, from a US standpoint this also made the WHO potentially vulnerable to 'capture' by more radical policies promoted by increasingly self-confident and independent-minded developing countries, rather than domination by Washington and its wealthier and more conservative co-thinkers.

With its emphasis on support for the world's poorest people and its explicit call for a 'New International Economic Order' (PAHO 2008: III), the Health for All 2000 policy was followed in the same year by a WHO challenge to the profits of the pharmaceutical corporations when it published a list of 200 cheaper 'essential' drugs. These were to be purchased and prescribed in preference to up to 5,000 branded drugs that were being sold at high prices to 'third-world' countries (Turshen 1999). This degree of independence made the WHO an obvious target for those who valued the freedom of the market above equity in health care or access to care for the majority of the world's population.

The US government, in particular, objected to the WHO's attempts to regulate the private sector and also to the WHO's (far from radical) efforts, through the HFA initiative, to reduce tobacco consumption. In 1981, the US became the only country at the WHA to oppose the new WHO international code on breast milk substitutes, arguing that it was 'an interference in global trade'. And in 1985, this growing antipathy culminated in the US, under the Presidency of Ronald Reagan, withholding its contributions to the WHO budget (Godlee 1994b). The WHO's central leadership has come under increasing pressure ever since to tailor the organisation's initiatives and policies to fit within the resurgent free-market ideology espoused by Reagan, Thatcher and their ideological successors, as well as the World Bank and the IMF.

Financial/economic pressure

As part of this pressure, the WHO's core budget has effectively been frozen since 1980, giving zero growth in real terms. By 2006–7, the regular 'assessed contributions' from member states amounted to just 28 per cent of the WHO's programme budget of $3.3 billion (WHO 2007: 20); in 2011, it had fallen to 25 per cent of $3.96 billion, with the WHO forced into making cuts in staff and programs (Nebehay and Lewis 2011); and the most recent figure is around 20 per cent (People's Health Movement 2011: 28).

This has meant that any significant new initiative has had to be funded through a rising level of 'extrabudgetary' contributions from the wealthier countries – funds and initiatives which are not controlled by the World Health Assembly (WHA). As a result of this new system, donor countries like the US, which had failed to maintain direct control democratically by winning a majority in the WHA, have been able to circumvent the apparatus and decide WHO policies on the ground by granting or withholding funding (Godlee 1994a).

By 1990, the WHO had been effectively sidelined as a major player in the provision of external assistance, with its levels of spending dwarfed by NGOs such as Oxfam and Save the Children Fund, and even by direct loans from the World Bank. Godlee found that in India, in 1994, the WHO's annual budget was just $7.5 million compared with $100 million available to UNICEF, the rival UN agency dealing with health and nutritional matters, with which the WHO was increasingly in competition for influence, despite the fact that UNICEF's rudimentary anti-HIV programme was dismissed as 'only condoms' (Godlee 1994c).

As Turshen (1999) argues, the various donors of extrabudgetary contributions are inclined to fund 'the disease of the day rather than long-term basic health care' and their contributions are given for only one year at a time, creating uncertainty and instability in any planning process. Large amounts of WHO time and resources then have to be allocated to the management of specific smaller-scale projects rather than offering more coordination, international cooperation and sharing of information.

The impact of the cash squeeze on the WHO was intensified by the refusal of its controversial director general to focus available resources on a more restricted range of key health issues for the developing countries where Health for All was farthest from being achieved. According to Godlee and other analysts of the WHO, its director general from 1988 to 1998, Dr Hiroshi Nakajima, carried much of the political criticism for the decline of the WHO's influence – despite the fact that this was partly a consequence of policy decisions taken before he took office.

One apparently perverse WHO response to the external pressure was to expand its top layers of directors and administration, adding to overhead costs, accelerating the decline in staff morale and further reducing the resources available for front-line project work. A third of its staff were based in Geneva – hardly the centre of global deprivation – incurring inflated overhead costs in one of the most expensive cities in the world (Godlee 1994b) and making it costly and difficult for delegations from the poorest countries to be involved in work at the centre. Donors began to make it clear from the early 1990s that they were increasingly reluctant to fund WHO projects without the prospect of a shake-up in the organisation, beginning at the top (Walt 1994, Vaughan et al. 1996). By 1996, the WHO was seriously in debt, but was itself owed $243 million of unpaid contributions from member states: it had to 'borrow' its entire internal reserve of $175 million to keep front-line operations afloat (Godlee 1996).

Turshen (1999) and other critics argue that the WHO's growing dependence on this additional revenue, and the way in which it has been effectively ring-fenced for specific programmes ('the disease of the day rather than long-term basic health care'), may have steered the organisation away from the influence of the poorer member states. Moreover, it has made the WHO increasingly subject to influence by other bodies – notably the World Bank, donor governments in the wealthier countries, and the drug companies – whose agenda can be seen as very different from the founding objectives of the WHO.

The impact of these external pressures on the WHO and its core programmes can be seen to some extent in the criticisms raised over the limited progress of its main central campaign. This impact is also apparent in concerns that the use of 'extrabudgetary' funds to run projects can lead in the opposite direction from the WHO's goals of equity and respect for the needs of the poorest.

The lack of satisfactory progress towards the target of Health for All by 2000 was questioned by a number of observers, not least in Europe, where, even in the more favourable circumstances of existing health-care systems and relatively high per capita incomes, the commitment of governments was 'patchy', yielding only 'moderate' signs of success by 1992 (Rathwell 1992).

While others such as Yach and von Schirnding (1994) endorsed the WHO principles, their focus was primarily upon the switch to primary care in the context of growing poverty in Sub-Saharan Africa, emphasising the need for health policies to be seen not as self-contained but as a key part of the wider 'development agenda'. A politically hamstrung WHO appeared to be emerging more as a lobby group for third-world countries than as an effective guiding and coordinating force orchestrating change on a world scale.

The WHO and health-system reforms

The WHO is not a homogenous political part, and its literature does not offer a coherent line of approach, especially when there are varying degrees to which researchers and analysts are influenced by external ideological pressures. As a result, WHO-sponsored debates reflect a rather more detached and critical approach than that of the World Bank to many key aspects of health-care reforms; but even while the debates have continued, the organisation's involvement in the process of reform since the mid-1990s has contributed to the pressure for change – at a time when the most powerful forces have been seeking to direct that change towards market-style measures.

Navarro is one of the critics who have stressed the potential political and ideological role which the WHO can play on behalf of neoliberal reformers, even while still being perceived by many as in some way outside of the overtly political arena (Navarro 2000). As we shall see, a number of studies have underlined the process of political evolution which some argue has transformed the WHO during the last quarter of a century: from its early role as the pioneering global promoter of public health, the WHO has been transformed into an organisation increasingly perceived as eclipsed by, or even an adjunct of, global bodies with alien agendas, such as the World Bank, the IMF and the giant transnational pharmaceutical corporations (People's Health Movement 2011).

The process of political softening within the WHO, if it has occurred, has not been an even one. But its results can be illustrated by a stark contrast. In 1995, its *World Health Report* focused relentlessly on extreme poverty as the 'world's biggest killer', pointing to the way in which 'the gaps between rich and poor, between one population group and another, between ages and between the sexes are widening.' (WHO 1995a: 1) It went on to warn that gains from recent immunisation campaigns were being 'eroded or even reversed by economic and social conditions' (1995a: 4). And (without naming the World Bank or the IMF as culprits) it also pointed out that structural adjustment policies aimed at improving the economic performance of poor countries had in many cases made the situation worse. The WHO sounded a warning that, while market forces alone could not achieve a rational and cost-effective system to deliver services:

> There is unease in some quarters that governments may be silently withdrawing from their responsibilities to provide care, acting instead as ring masters, while other actors do the work...
>
> (1995a: 42)

A WHO position paper on social determinants of health in the same year contained an explicit rejection of market forces and privatisation, with a scathing critique pointing to the growing inequalities flowing from globalisation (WHO 1995b).

But that was soon no longer WHO policy. A radically different approach to the question of the roots of ill health can be found in the *World Health Report 2000* (*WHR 2000*), which – as Navarro (2000) has shown – makes the link not between ill health and poverty, but ill health and health spending:

> Thus if Sweden enjoys better health than Uganda – life expectancy is almost exactly twice as long – that is in large part because it spends exactly 35 times as much per capita on its health system.
>
> (WHO 2000: 40)

Navarro (2000) challenges this unsupported claim that medical treatment and spending on health care are alone likely to reduce mortality and morbidity levels, along with a number of the *WHR 2000*'s other fundamental assumptions, which we will return to below. But it is clear from this change of emphasis that the WHO has begun to position itself differently in relation to the main global organisations and governments deciding health-care policy.

Exactly when this change of line took effect is hard to pinpoint. During 1996, the WHO in Europe conducted an extensive debate – later published – on the various models of 'health reforms', in which a range of authors reviewed the options and came to a generally critical conclusion, summed up by the editors thus:

> The cross-national evidence... indicates that reforms have been less successful when they have focused on the application of market-style incentives to individual patient-based demand...
>
> (Saltman et al. 2000: 401)

The same debate also came up with a negative balance sheet on the other main policy fetish of the neoliberal reformers: the introduction of 'cost-sharing' schemes or exclusion of particular treatments from publicly funded packages of care:

> Cost sharing may reduce the utilization of services initiated by the patient, but such reductions may not be very effective in achieving cost containment.
>
> (Saltman et al. 2000: 403)

The Ljubljana Charter

These conclusions – effectively a (fairly timid) restatement of the WHO's long-standing commitment to social solidarity and equity in the provision of health care – will have done nothing to endear the WHO to the British and US governments of the day. Indeed, there was evident disapproval from the neoliberal camp.

At the WHO-sponsored conference in Ljubljana in June 1996, while ministerial delegations from the other 50 WHO European member states lent general support, the British government's representatives resorted to the undignified manoeuvre of absenting themselves from the final stages of debate – to avoid lending their support to a Charter based on the findings (Richards 1996). Britain's Conservative health minister, Gerald Malone MP, subsequently avoided offering any explanation of the delegation's behaviour and made no explicit attack on the Charter itself, dismissing it as proposals for Central and Eastern Europe and the former Soviet Union (Hansard 1996).

Although not binding on the WHO as a whole, the outcome of the Ljubljana conference did represent the consensus view of many of the WHO's wealthiest European member states, embodying a substantial proportion of the OECD countries. It was a significant arena in which to lose the argument for greater use of market-style methods and, as an event sponsored (and the results published) by the WHO, it clearly will have been seen as maintaining a line counterposed to that of the World Bank.

In the same year, Klugman and Schieber (1996), reflecting the World Bank's point of view, approvingly pointed out the extent to which a single market-style model could increasingly be seen at the centre of most health-system reforms in the aftermath of the fall of the Berlin Wall:

> Virtually all former socialist economies, middle income Latin American countries and western industrial OECD countries are separating provision from finance, having money follow patients in the context of an overall global budget.

By contrast, the Ljubljana Charter stressed very different values. It insists (para 2) that a criterion for promoting any form of health-care or health-system reforms is that they 'should first and foremost lead to better health and quality of life for people' (WHO Europe 1996). And while it recognises the need for cost-effectiveness (5.3), and the need for sound financing, it also restates the objective of 'universal coverage and equitable access by all people to the necessary care' (5.4).

The World Bank, and especially the British government of the day, still embroiled in the implementation of its own controversial market-style reforms and rejecting calls for their effectiveness to be evaluated (Lister 2008a), would not have been keen to endorse the Charter's declaration that:

> Major policy, managerial and technical decisions on development of the health care system should be based on evidence where available. Reforms must be continuously monitored and evaluated in a way that is transparent to the public.
>
> (6.1.2)

Nor would the government that pushed through the privatisation of many non-clinical support services in British hospitals, on the basis of insisting that management accept the cheapest available tender, have welcomed the Ljubljana Charter's proposal that quality of care, not cost, should be the key criterion:

> Wherever market mechanisms are appropriate, they should favour competition in ensuring quality and in using scarce resources.
>
> (6.1.3)

A new spin on 'primary care'

However, while the Charter's rejection of the market system would not have gone down well, it is important also to note that the British government had already taken on board one of the other planks of the HFA platform which was again part of the Ljubljana Charter: the focus on 'primary care' – even if this is translated to mean something very different from the WHO/Alma Ata approach. In Britain, this took the form of the call from the early 1990s for a 'primary-care-led NHS', which was in turn used as a way to justify using family doctors and primary-care staff as a cheap and cheerful replacement after closures and rationalisation of hospitals: but also to promote the controversial plan to make larger GP practices into 'fund-holders', wild cards in the new internal market, free to buy health care for their patients from NHS or private-sector providers of their choice (Lister 2008a).

It is hard not to see potential problems and weaknesses in the Charter's insistence – even in the context of relatively advanced economies and developed health-care systems in Europe – that resources had to be taken from hospitals and redirected to 'primary care' without any clear definition of what type of alternative system was being proposed, or how it could be organised and funded. What was little more than an untested theory was now being imposed as a fixed model, albeit through a watered-down phrase from the WHO model for care in developing countries. Nevertheless, the Ljubljana Charter was quite emphatic on the need for:

> Well-designed strategies [that] are needed to shift working capacity from acute hospital care to primary health care, community care, day care and home care, whenever necessary.
>
> (6.3.2)

This is not the only potential weakness in the Charter: there are also signs of inconsistency in its call for greater decentralisation of health-care management. On the one hand, it was urged that individual health-care institutions 'should enjoy the maximum possible autonomy' in managing their resources – but on the other, it was said that this must be 'consistent with the principles of an equitable and efficient health-care system.' (6.5.2) The British market-style reforms had shown that the balance between these two objectives is not easy to strike, especially if the 'autonomy' is also interpreted as the freedom to compete for funds and human resources against other similar institutions (Lister 2008a, Leys and Player 2011).

Despite these apparent weaknesses, the adoption of the Charter was viewed as a step forward by some of those opposing market-based reforms. As Vienonen and colleagues pointed out three years later:

> Since 1996 the Charter and the analysis associated with it have been used by health sector politicians, administrators, professional groups and grass roots organisations in support of their arguments with ministries of finance and particularly with proponents of unrestrained privatisation.
>
> (Vienonen et al. 1999: 46)

But in the aftermath of Ljubljana, while some enthusiasts for public-sector provision and opponents of market-style measures were invoking the 1996 decisions, the direction of the WHO appears to have changed substantially and abruptly. If the seeds of this change had been sown through the prolonged political and financial pressure on the WHO, they appear to have begun to germinate more strongly just after the 1998 change of leadership within the WHO and the appointment of the former Norwegian Prime Minister Gro Harlem Brundtland as director general.

World Bank adjusts its line

In part, the change of line also reflected an accommodation by the WHO to political developments already implemented within the more established health-care systems. But another major influence seems to have been the World Bank itself, which (as we will examine in more detail below) had moved increasingly from its original post-war role – in which it had largely ignored health issues and simply funded development projects – to the elaboration of detailed policies and engagement in efforts to shape health-care systems in developing countries. It is clear from some of the changing rhetoric of its pronouncements and from the research it sponsored that the Bank was looking for ways to present itself as a less-aggressive, more-caring force on issues of social policy, in contrast to its harsh 1993 line of user fees and minimal care in poorer countries[1] (Abbassi 1999f).

Buse and Walt have also commented on the political convergence, since the late 1970s, between the UN and its agencies on the one hand and the World Bank on the other, noting that:

> Entente between private-for-profit (corporate) and public sectors in particular was the result of a number of changes in the context of international cooperation on health. First the 1990s were marked by an ideological shift from 'freeing' to 'modifying' the market. ... [Since then] most advocates of free markets have moderated their position, seeing a continuing role for the public sector,

---

1   The WHO's *World Health Report 1995* specifically challenges the Bank's 1993 proposal that 'in poor countries there should be no complex heart surgery, no treatment other than pain relief for cancer, no provision of expensive drugs for HIV/AIDS and no intensive care for premature babies.' Rather mildly, the WHO responds: 'This proposal was criticised as applying a balance-sheet mentality on health care' (WHO 1995a: 44).

particularly within the area of health, where markets are often inefficient and equity is harder to achieve.

(Buse and Walt 2000a: 551)

Among the factors driving this accommodation from the other side was the financial weakness of the WHO (with frozen budgets and under pressure from the wealthier member states), coupled with WHO recognition that many programmes were dependent upon the use of drugs and vaccines developed and controlled by the private sector, especially pharmaceutical corporations. For their part, some key corporations, notably the drug companies, perceived the commercial advantages of being seen to work in 'partnership' with widely respected global organisations.

The relationship between the Bank and the WHO become much more overtly close. An example of this was the WHO technical seminar held in July 1997 to discuss a presentation by the Bank's Principal Economist, Dr Alex Preker, on the 'new strategy of the World Bank'. The Bank was seeking to enlist the credibility of the WHO's expertise on public health issues, while upholding its own economic views. The subsequent published summary reports (without comment) that:

The need for strong collaboration between WHO and the World Bank was stressed. In many areas, particularly disease prevention and control, the World Bank indicated that WHO has the best international technical capacity, while in other areas, such as in the development of health-system policies, an enhanced integration of the strategies of both organisations at the country level would be most effective.

(Feachem and Preker 1997)

Whose agenda?

Although the financial and ideological pressures that had been brought to bear on the WHO have been discussed above, there had not until this point been a great deal of obvious convergence in views between the leading global force for neoliberal reforms, cost-sharing and privatisation, on the one hand, and the post-Ljubljana WHO with its renewed opposition to such policies, on the other. The big question was therefore: on whose agenda might the suggested greater level of integration and joint working be based?

A clue to this can be found in the summary of another WHO HFA 21 technical seminar, on 'Health Financing in Developing Countries: Issues, Evidence and Options' and held in January 1997. In it, Professor Dean T. Jamison:

presented work in progress by Dr Feachem [then head of the World Bank's Health, Nutrition and Population programme] and himself. He emphasised that country data on health outcomes and lessons learned from OECD countries could be utilised to guide policy makers in developing countries in choosing between options to finance the health care system.

(Feachem and Preker 1997)

While this makes clear the eagerness of WHO and World Bank academics to transfer political and organisational structures from the first world to the third, and raises doubts over the appropriateness of doing so, the conclusion of the summary is even more categoric: one of the 'lessons' which the seminar agreed should be transferred was the establishment of a market-style approach, with competition between providers. Within this, the private sector should be welcomed:

> Health care markets are not really competitive markets. ... Nevertheless competition between providers should be stimulated, for instance in a capitated system, that gives, when required, the necessary information (e.g. on provider performance) to consumers. Such a system would welcome the private sector, but within a framework of strong government regulation and a publicly financed system.
>
> (Feachem and Preker 1997)

With policies like these, despite any reservations it may have had about the direction of health reforms, the WHO could play a useful role for the World Bank – by promoting a debate which kept open the door for market-style solutions or for an increased role for the private sector. The impact of the WHO's promotion of such debates would be even greater in the developing countries, where there was much less in the way of a well-established pre-existing health-care system with sufficient political leverage to block the imposition of 'reforms'.

However, in there were warnings – albeit low-key – that 'reformers' were in danger of making serious mistakes, with the publication of the (edited) WHO-commissioned background papers for the Ljubljana conference. These raised serious doubts over the long-term effectiveness in Europe of many of the key reforms advocated by the neoliberal lobby – market-style reforms such as decentralisation, cost-sharing and rationing of services (Saltman et al. 2000). The critique was neither strong nor consistent.

The WHO: change at the top

The increasingly close working relationship between the WHO and the World Bank and other organisations promoting neoliberal policies developed even more after Dr Gro Harlem Brundtland was elected WHO director general in 1998. Brundtland consistently emphasised her determination to work alongside the private sector and her quest for 'partnership' with the World Bank and other global agencies. Sometimes, as in her 1998 speech to the WHO Regional Committee in Harare, she combined this with an emphatic statement that markets alone cannot deliver the public-health agenda:

> Markets have failed to achieve similar success in health. In general terms the private sector may be good at allocating resources cost-effectively. But the private sector – private industry – will never become the key provider of primary health stations or the guarantor of securing health services to the poor. Neither will it assure universal access. ... Only the public sector can guarantee basic universal rights.
>
> (Brundtland 1998a)

However, a few sentences further on in the same speech, appearing to have borrowed from the speech book of Tony Blair, she added the qualification that the public sector may 'guarantee basic services' – by buying them from private providers.

> We need to reach out. Provision of government financed services must come from the most efficient source. That may mean providers from the private sector. From NGOs. Governments should seek to engage capacity wherever it may be in meeting [their] responsibility of universal care.

Brundtland reached out repeatedly to the private sector in building a new leadership to take the WHO down her chosen path. On taking office on 21st July, she was swift to appoint ten new people to a new cabinet of top-level advisors, including Dr Michael Scholz, a senior figure from the pharmaceutical industry, who was seen as providing a new 'liaison' between the industry and the WHO (Godlee 1998).

A leading light from the World Bank, the former director of its Health Nutrition and Population (HNP) sector, Richard Feachem, took over as Editor in Chief of a remodelled *Bulletin of the World Health Organization*. Feachem's appointment was controversial, not least because of criticisms raised by the World Bank's own Operations Evaluation Department (OED) of the poor performance of HNP programmes during the time Feachem had been in control. The OED was especially concerned about the HNP's inadequate analysis of the factors that lead to ill health among the poor – suggesting a very different set of assumptions from the public-health perspective of the WHO (Gershman and Irwin 2000, Johnston and Stout 1999). Nevertheless, the new magazine began monthly publication in 1999, becoming much more overtly political and focused on the various issues of reform (Feachem 1999).

The Bank's team take over

More personnel were also recruited from the World Bank to help boost the limited numbers in the WHO focused on health economics. The Bank's people predictably brought many of the Bank's ideas with them: the scale of the resultant change in the WHO's political stance can be seen from the abrupt change of tone and position in *WHR 2000*.

The report's principal authors included two heavy-hitters from the World Bank, Philip Musgrove and Alex Preker, and the conceptual framework was developed by Christopher Murray, together with upwardly mobile Mexican health academic and World Bank consultant Julio Frenk (appointed Health Minister in Mexico from 2000 to 2006, and then a potential neoliberal contender for the WHO director general position), who also chaired the report's steering committee.

The change was dramatic. Out went primary health care, universalism and a focus on public provision: in came 'selective universalism', 'primary care' as a cheap, second-tier option, and 'stewardship' as a polite way to describe the commissioning of services from private and other providers. Along with these came the notion of 'Global Public Private Partnerships', initially with the drug companies, but with the option to link up with others offering sufficient money. Moreover, a controversial new measure of 'equity' in the funding of health care was introduced together with an even more controversial 'league table' of health systems, which appeared to favour those closest to the neoliberal approach (WHO 2000).

Brundtland's 'partnership' approach with the private sector brought the inclusion of other leading representatives of the pharmaceutical industry in the WHO's working parties, including the Tobacco Free Initiative and the HIV/AIDS campaign. In 2000, Buse and Walt discussed the emergence of 'Global Public–Private Partnerships' in two articles in the WHO *Bulletin* (Buse and Walt 2002a, 2000b).

In March 2001, giving a lecture improbably titled 'Globalisation as a force for better health' at the London School of Economics, Brundtland pressed further along the same path when she outlined an apolitical appeal to the 'enlightened self-interest' of big capital, which she argued would 'compel':

> industrialised country governments and private corporations to do what it takes to drastically reduce the current burden of disease in the developing world.
>
> (Brundtland 2001a)

The following month, Brundtland launched a WHO/WTO workshop on differential pricing and financing of essential drugs, apparently oblivious to the fact that the meeting took place in the midst of what was already a growing worldwide revolt against both globalisation in general and the WTO in particular. Since the Seattle demonstrations, the WTO was increasingly seen as a US-dominated front organisation pressing home the neoliberal agenda; whereas Brundtland described the WTO in wholly positive terms: 'We need WTO as an effective and fair forum for negotiating trade rules and resolving disputes.' (Brundtland 2001b) In May 2001, Brundtland spelled out an even wider and less-focused agenda for partnerships with almost any global agency, citing work with the OECD, the EU and many more organisations with very different aims and objectives, including USAID, the most explicit proponents of private-sector solutions:

> We have placed large emphasis on partnerships – reaching out has become one of the key policies of WHO. We have strengthened our links with the IMF, the World Bank, the World Trade Organisation, our UN partners in UNICEF, UNFPA and UNDP. ... We have stepped up our partnership with bilateral cooperation agencies like USAID, which we consider partners, not just donors. We have organised round tables with private sector industry and have undertaken several initiatives in partnership with corporations and foundations.
>
> (Brundtland 2001c)

We will return below to this issue of partnership and some of the implications and potential dangers that have been identified by critics of the policy; but it is clear from Brundtland's speeches and personal involvement that the change of emphasis and rapprochement with the World Bank was a deliberate WHO policy, not a series of accidents or coincidences.

WHO independence

It could be argued that one of the reasons why the WHO is an attractive partner for the World Bank is because it is seen as having a degree of independence, together with a brief for public health rather than a brief to improve the balance sheets of big capital. A WHO which openly embraced neoliberalism and the World Bank's own undiluted free-market rhetoric would immediately lose its credibility in many developing countries. It should be no surprise, therefore, that the WHO's *World Health Report 2000* (WHO 2000) discusses ways of mitigating the damage (such as perverse incentives, exclusions and adverse selection) that can arise from the introduction of more market-based systems of health insurance. Nevertheless, it still managed to give a kind of retrospective endorsement to Margaret Thatcher's market-style reforms by echoing the famous claim of Conservative ministers that a system is good if 'the money follows the patient'.

In some parts, *WHR 2000* held on to traditional WHO positions, taking a strong line against the imposition of user fees and the objective of 'full cost recovery', explicitly challenging the stock neoliberal assumption of moral hazard, although ending limply, leaving open the option of arguing that 'there is no alternative':

> Free-of-charge services do not translate automatically into unjustified over-utilization of services. ... Because of the desirability of separating contributions from utilization, out-of-pocket payment should not be used unless no other alternative is available.
>
> (WHO 2000, Chap 4: 4–6)

A system which requires individuals to pay at the point of treatment would act most consistently to deter the poor and has the effect of 'indiscriminately' reducing demand, the report argues. The implications for public health could be serious:

> Some important health interventions would not be financed at all if people had to pay for them, as is the case for the public good type of interventions discussed in Chapter 3.
>
> (WHO 2000)

However, the most far-reaching political debate over the evolution and role of the WHO was triggered by two changes in WHO policy that were embodied in *World Health Report 2000* (WHO 2000):

- The decision to synthesise some of its routinely published statistical information into a direct comparison between different national systems
- The decision to embark on a process of building 'Global Public Private Partnerships'.

The *WHR* attempted (albeit in an Appendix rather than in the main body of the report) to rank 191 health services from all over the world in a single league table – based on contentious calculations of 'healthy life expectancy' for the country's population, 'responsiveness' of the service to patients and the 'fairness' of the financing system. It triggered a wave of angry responses.

While a few struggled to find positive aspects in the *WHR* findings or at least in the likely consequences of their publication (McKee 2001), those offended by the conclusions and/or the methodology employed by the *WHR* ranged from the aggrieved governments whose health-care systems came unexpectedly low on the list (notably Brazil, which came 125th (Almeida et al. 2001)) to World Bank neoliberals who ridiculed the 'counterintuitive' and 'seriously flawed' fairness indicator (Shaw 2002, Wagstaff 2002). Other critics on the left included enthusiastic proponents of equity in health care (Braveman et al. 2001).

So serious were the shock waves generated by the WHO's 2000 report that publication of a second, updated version, due in October 2002 (PAHO 2001b, 2001c) was postponed to late 2003 (Brown 2002). A full-scale debate over the methodology for any future comparisons between systems was opened up on the WHO website.

Gaps in data

While some of the anger focused on the very large gaps in the data used for the comparisons, the use of ten-year-old data (Landmann Szwarcwald 2002) and the fact that these gaps were covered over by the way in which the WHO league table was drawn up, there are more far-reaching debates over the adequacy of some of the statistical measures which the WHO has borrowed from health economists.

The gaps in data were extremely large. Almeida et al. (2001) point out that there were no data available for the WHO to construct its 'index of inequality' for 133 of the 191 countries (70 per cent), while 'responsiveness' data were unavailable for even more (161, or 84 per cent) and only 21 of the 191 countries (11 per cent) supplied data to construct the index on fairness. There were some countries for which no data at all were available on which to base a score, and therefore their ranking order was based purely on 'imputed data'. Almeida et al. argue that the result was seriously flawed:

> Because all the measures are new, and imputed values for the 70–89% of countries without data were based on new methods involving multiple non-standard assumptions, readers deserve to know the underlying assumptions, methods and key limitations, which were not adequately acknowledged...

Other criticisms include the fact that the WHO report claims to have drawn on 1,791 responses, but admits that these came from only 35 countries, and has failed to show how representative these responses may have been; and that 26 of the 32 documents cited as the basis for the methodology of the report had only been published as internal WHO documents and not subjected to peer review. To make matters worse, the calculation of 'responsiveness' of health services excluded any weighting for the accessibility of services (Van der Stuyft and Unger 2000).

Navarro (2000) also took the *WHR* to task for its counterintuitive positioning of the Spanish health-care system as third best major country in Europe in the overall league tables (after France and Italy), at the very time of widespread public discontent and protests by Spanish people over failures in the system. Indeed, Spain emerges in the WHO's own figures as one of the least 'responsive' of all the European health services.

Navarro draws a link between the *WHR*'s contrived selection of statistical data and lop-sided findings (in which Colombia, with its very limited insurance-based managed-care health system, emerges as the 'best overall system' in Latin America), on the one hand, and political and ideological concessions by the WHO to US neoliberal economics and the World Bank, on the other.

Navarro also warns against seeing the WHO as apolitical or neutral, stressing that it can play an ideological role, and condemns the way in which, with no serious evidence or discussion, the *WHR* declared the long-standing WHO policy of promoting services based on primary care to be 'at least a partial failure'.

A different line of criticism points out that using statistics to measure the average level of health in a population is a reductionist retreat from the WHO's often-quoted definition of health as 'a state of complete physical, mental and social well-being and not merely the absence of disease' (Van der Stuyft and Unger 2000).

Dahlgren (2000) pointed to the explicit World Bank input and role in these WHO debates in the form of WB statistician David Gwatkin and questioned the extent to which the Bank's policies are compatible with the WHO's proclaimed objectives. We will return in subsequent chapters to a closer examination of the evolving politics of the Bank and the extent to which they are a factor in the reforms that are taking place.

A retreat from equity?

Indeed, the barrage of criticism of *WHR 2000* serves to underline the extent to which the collection and selection of ostensibly 'objective' statistics can be – or be *construed* to be – highly political, reflecting a clear ideological standpoint and potentially supporting one of a number of vested interests in the debate over health-system reforms.

Critics pressing for greater equity in health systems, for example, have questioned the *WHR*'s peculiar definition of health-care financing as 'perfectly fair' if all households pay the same proportion of their non-food spending on health services – irrespective of how much money (if any) different households may have left over after paying for food (WHO 2000: 36, Murray and Frenk 2000). Almeida et al. point out that this reflects:

> The questionable view that it would be 'unfair if rich households pay more as a share of their capacity [than poor households]' since 'simply by paying the same fraction as poor households they would be subsidising those with lower ability to pay.'
>
> (Almeida et al. 2001: 1,694)

The authors go on to argue that under such criteria it could be deemed 'fair' if two households, one with a $500 income and one with $100,000 (each after paying for food), both paid 10 per cent of their 'disposable income' on health care. But the low-income household would have little or no disposable income at all – and may even be forced to sell assets to raise the equivalent of 10 per cent, while the wealthier household could easily spare its share of the health budget. Such a policy would therefore be far from 'fair'.

Another key weakness in the *WHR 2000* approach is that it takes no account of health need. The poorer household is likely to suffer poorer health and thus require more health care – but may well be less likely to buy it because it could not afford the costs. By contrast, the wealthier household, though suffering less ill health, may make more use of health-care services, including some hospital and specialist services which are unavailable to poorer people, especially to the rural poor.

The *WHR 2000* policy reduces 'fairness' to the abstract question of sharing the burden of funding health services – and appears to come down against progressive taxation… as a measure that is unfair to the rich. To confuse matters even more, Almeida et al. point out that the *WHR* offers an index of fairness which runs from zero (maximum inequality) to one: but no less than 147 countries (over 75 per cent) score 0.9 or above.

Braveman et al. (2001) accuse the *WHR 2000* (and by implication the WHO leadership which promoted it) of undermining efforts to achieve greater equity in health between and within nations. But they also argue that the WHO's controversial measures of inequality are ineffective as a means to guide policy or intervention, not least because they do not differentiate between different social groups within a country, rich and poor. As a result, they argue:

> A minister of health whose country ranked poorly on the Report's inequalities measure would have no idea where to begin to look to tackle the disparities.

While under fire on this issue from its more radical potential supporters, as well as facing continued criticism from the hard-line advocates of neoliberalism, the WHO has also embraced the prevailing notion of a 'partnership' between the public sector and a private sector which tends to rely heavily on the imposition of charges – either for direct revenue and return on investment or as a means to persuade wider (more prosperous) layers of society to pay out in advance for medical insurance schemes.

The *WHR 2000* explicitly criticises the 'complete omission of private finance and provision of care from the Alma Ata Declaration' and praises 'third generation' reforms which try to make 'money follow the patient' (WHO 2OOO: 15). It echoes the World Bank's stock argument that an unequal share of publicly funded services are appropriated by the rich (ibid.: 16) before stressing that publicly guaranteed or regulated services do not necessarily have to be publicly provided:

> The idea of responding more to demand, trying harder to assure access for the poor, and emphasising financing, including subsidies, rather than just provision within the public sector, are embodied in many of the current third-generation reforms.
>
> (WHO 2000: 16)

This is very clearly a substantial change of line by the WHO, softening what many saw as its long-standing line of pressing for public provision of public health and embracing the market model and many of the arguments propagated by the World Bank and neoliberal advocates of increased private-sector provision.

'Partnerships'

However, as Buse and Walt have pointed out, a different adaptation to the pressures of the market, and an echo of the politics of the 'Third Way', can be found in the emerging UN and WHO concept of 'Global Public Private Partnerships' (Buse and Walt 2000a: 551). Around 70 such partnerships were identified, many of them involving drug companies and research projects (Buse and Waxman 2001).

This stance has also been controversial among NGOs and within the WHO's own structures. Critics pointed out that the WHO, with its global budget then standing at $1.7 billion, was potentially vulnerable to political and economic pressure from much wealthier drug companies and private corporations, making any 'partnership' profoundly unequal (Hardon 2000). They questioned the altruism of the corporations concerned and pointed to the potentially valuable commercial, political and public relations advantages that could be secured by large private companies that could be seen to be working alongside the UN, the WHO and health NGOs.

From the start, there have been genuine concerns that the involvement of the WHO and NGOs in a 'partnership' framework dominated by big business could turn out to benefit business interests rather than the world's poor. Policies emerging from such 'partnerships' are seen as likely to revolve around the use of more costly, modern (patented) drugs and vaccines than cheaper generic alternatives and, in the case of immunisation campaigns, more likely to concentrate on areas of proven success – the 74 per cent of the target population already covered by immunisation – rather than attempting to penetrate the more needy areas, the 30–40 per cent who do not yet receive any preventative treatment. As one critic argued:

> Today vaccination policies seem to have shifted towards public–private partnerships and away from equity. ... In vaccination programmes the focus now appears to be creating markets for new vaccines. ... Unlike earlier vaccine campaigns, these initiatives spend little time discussing sustainability.
>
> (Hardon 2000)

There are also fears that the privately backed immunisation campaigns, using the latest vaccines, could result in a reduced local capacity to produce vaccines and a rejection of local generic products by a sceptical public convinced that the cheaper product is inferior.

Treatment versus prevention

In the case of HIV/AIDS, there was a parallel concern that the main interest of the pharmaceutical companies is the *treatment* of the epidemic – using drugs which remain expensive in third-world terms even after large discounts – rather than the prevention of its further spread. Even where drugs are donated, this is not sufficient to create an effective 'partnership' capable of tackling HIV/AIDS: only a combination of preventative health-education campaigns and the establishment of a health-care system able to give long-term support can answer the problem (Schulz-Asche 2000).

The ethics and longer-term implications of the 'partnership' with the private sector are therefore at the centre of a debate that has continued within and around the WHO. But even if the corporations were not directly involved in the new partnerships, it is clear that the WHO, as an international body dependent upon the patronage of US and other pro-market governments, remains subject to substantial political pressures: it would be remarkable if it were able to avoid reflecting these pressures in its political agenda and debates.

However, the links with private corporations raise suspicions over their motives and the possible adoption of some of their less-savoury practices. The ethics – and the longer term effectiveness – of the immunisation and other programmes promoted by the WHO, alongside UNICEF and the World Bank, have occasionally been challenged by angry critics, often from bitter experiences in developing countries (Banerji 1999, Schreuder and Kostermans 2001). Banerji decries global programmes on immunisation, AIDS and tuberculosis in Asian countries, which he describes as 'astonishingly defective' in concept, design and implementation. Ncayiyana (2002) is also critical of the way Africans have been used to test drugs from which they will never benefit: 'either because the drugs are too costly, or because they are designed to treat conditions that largely affect industrialised nations.'

Tessa Tan-Torres Edejer provides a similar, if slightly less sharp critique of the problems of securing long-term supplies of anti-AIDS drugs after research programmes are completed in developing countries (Edejer 1999). She quotes a participant in a drugs study in Guatemala who faced the need to fund two costly drugs from a triple cocktail if he was to continue feeling the benefit he had experienced during the trial. While arguing that 'the "scientific colonialism" that characterised earlier North–South research collaborations has slowly been transformed', Edejer goes on to question the ethics of using placebo-controlled trials of drugs on perinatal transmission of the HIV virus in developing countries where the standard package of care did not include the use of AZT. She also warns that despite the good intentions of the north–south partners, 'clashing agendas and values persist'.

Missing infrastructure

Schreuder and Kostermans (2001) point out that although crash programmes of immunisation organised through National Immunisation Days in some southern African countries appeared effective, they do nothing to strengthen the necessary infrastructure of primary-care services because they tend to be organised from above and from outside to satisfy the demands of external donor countries. Consequently, the longer-term results are a reduction in the level of routine immunisation coverage. This, they argue, refutes the stock WHO argument that NIDs help promote immunisation and public health.

The same authors also argue, in more radical terms than the WHO, that the full costs of seeking to eradicate diseases should be carried by the wealthier countries:

> Since the industrialised countries benefit most from eradication, they should take responsibility for covering the needs of those countries that cannot afford the investment.
>
> (Schreuder and Kostermans 2001)

Another sharp criticism of the new style of WHO policy was Lockwood's review of its 'leprosy elimination' programme. She argued that the apparent, dramatic fall from 5 million to 0.7 million in the numbers of registered leprosy patients between 1985 and 2001 was largely due to a change in the definition of a leprosy patient, to include only those receiving multi-drug therapy. Far from leprosy being 'eliminated', there were 719,300 new patients registered as suffering from the disease in 2000, with numbers actually rising in the worst-affected countries (Lockwood 2002).

Lockwood went on to challenge some of the new methods used by the WHO in tackling the disease, which involved far less patient contact and monitoring, and a halving of the length of a course of multi-drug therapy from two years to one ('despite evidence that patients with high bacterial loads are at greater risk of relapse'). She argued that these changes were based on no published evidence of effectiveness – but that when they were challenged on the Global Alliance to Eliminate Leprosy by the ILEP (the international umbrella organisation of NGOs fighting leprosy), the ILEP was excluded from the 'partnership'. Significantly, the partnership still included the drug company Novartis. She warned that the WHO rhetoric about having 'eliminated' leprosy may lead governments to wind up their own control programmes. And she asked who would pay for the drug treatments that would be necessary after 2005, or train the staff who would still be needed to care for leprosy sufferers 'for many years to come'.

The return to primary health care

By 2003, Brundtland's period of office in the WHO had come to an end and the first signs emerged of a change of direction. *WHR 2003* shifted the emphasis back to primary health care, declared a global emergency on the slow progress in treating HV/AIDS and invoked the ideals of Alma Ata. Partnerships with the private sector were relegated to the background and only referred to in the context of the initiatives to combat Polio.

In 2005, a key document analysing progress and the lack of it in achieving the Millennium Development Goals for health by 2015 reflected a mixed approach. Discussions on involving the private sector and a refusal to rule out user fees ran alongside a stress on the need to combat poverty, strengthen health-care systems and make them more equitable, and address wider 'social determinants':

While the relationship between health and 'social determinants' – such as income and employment – is well documented, this chapter looks at whether and how developing country governments can use a range of policy levers across government to the benefit of health. Addressing health within a broad developmental framework must, of course, be carefully balanced with support for development of 'pro-poor' health systems...

More equitable health systems are prerequisites for achieving the MDGs. They also contribute to social protection, the empowerment of marginalized groups, and the fulfilment of human rights, and are therefore central to poverty reduction efforts.

(WHO 2005b: 45)

Achieving greater equity requires solutions beyond health care, and health-care interventions other than market-style reforms and partnerships with the private sector. In 2005, the WHO went further and set up a Commission on Social Determinants of Health, which in turn established a Global Knowledge Network conducting research and pulling together expertise on a variety of aspects of social determinants in the context of globalisation of capitalism from a wide range of academics, activists, professionals and civil society organisations. This reported in 2008, the 30th anniversary of the Alma Ata conference.[2]

Moving in the same direction, the 2006 WHO document 'Engaging for Health' raised the need for action not simply through health care and health systems, but to impact on the (social) determinants of health, including poverty, diet, lifestyle issues (alcohol and tobacco) and climate and environmental issues:

The action required to tackle most of these determinants goes beyond the influence of ministries of health, and involves a large number of government and commercial responsibilities. If these determinants are to be dealt with effectively, therefore, the boundaries of public health action have to change. Governments, especially health ministries, must play a bigger role in formulating public policies to improve health, through collective action across many sectors.

(WHO 2006b: 18)

---

2   The 13 topics covered were: Globalisation and health: pathways of transmission, and evidence of its impact; Trends in global political economy and geopolitics post-1980; Globalisation and policy space; Globalisation, labour markets and social determinants of health; Trade liberalisation; Aid and health; Globalisation, debt and poverty reduction strategies; Globalisation, food and nutrition transitions; Globalisation and health systems change; Globalisation and health worker migration; Globalisation, water and health; Intellectual property rights and inequalities in health outcomes; and Globalisation, global governance and the social determinants of health: A review of the linkages and agenda for action. The project's findings were synthesised in *Towards Health-equitable Globalisation: Rights, Regulation and Redistribution, Final Report to the Commission on Social Determinants of Health* (Labonté et al. 2007) (Labonté-edited versions of the papers were subsequently published in the volume *Globalization and Health* (Labonté et al. 2009)).

Reforms rejected

The Commission's eventual report 'Closing the Gap in a Generation' (WHO 2008a) was seen by some as a diluted and less-radical version of many of the interim findings and specific papers produced in the process; but it still represented a considerable advance from the political prostration to neoliberalism of the Brundtland-led WHO. The Commission argues against the prevailing line of recent health sector reforms, warning that they are commercialising and fragmenting health care and promoting a narrow technical/medical focus that undermines primary care. It argues in favour of universal health care funded from general taxation or mandatory insurance, and opposes user fees. There is little comfort for the World Bank or the fundamentalist advocates of private-sector and market solutions in the Commission's firm statement that:

> The Commission considers health care a common good, not a market commodity. Virtually all high-income countries organize their health-care systems around the principle of universal coverage (combining health financing and provision). Universal coverage requires that everyone within a country can access the same range of (good quality) services according to needs and preferences, regardless of income level, social status, or residency, and that people are empowered to use these services. It extends the same scope of benefits to the whole population. There is no sound argument that other countries, including the poorest, should not aspire to universal health-care coverage, given adequate support over the long term.
>
> (WHO 2008a: 12)

They may well aspire, but the chances of the world's poor achieving even the modest and focused goals of the MDGs appeared to be slim at best in a European Report on Development produced by a team of researchers in September 2008. Summarising World Bank and UN reports in that year, it assessed progress as 'good on poverty and gender parity' but then conceded that 'progress has been slow' and that 'most countries are off-track on most MDGs, even those that have seen the greatest growth.' Donors were to spend less time and energy measuring progress on MDGs and more learning what was working (Bourguignon et al. 2008).

Also in 2008, *The World Health Report 2008 – Primary Health Care (Now More Than Ever)* brought together a new team and again made explicit reference back to the values and ambitions of Alma Ata, identifying trends that 'undermine the health systems' response' which included 'Hospital-centrism: health systems built around hospitals and specialists', 'Fragmentation: health systems built around priority programmes' and 'Health systems left to drift towards unregulated commercialization' (WHO 2008b).

At the same time, a new body focused on the financing of health systems to achieve the health MDGs in low-income countries was at least beginning to confront some of the political and other obstacles. The High Level Taskforce on Innovative International Financing for Health Systems identified a number of constraints: one working group focused on issues including the lack of detailed and context-specific health-systems knowledge, a lack of consensus on the best approaches to service delivery or the benefits from interventions, and difficulties even quantifying the size of the cash gap to be bridged. A second working group noted the small evidence base for many innovative finance mechanisms and inadequate experience in using international investments to improve maternal and child health. There were disagreements over 'the potential role of the private sector, the rights-based approach to health, and the move to results-based aid' (Fryatt et al. 2010).

No politics please, we're the WHO

By contrast, *WHR 2008* remains doggedly apolitical in its approach to problems which at root centre on political and ideological decisions and policies. There is plenty of talk about poverty and low pay, but nothing about the rich, the system that keeps them rich and makes them richer by keeping others poor, the massive global problem of tax evasion by the rich (Mathiason 2012) that starves health care and education of vital resources, or the growing concentration of wealth in the hands of this small minority. There is discussion of economic 'growth and stagnation' but none on the system that ensures the benefits of growth are enjoyed by the wealthiest, while the miseries of stagnation and recession are dumped onto the poor and those on middle incomes.

There is little reckoning with the reality that, while the wealth of the super-rich continues to grow, there were actually more relatively poor people in 2008 than 1981 and that the numbers deemed to be living in absolute poverty have only apparently reduced because of a marginal improvement in living standards in China (Chen and Revallion 2012). There is no discussion of the power of transnational companies, their demands on governments of low-income countries, their impact on the environment and their powerful lobbying – overt and covert – against increased taxation.

The *WHR 2008* warns of what it calls the 'drift towards unregulated competition', but the word 'neoliberal' does not appear at all and there is no reference to the neoliberal pressure on governments everywhere to reduce regulation, privatise public services and unleash competition – which means that far from being a 'drift', all these things are in fact a conscious policy.

The document again rehearses the lack of resources for health in the poorest countries and the extra resources needed to meet the MDGs: but it does not even mention that all of this and more could easily be generated through relatively modest progressive taxation on corporations and the super-rich, and even the poorest low-income countries could raise additional money through turnover taxes on the multinationals that exploit their natural resources. There is no mention of capital flight, snatching far more from the poorest countries than aid packages pump in. In fact, as the People's Health Movement have correctly pointed out, whatever the reason may be (and the WHO is still under heavy pressure from powerful governments and institutions wedded to neoliberal policies), the element of Alma Ata that has been completely eradicated in the WHO, especially since 2000, is its commitment to a 'new international economic order' (People's Health Movement 2011).

Even on the issue of primary health care (PHC), the WHO has clearly retreated, even in the document that explicitly harks back to Alma Ata. Although the document seeks to argue that PHC is far more than simply a cheap and cheerful provision of scaled-down services by less-qualified staff to the poor in low-income countries (WHO 2008b: xiv), time and again it refers simply to 'primary care' in ways that make clear it is envisaged as a version of health services rather than the combined, proactive and community-based model of PHC (People's Health Movement 2011).

Radicalism missing

The verbal nod that is made to the iconic values of Alma Ata fails to raise the WHO even to the radicalism of some World Bank literature since 2006, which has openly discussed and weighed the possibilities of a variety of alternative ways to raise the money needed to resource the MDGs – through a 'Tobin tax' on speculation, a tax on airline travel or other carbon taxes, and other bold, if unlikely suggestions (Gottret and Schieber 2006). The WHO bemoans poverty and inequality, but has no suggestions on how to tackle them, other than abstract appeals to 'global solidarity' – which is clearly in desperately short supply in today's global banks and boardrooms.

The Bank has also taken a much sharper critical approach than the WHO towards the delivery of health services through top-down 'vertical programmes' run by 'global public–private partnerships', including major donors and often the WHO, warning of the possible negative consequences, which include undermining existing health systems and services, luring away scarce health professionals and leaving behind unsustainable bills and obligations (Gottret and Schieber 2006). The WHO in 1995 shared these criticisms and, at that time, proclaimed this style of delivery a thing of the past:

> Although in the past special programmes for specific diseases – immunisation for example – have produced truly impressive results, it is no longer sustainable or cost-effective to set up self-contained taskforces for individual illnesses. Fragmented and duplicated health care services jeopardise the effective use of available health resources, and the continuity and sustainability of services. It makes no sense for doctors and nurses to vaccinate children if at the same time children die because they do not have antibiotics against pneumonia or oral rehydration therapy for diarrhoea. It makes no sense if nurses give superb care to infants but ignore the fact that a mother has malaria. ... Integration is the key to effective delivery of care.
>
> (WHO 1995a: 43–4)

The radicalism is gone, as the WHO has been sucked into 'partnerships' with drug companies and donors with greater resources, but which are wedded to vertical programmes and single-disease campaigns (See Chapter 5 below). Further documents, discussions and conferences on the Social Determinants of Health since 2008, culminating in the Rio Summit in 2011, have served to underline rather than overcome the limitations and timidity of the WHO position. As Ted Schrecker regretfully observes:

> Beset by budgetary constraints even more acute than usual, and by intense opposition to the agenda from elements of the medical profession both outside and (one suspects) within the organization, WHO is ill equipped to carry the agenda forward. The World Conference on Social Determinants of Health, to be held in Brazil in October 2011, appears directionless and sometimes seems nothing more than a ritual response to a generic World Health Assembly resolution responding to the Commission's report.
>
> (Schrecker 2011a)

In the meantime, the WHO's highly controversial pronouncement of a 'pandemic' of swine flu – which many have regarded as ill-judged and based on a new, flawed set of criteria – and the ensuing hue and cry which resulted in the squandering of huge sums on anti-viral medicines of dubious efficacy, many of which were wasted and destroyed unused, undermined confidence in the scientific credibility of the organisation. Revelations and allegations over the links between key members of the scientific committee that made the pronouncement and major drug companies which stood to profit handsomely from preparations for a pandemic have further added to this (Cohen and Carter 2010), even though a WHO inquiry has declared that, despite some errors in the day-to-day decisions during the crisis, all had been done properly (WHO 2011). One real problem for the WHO is that governments and rival international institutions seeking to discredit some of its more radical messages on social determinants of health – and other proposals for progressive action they find uncomfortable – are able to seize on incidents like this, and it can take a long time to rebuild credibility once it has been called into question.

Fatally weakened

Overall, more than 60 years after the WHO was established, it is hard to disagree with the 2005 summary by the first *Global Health Watch* that the WHO is fatally weakened by 'Woefully inadequate resources, poor management and leadership practices, and the power games of international politics' (People's Health Movement 2005). Three years later, *Global Health Watch 2* argued that 'Instead of being funded as a democratic UN agency, [the WHO] is in danger of becoming an instrument to serve donor interests' (People's Health Movement 2008).

The latest *Global Health Watch* stresses the consequences of the lop-sided funding structure of the WHO, which leaves most of its funding dependent upon 'voluntary' donations from key member states. This enables them to apply pressure and effectively circumvent the more democratic accountability of the WHO to the annual World Health Assembly. It is impossible for the WHO to exercise much greater independence, or to have any ability to challenge retrograde policies and decisions by the international financial institutions (Bank, IMF) or the US or other governments, without a drastic change in this funding system:

> Clearly, there is a need to develop a sustainable financing and strategic plan for the WHO that is premised on increased assessed contributions of member states,

with a view to securing the independent role of the WHO, its continuing and expanding role in providing stewardship in dealing with global health issues, and to reversing the present 20:80 division in the WHO's finances.

(People's Health Movement 2011: 244)

While the GHW suggestion would obviously go a long way to putting things back into balance, the chances of it being implemented are remote at best. In the real world, in which pressure is exerted, often behind the scenes, through decisions on funding, the biggest member contributions and external donors almost inevitably call the shots. It's not clear how the WHO could ever attain a level of accountability and democracy that is higher than its principal funders want it to have, or achieve a level of authority that would enable it to call to account the conduct and policies of member states, or drug companies with which it is working in 'partnership'.

Equally, given the tenuous level of democratic accountability within member states on their links with the WHO, and the attitude taken by many of their governments in relation to control of the WHO, it is hard to identify a mechanism that could force the large-scale increases in assessed contributions required to reverse the current situation and give stability to 80 per cent of funding, especially if that would have the effect of reducing that member state's influence over WHO policy.

Despite severe problems and attempted interference, especially from the US, the WHO over the years has been able to do some useful work, promote some important and progressive ideas, and share valuable information. The efforts of Brundtland and ideologues from the Bank never completely succeeded in transforming it simply into a vehicle for neoliberalism or a front for collaboration with the big pharma companies – the level of awareness and commitment to the WHO's progressive values was too high and every attack was resisted from within as well as by activists and academics outside the organisation. The politics of *The World Health Report 2000* were challenged and much of the neoliberal poison was neutralised. But damage has been done: the WHO's usefulness has been impaired and it has not been able to deliver on the progressive mandate from Alma Ata.

'Universal health care'

As this book is written, the 2012 World Health Assembly and the WHO's Director General Margaret Chan have again committed themselves to promoting the goal of 'universal health care'. A series of articles on this theme in the *Lancet* include two editorials co-authored by the same David de Ferranti who first promoted the World Bank's policy of imposing user fees, this time arguing quite clearly for a very different approach. Although in one article the notorious World Bank 1993 Word Development Report *Investing in Health* (which called explicitly for a two-tier global system with only minimal health-care provision in the poorest countries) is presented in a positive light (Frenk and De Ferranti 2012), and each of the *Lancet* papers insists upon a role for the private sector, the dogged promotion of user fees for treatment appears to have been dropped:

For a long time getting health care has meant first paying a fee to the provider – a practice that effectively burdens sick and needy people, a small and vulnerable section of the population, with most of the health-care costs...

(Rodin and De Ferranti 2012)

It would seem, therefore, that if there has been this sea change among some of the former hard-line advocates of fees, there could be a little more robust and radical approach from the WHO. Rather than simply welcoming the signs of progress towards the new common goal, it could question and challenge the extent to which the private sector has any useful role to play in the move towards universal coverage, and explore the extent to which the phrase 'universal coverage' actually represents a shared approach – and is accompanied by sufficient resources to ensure that those most in need can access care in practice, not just in theory.

There are reasons to doubt the extent to which this is already happening: research by Savedoff and colleagues has shown that, in nine developing countries in Africa and Asia that are implementing national health insurance models, out-of-pocket spending as a percentage of health expenditure has fallen by only 3–6 percentage points, and OOP payments therefore remain higher than the level recommended by the WHO to avoid impoverishment. This will inevitably exclude millions of people from enjoying 'universal access' and has happened despite increased government spending on health. The authors further argue that developing-country governments 'would benefit from common, comparable standards for measuring key outputs and outcomes of universal coverage reforms' (Savedoff et al. 2012). Similar conclusions emerge from the studies by Lagomarsino and colleagues (2012).

More pressure needed

In countries where universal systems have been in place for some time, inadequate resources and inequalities in provision between rural and urban areas stand as an obstacle to access, most notably for the poorest and least mobile. These are issues the WHO should be actively raising to ensure that the momentum towards progressive solutions continues: but there is little sign of this approach.

Rather than expect it to transcend limitations that have very real and long-standing material and political roots, it would seem more useful to use the WHO and its structures where this helps to advance knowledge and do progressive work – and to look to other ways (such as the People's Health Movement, in alliance with civil-society organisations, progressive NGOs and so forth) to organise to do the things the WHO can't or won't do.

An alternative global centre is needed to campaign consistently for implementation in every country of the right to health, progressive health reforms and primary health care, and mount a challenge to the logic of global capital and neoliberalism and the drive to privatise and commercialise health care. On past form and in the foreseeable future, it's not likely that the WHO will be that centre.

Chapter four

The World Bank and the International Monetary Fund (IMF)

Those who know the Bank expect criticism from both ends of the political spectrum. Critics on the far left accuse the Bank of being a tool for the spread of international capitalism. Those on the right complain that it is not. Of the two, the leftists seem to have the better factual grasp of what the Bank actually does.

(De Ferranti 2006)

Historical origins

The World Bank is one of the principal organisations established after the Second World War to assist with the reconstruction and development of capitalism.[1] This gives it a unique influence in the shaping of policies in developing countries – but also means that its influence in the health sector is to reinforce private-sector and market models, and to do so with massive resources at its disposal to build up a body of research and argument to support this approach.

While the IMF, which was established at the same time, was charged with the task of extending loans to relieve balance-of-payments deficits and ensure stable currencies and economies, the Bank's role was to lend for long-term development. Beginning with the reconstruction of war-torn Europe and then focussing on industrialisation, it was not until the 1980s that the Bank's focus (and influence) began to concentrate on the poorest developing countries. More recently, the Bank has embraced poverty reduction as its overarching goal, emerging as 'the world's foremost development agency' (Williams 1994: 101). However, Williams also notes that, unlike many NGOs and other organisations focusing on development:

> The World Bank has never pretended to be anything other than a capitalist enterprise with a commitment to free trade, the optimisation of investment flows and the support of free enterprise.
>
> (1994: 111)

---

1   The 'Bank' explains on its website that it is in fact a group, made up from five linked institutions: the International Bank for Reconstruction and Development (IBRD), the International Development Association, the International Finance Corporation (IFC), the Multilateral Investment Guarantee Agency and the International Centre for the Settlement of Investment Disputes. The first three of these are the most relevant to the development and implementation of health-care reforms.

It now covers 184 member countries, although its internal structure has left it vulnerable to veto and to domination by the most powerful of the wealthy countries. Its governance arrangements have continued largely unchanged until recently, reflecting the Bank's reliance on the wealthy industrialised countries for its funding, long after the funds from these donor countries diminished to a small share of the Bank's lending. Most of the Bank's working capital is raised through loans on the financial markets and from interest payments on the billions already extended in long-term loans (Christian Aid 2003), requiring it to maintain its 'triple A' credit rating and to operate as a bank, offering loans and not grants.

A 2006 report from Social Watch, an organisation linking over 300 civil-society groups across more than 60 countries, concluded that multinational financial agencies were 'increasingly becoming a burden' to the poorest countries, taking more money from them in payments and interest than they lend. Since the 1990s, 'net transfers (disbursements minus repayments minus interest payments) from the World Bank's International Bank for Reconstruction and Development (IBRD) have been negative.' (Social Watch 2006: 14)

Only the poorest of the developing countries, with the fewest alternative options for raising funds for development, are still trapped in this relationship with the Bank. All of the major emerging market economies, with the sole exception of Turkey, paid off their loans to the IMF and the Bank some years ago. But while it supplies funds to the poorest countries, the Bank has remained in the grip of the wealthiest. The US alone has 17 per cent of the votes, while just 15 per cent is required to block a decision by either the World Bank or IMF boards. Five of the world's richest G7 countries, none of which borrows from the Bank any more, share over 20 per cent of the votes, while the world's 80 poorest countries have a combined voting strength of just 10 per cent on the Bank's board and the combined voting strength of 50 African countries is less than half that of the US.[2] Only European members and the US can nominate candidates for the top job in either the Bank or the IMF: it has become a carve-up, with the Europeans heading the IMF and the Americans heading the Bank.

Tradition defied

This continued domination was emphatically demonstrated in 2012 when, in a rare show of unity, all 54 African states defied tradition and backed a rival candidate (the Nigerian finance minister and former World Bank managing director Ngozi Okonjo-Iweala) to be the Bank's president. This went all the way to a vote-out which saw her defy US pressure to stand down, but the result was a formality: the little-known US nominee, South-Korean-born Jim Yong Kim, was predictably appointed to take over from American Robert Zoellick as the Bank's president in July 2012. However, there is now even greater pressure on the Bank to reform itself and to make more than token gestures towards the inclusion of the world's poorest countries in the

---

2   In the IMF, which describes its 184 member states as shareholders, just five countries – the US, Japan, Germany, France and the UK – hold 29 per cent of the votes.

decision-making process. A new seat on the Bank's board has been created for a Sub-Saharan country, but dissatisfaction with the Bank has led to growing interest – especially among African countries – in borrowing from other sources, including the African Development Bank and the Chinese government, who have now overtaken the Bank as the biggest lender to developing countries (Dyer et al. 2011).

Even this summary gives an exaggerated view of the level of accountability and democracy in the Bank. In practice, the influence of executive directors in the operational running of the Bank has been marginalised since 1947 and all of the Bank's presidents have been US citizens (Williams 1994, Woodward 2006).

Alongside the Bank, the other Bretton Woods global body, the IMF, has also acquired a reputation for imposing its will on developing countries without reference to the views (often involving active protests) of their populations and failing to play a useful or progressive role in providing multilateral finance (Development GAP 1999, Tan 2006).

There is no denying that both of these powerful institutions have played a significant role in shaping the development (or lack of it) in health care since the 1980s. In 2001, the World Bank itself employed 10,587 people originating from 160 countries, made loans totalling $17.3 billion and guaranteed investments in 28 countries worth another $2 billion (Pincus and Winters 2002). And this influential role is also reflected in the development of policy, theory and ideology: the Bank is a major sponsor of research – giving a real incentive for academics to adopt an approach that is likely to appeal to the Bank.

Research millions

By the late 1990s, the Bank was spending around $100 million each year on research, commissioning work from hundreds of academics and professionals, and publishing hundreds of reports each year on a wide range of social policy issues, including health care (Caufield 1997). More recent figures show direct Bank spending still in excess of $50 million each year, with many more well-resourced projects involving the Bank also drawing in researchers and consultancies in search of generous funding, publication and prestige. However, an evaluation of the quality of this research (between 1998 and 2005) by a top team of academics (Banerjee et al. 2006) came up with a series of withering criticisms, noting that a 'great deal' of expensively commissioned research is 'undistinguished and not well directed either to academic or policy concerns'. It noted that there was remarkably little work co-authored by non-Bank researchers from developing countries and that researchers were chosen by teams of Bank staff working in the specific country who were looking for a particular answer or for someone known for not rocking the boat (Heighway-Bury 2007).

The Bank has also developed an image of itself as a 'knowledge bank' (Pincus and Winters 2002), running a 'Flagship Program' for training the top managers and civil servants running health services in developing countries and Eastern Europe, thus schooling them in the assumptions and values of the Bank. Trainees receive an intensive, four-week course in Washington, at the end of which participants are expected to be able to 'speak a common language about dimensions of health-care reform and sustainable financing options' (World Bank 2010). The Bank also runs its own pedagogical arm, the World Bank Institute, which 'imposes institutional viewpoints on development theory and practice upon developing country government officials' (Sharman 2010). Given the Bank's reluctance to accept criticism and its continued failure to cultivate strong and independent critique and analysis, such programs will tend to reinforce the views that already cohere with the prevailing policies of the Bank itself, and thus to train and elevate policy-makers and leaders in developing countries who also share the Bank's predominant ideological and policy preferences.

The Bank's influence is in any event only partly based on policy and ideology, whether this is imposed by duress or consent: it also has very powerful material influence, especially through its role in deciding whether or not to grant loans which are vital to enable LICs to implement health programs. Though its first lending for health services was not until 1980, the expansion of the Bank's role in this area was rapid. By the end of that decade it was the largest funder of health-sector activities, having overtaken the WHO and lending an average of $1.5 billion per annum in the early 1990s (Walt 1994). Since 2006, it has lent $26.3 billion for health and social services, averaging over $4.5 billion per year, with loans of more than $6 billion each year since 2009 (World Bank 2012b).

The Bank adopts a health policy

In 1985, the Bank published a major document, *Paying for Health Services in Developing Countries: An Overview*, arguing the case for user fees for health care (de Ferranti 1985). This was followed by a more developed neoliberal policy in an official Bank document, *Financing Health Care: an Agenda for Reform*, which combined arguments for user fees with a concerted argument for a reduced role for the state and increased reliance on market mechanisms and the private sector (World Bank 1987).

Perhaps the most influential policy document shaping health policy for developing countries in the 1990s was the Bank's 1993 *World Development Report* (*WDR*). This effectively proposed the consolidation of a two-tier global health system, in which the wealthy countries would still be able to spend as much as they wished whilst publicly funded hospital care in developing countries would be reduced to a rudimentary minimum or privatised. The same report itemises and estimates the costs of a 'minimum package' of public health and essential clinical services for the poorest developing countries.

The Bank estimated the cost of this minimal – largely educational rather than health care – package at $12 per head of population per annum in 1990 prices for the low-income countries. This low figure could only be achieved by strictly limiting the range of health-care services to be provided, stipulating it to be a 'minimum package of clinical services'. The Bank warned that 'government-run health systems in many developing countries are overextended and need to be scaled back.' (1993: 108)

Despite increasingly critical reports on the failure of the 1993 policies to deliver even the 'essential package' (Colgan 2002) and mounting evidence of the negative impact on equity and access flowing from the imposition of user fees (Creese 1997, England et al. 2001, Nanda 2002), the World Bank continued to press low- and middle-income countries in this same direction throughout the 1990s. However, there is little evidence of success in delivering the proclaimed objectives, just as there is little if any evidence that Bank–IMF economic prescriptions succeeded on the economy. Indeed, Weisbrot points out that the economic policies imposed on the same developing countries in the same period by the World Bank and/or IMF in the guise of 'structural adjustment' have also proved to be an unquestionable failure: growth in GDP per capita in Latin America had been about 7% in the two decades of neoliberal policies to 2006, whereas the 20-year period 1960–80 had brought growth of 75%. The failure was most evident in Africa, where income per head had fallen by 15% in the 25 years from 1980, compared with 34% growth during 1960–80 (Weisbrot 2001: 6; 2006).

This further drop in living standards has also had negative consequences for health. A background paper assessing the evidence of the impact of these policies on health outcomes, prepared for the Commission on Macroeconomics and Health, found mixed results – although a preponderance of empirical studies were negative, including almost all of those looking at the outcomes for Africa (Breman and Shelton 2001).

By 1999, however, in an apparent change of emphasis amid growing signs of system failure in key areas, the Bank's *Annual Report* argued that its task would now be to work with countries:

> to help protect public expenditures in crucial areas in the social sectors; protect access to basic social services especially for the poor, improve social insurance...
>
> (cited in Petchesky 2003: 145)

The turn of the century produced a limited ideological retreat by the Bank, even on the basic approach: *The World Development Report 2000/2001: Attacking Poverty*, even admitted openly that 'markets do not work well for poor people' and praised countries such as Costa Rica, Mauritius and Morocco that had spent less on debt servicing and more on health, education and infrastructure. It singled out the health gains made in an earlier period by different policies in the Indian state of Kerala – even though these have since been undermined by a change of government and the adoption of neoliberal policies (cited in Petchesky 2003: 147–9). But the main lines of policy remained intact, as did the Health Strategy developed by the Bank's Health, Nutrition and Population division in 1997 (World Bank 1997).

Conditionalities and user fees

Pressure was brought to bear on the Bank to change. In 2000, a group of US NGOs managed to press Congress to threaten a withdrawal of US funding if either the IMF or World Bank continued to make user fees for health or for education a condition of loans to developing countries (Weisbrot 2001). While this was not fully or immediately acted upon,[3] it did secure a shift away from a full-scale policy of proposing user fees and open up some discussion of exemption schemes. Eventually, in its 2004 *WDR*, the Bank proclaimed that it now had 'no blanket policy' on user fees (Hutton 2004). In the same year, *WDR 2004* for the first time highlighted some of the gains that had been made by health systems that had not been implementing the Bank's strategy and did not apply fees, such as Cuba.

In 2005, the World Health Assembly passed a resolution calling for user fees to be abolished. A 2007 letter from Paul Wolfowitz to 60 NGOs agreed that user fees may pose a barrier to poor people seeking essential services and stressed the Bank's willingness to help find alternative financing to compensate for lost revenue if fees were abolished (Wolfowitz 2007). But there was clearly no enthusiasm for the new policy. Eventually, the Bank's 2007 'Strategy for Health Nutrition and Population Results' [sic] grudgingly conceded that:

> Upon client-country demand, the Bank stands ready to support countries that want to remove user fees from public facilities *if*: (a) the lost revenue from user fees can be replaced with resources that reach the facilities in a timely and fiscally sustainable manner over the long-term; (b) effective public financial management systems ensure that such financial transfer replacements will effectively reach the health facilities that need them the most and in the context of the appropriate incentive framework for the provision of services to the poor; and (c) that resource replacements will be used to pay for the delivery of effective quality services for the poor, provided at the health facilities.
>
> (World Bank 2007b: 50)

Earlier, in what appeared to be a change of direction, the Bank in 2000 launched a new policy of Poverty Reduction Strategy Papers (PRSPs) to replace the highly controversial Structural Adjustment Programs (SAPs) in the poorest countries, the bulk of which had been seen to have had a negative impact on health. A 2001 review of 76 articles studying the effects of SAPs on health found that 45 per cent drew negative conclusions and 20 per cent neutral: only 8 per cent recorded positive results (Breman and Shelton 2001). The new PRSPs were supposed to create planning frameworks giving the lowest-income countries much more control and 'national ownership' of the strategies, although the process of negotiation was always to include 'external development partners' alongside 'domestic stakeholders' (IMF 2012). The concept of PRSPs was endorsed by the 2001 WHO Commission on Macroeconomics and Health, but in the same year another WHO review of 10 countries implementing PRSPs found that the composition of teams included members of ministries such as finance, economics and planning, but excluded health and other social sectors, with the process dominated by the IMF and World Bank (WHO 2001).

---

3   According to Stiglitz (2002: 52), the President signed the law requiring the US to oppose proposals for user fees 'but the US executive director [at the IMF] simply ignored the law, and the secrecy of the institutions [IMF and World Bank] made it difficult for Congress – or anyone else – to see what was going on.'

Poverty strategies that ignore health

The resulting schemes have been strongly criticised. When Laterveer and colleagues assessed 23 PRSPs, they found they made little reference to health, particularly for the poor (Laterveer et al. 2003). A WHO review of 21 PRSPs found that health was approached from a narrow perspective; 18 argued explicitly that improving health assists with economic growth, one consequence of which is that health becomes seen as an adjunct, even a by-product, of economic policy, rather than policies being shaped to improve health. All 21 PRSPs featured health in their strategies, all provided some national health data and 15 discussed financial barriers, such as user fees which prevent the poorest from accessing health care, although most assumed that some form of exemption system would be the solution. Few discussed the barriers obstructing poor women from accessing reproductive health care (Dodd et al. 2004). In 2005, with 'the PRS approach' rolled out to 49 countries, another review conceded that 'a major criticism of PRSPs however is that they are generally not formulated as an operational framework for reaching the MDGs': but nonetheless it concluded that the PRS 'can and should be the operational framework for scaling up results to meet the MDGs' (IMF and World Bank 2005).

One difference in PRSPs is that they make less reference to the government spending cuts and privatisation that had been central to earlier SAPs. Other critics have argued that despite the deceptive rhetoric, PRSPs effectively replicated the failed model of SAPs (Bond and Dor 2003, Verheul and Rowson 2001). Despite the criticisms, the Bank and the IMF have persisted with PRSPs. By 2003, 32 countries had produced full PRSPs and, by 2012, 110 PRSPs had been circulated to the IMF's Executive Board, as well as a further 57 'interim' PRSPs (IMF 2012). However, the profile of the schemes has fallen and updates are hard to find on the progress being made. The Bank's website in May 2012 offered no updates more recent than 2005.

Conditionalities and the drive to privatisation may have appeared to be sidelined in PRSPs but they were certainly still very much alive in the Bank–IMF negotiations over the cancellation of debts for 23 Heavily Indebted Poor Countries (HIPC). The cancellation was supposed to reduce their debt service payments by an average of 1.9 per cent of GDP (Gupta et al. 2001). Significantly, HIPC countries were required to make improvements in immunisation and health-care delivery, including steps to slow the spread of AIDS, *before* they could receive the promised financial reward. Many were kept waiting. In the case of Malawi, the process dragged on for years from 2000, with the IMF accusing the government of 'overspending' – despite the fact that it was attempting to compensate for the loss of donor support. Malawi also fell victim to limits on the proportion of public spending that could be used to pay public employees (Fontana 2005).

But the conditionalities have been contested, including opposition from an unlikely quarter: in 2006, the British government, which gave the Bank £1.3 billion in 2005, having been strongly lobbied by NGOs, openly criticised the strategies outlined by the Bank's then president, Paul Wolfowitz, and threatened to withhold payments unless the Bank dropped its requirement that poor countries liberalise their economies and privatise public-sector enterprises (Elliott 2006).

IMF under pressure

These signs of division over Bank policy came at a time when the authority and the economic power of the IMF were also under threat. The IMF's long-awaited promise of reform to the voting strengths of different countries (Hujer and Reiermann 2012) may be attributable to an eagerness by the US to divert attention and discussion away from possibly more serious economic questions. These could include the massive expansion in the US current-account deficit, standing at $900 billion or 6.5 per cent of US GDP, while China is just one of a number of Asian countries that have accumulated huge surpluses. China's surplus is likely to reach 10 per cent of GDP in 2007 (Guha 2006). In any event, the IMF itself has been facing a mounting financial crisis as a growing number of countries pay off their outstanding loans, with many of them vowing never again to borrow from the IMF, with its punitive strings attached to loans. In 2006, the Fund's lending fell to the lowest level for 25 years amid warnings that the level of income from repayments was set to fall below the Fund's rising annual expenditure (Wolf 2006).

With most emerging market economies running surpluses, the first low-income countries released from long-standing debts, and new potential lenders emerging on the world market, the power of the IMF to dictate policies appeared to have been drastically reduced. Thailand's then Prime Minister, Thaksin Shinawatra, for example, while repaying the final instalment of a $17.2 billion IMF loan two years early in 2003, declared in a live TV broadcast that Thailand would 'never again fall prey to world capitalism' (Giles 2006).

But in the event, the dramatic and massive financial collapse of Lehman Brothers and key banks in the US and Europe has lent the IMF a lifeline (Weissman 2009). In 2012, its lending levels are once again as high as they have ever been, new lines of credit have been established, and an arrogant international agency has again begun systematically to impose more of the same kind of brutal 'conditionalities' on loans that have been criticised since the days of Structural Adjustment Programmes (Molina and Pereira 2008).

One remarkable common factor in the IMF's various proposals to constrain spending and raise interest rates in the already troubled countries is the call for a freeze on the pay of public-sector workers; and one consistent omission is the lack of any requirement to raise taxes on the banks or big business – domestic or multinational. In 2009, the Fund was still hard at work trying to press-gang governments into implementing policies that would impact brutally on public-sector workers and on the poor: Pakistan's government, required by the IMF to cut the fiscal deficit from 7.4 per cent of GDP to 4.2 per cent, was pressed to slash public spending, bump up electricity prices by 18 per cent and eliminate tax exemptions. Hungary was told to cut its deficit by freezing public-sector pay and capping pension payments. A public-sector pay freeze was also prescribed for Ukraine. And while IMF chiefs made speeches proclaiming the need for fiscal stimulus, nine countries seeking loans were pressed to slash public spending (Muchhala 2009).

The iron laws of neoliberalism still have a consistent enforcer in the IMF, and working people and the poor are still paying the price – through policies which prop up the system that has exploited them and made them poor, widening further the inequalities and exacerbating the social conditions which have condemned hundreds of millions to chronic ill health.

The Bank since 2004

The Bank's formal decision to adopt 'no blanket policy' on user fees in 2004 has not stopped continuing efforts by campaigners to force the pace and ensure fees are lifted. In 2005, greater weight was added to the argument by the findings of the multi-agency Equitap project, which studied health-care systems in 16 Asian countries,[4] exploring equity in payments, delivery of health services, protection against catastrophic impacts and health status (Rannan-Eliya and Somanathan 2005b). The project did not examine specific projects and schemes, but health systems and noted patterns which applied in similar systems. Among its conclusions was the general observation that:

> The ability of countries to reach and protect the poor varies considerably not by level of economic development, or even levels of public spending, but by type of health system. Health systems with similar attributes perform similarly, even at different income levels, showing that failure to reach the poor is not an inevitable outcome of low levels of national income, but of how health services are organised and delivered...
>
> (Ibid.: 2)

The report also refutes the notion that public health measures alone could deliver the improvements in health status required to meet the MDG targets and, noting that 'poverty is universally bad for your health', stresses the positive role of health care in delivering health outcomes:

> It should be stated emphatically that (a) no low-income developing country population has been able to achieve good health outcomes without achieving high levels of access to and use of medical services; and (b) there is considerable empirical evidence that medical services do produce health improvements, and are responsible for the bulk of health improvement in the developing world in the past fifty years...
>
> (Ibid.: 4)

The conclusions from the Equitap research serve almost as a point-by-point refutation of World Bank nostrums, in particular its focus from 1987 on the imposition of user fees:

> Most of the countries where the poor do worst are ones which either continue to maintain significant user charges in government facilities (China, Vietnam,

---

4   The countries covered were Bangladesh, Nepal, India, Sri Lanka, Thailand, Vietnam, Malaysia, Indonesia, Philippines, China, Kyrgyz, Mongolia, Hong Kong, Taiwan, Japan and Korea.

Indonesia), or which tolerate a high incidence of informal fees in government facilities (Bangladesh, parts of India). Official user charges either deter the poor from seeking care, or sustain institutional cultures that legitimate the charging of unofficial fees by health service providers.

(Rannan-Eliya and Somanathan 2005b: 11)

Even more explicitly, the report echoes those who have consistently argued that the imposition of fees works most overtly to limit access for the poor:

It is a legitimate question given this experience, whether any pro-poor health strategy can be considered realistic as long as official policy continues to maintain user charges for health spending.

(Ibid.: 11)

Against those who immediately react against universal provision and the abolition of fees by arguing that such systems are not sustainable in developing countries with limited government budgets, Equitap's findings suggest it need not be expensive – just a question of how limited funds are spent:

Most low and middle-income countries in Asia report government spending on health of the order of 0.9–2.0% of GDP. As Sri Lanka, Philippines and Thailand show, it is possible to mitigate the worst inequalities with government expenditure levels of less than 2% of GDP (spending in Sri Lanka is less than 1.7% of GDP, and total spending less in dollar per capita terms than in India).

(Ibid.: 12)

Moreover, rejecting the neoliberal view that insurance-based and privately provided systems (markets) are inherently superior, the Equitap findings offer a convincing endorsement of tax funding:

It is not the case that tax-funded public delivery systems are doomed to failure in reaching the poor. Although many do fail, it still remains the case that the only low and middle-income countries in Asia which are successful in reaching and protecting the poor are ones that rely solely or predominantly on tax-funding (even Thailand's social insurance system is 65% funded from taxation), and on public sector delivery.

(Ibid.: 12)

As a further blow to the 1993 Bank notion of providing only an 'essential package' with minimal provision of hospital treatment, Equitap's findings suggest that the poor can be best protected against catastrophic costs by a system that invests in hospital care, where the costs would otherwise be higher:

The successful systems are structured to ensure effective access to the poor, both by eliminating financial barriers, and also by ensuring geographic barriers to access are removed for the rural population through provision of many facilities. These systems also allocate a much larger share of public spending to hospital and inpatient services, thus ensuring that they provide substantial risk protection (Sri Lanka, Kerala, Malaysia, Thailand).

(Rannan-Eliya and Somanathan 2005b: 12)

These serious blows to the credibility of the Bank's established policies have not led to an immediate shift of position, but since 2005 there has been increased focus on 'health systems strengthening' and also substantial Bank-sponsored research on methods of health systems financing (Gottret and Schieber 2006, Gottret et al. 2008).

2007: time for a new strategy

In 2006–7, the Bank conducted extensive discussions and adopted a new strategy, now centred on strengthening health systems and focusing more clearly on improving results for the poor (World Bank 2007b). However, this change appears to have been only partially successful, with many of the Bank's leading managers reportedly lacking any understanding of the new approach and struggling to implement it. This weakness appears also to help explain the failure of the Bank, along with the largely unreformed IMF, to respond in any way positively to the radical proposals from the WHO's Commission on the Social Determinants of Health (WHO 2008a) and its embarrassed evasion of the sharp critique raised by a joint initiative of British NGOs asking for evidence that the Bank's favourite policy of promoting health insurance in low-income countries actually works (Berkhout and Oostingh 2008).

Weak management and a lack of clear grasp and commitment of equity issues were also factors in the scathing report on ten years of the Bank's HNP projects to 2008, conducted by the Bank's own Independent Evaluation Group (IEG). It found that few of the 220 projects – which had cost almost $18 billion – had satisfactorily met their stated objectives, with only a handful rated highly satisfactory. Outcomes were rated moderately satisfactory or better in 66 per cent of cases, but with only 27 per cent of projects in Africa achieving satisfactory outcomes. Monitoring, which had been criticised in previous evaluations, remained 'weak' and the evaluation of projects was 'almost nonexistent'. The Bank's work on health was characterised by 'irrelevant objectives, inappropriate project designs, unrealistic targets, inability to measure the effectiveness of interventions.' Only half of the projects were explicitly pro-poor and fewer than one in six (13 per cent) had a specific poverty-reduction objective (World Bank 2009a).

But the performance on the new Strategy was if anything even worse, according to a subsequent IEG report that weighed up progress on the policies adopted almost 20 months earlier. It found that, despite being set the task of improving the percentage of projects rated satisfactory from 66 to 75 per cent, this had fallen to just over half (52 per cent) of the projects surveyed – and even fewer (only 25 per cent) of the African projects were rated satisfactory (World Bank 2009b). It's clear from the opaque and convoluted language being used in their policy documents that many Bank employees were struggling with the basic concepts of targeting services at the poor, removing obstacles to access to care, and opening up hospital and other services, along the lines spelled out by Equitap. The clash between this approach and their instinctive neoliberal assumptions has been too difficult for them to reconcile.

Among the six confusingly written 'rules of thumb', designed to offer an idiot's guide for confused bank staff (World Bank 2009b: 12), were:

- 'Delink payment from utilization of health services by the poor at the point of service delivery'
  [At face value, this would seem to imply abolishing user fees and investigating options for pre-paid insurance]
- 'Reduce the distance between the poor and services'
  [i.e. ensure services are located close to centres of low-income population]
- 'Close the gap between need and demand by the poor'
  [i.e. find ways to ensure that those needing treatment seek access to services].

A chorus of critiques

NGOs and campaigners were also stepping up criticism of the Bank's continued reliance on the private sector to deliver expanded and improved services, even in Africa where the levels of conventional private-sector investment remained chronically low. A scathing critique from Oxfam (Marriott 2009b) triggered an unconvincing response from the Bank, indicating a continued insistence on ways of working that were still being discredited (World Bank 2009c). 2010 also brought further criticism from TB campaigners of the Bank's persistence in organising work around ineffective 'Sector Wide Approaches', which had failed to deliver effective services to combat TB (Skolnik et al. 2010, Aid Watch 2010). There has been a slight weakening of the iron resolve to rely on the private sector, in the form of an article by a Bank health economist in the *Times of India* arguing that government provision of health care is the best option, at least for rural areas in India (Marriott 2011).

Further critique by Oxfam and other NGOs (Berkhout and Oostingh 2008) has shown the limitations of some of the trumpeted 'health insurance' schemes, in West Africa and other low-income countries, that leave the poor with only the most minimal health cover and exposed to risk of catastrophic health costs through co-payments. After Oxfam's powerful 'Your Money or Your Life' broadside against user fees (Marriott 2009a), a moment of rare celebration came late in 2011 with a World Bank statement welcoming a project in the Lao PDR to deliver free maternity care in two districts – and a renewed tranche of Bank funding to make it possible. As might be expected, the free services have attracted an increased number of women to give birth in proper health facilities, but it is still unclear whether the Bank will continue to support such initiatives elsewhere (Marriott 2011). The US-based NGO Partners in Health has initiated a campaign to eliminate user fees, more than a decade after the US Congress voted to oppose them and eight years after the Bank declared it had 'no blanket policy' to impose them (Marriott 2012b).

The Bank still lacks credibility as an honest player in the fight against poverty and inequality, and its efforts to present a new image in the twenty-first century appear to rely heavily on its new president, Jim Yong Kim, the first doctor and scientist to be president and the first with development experience. Kim has made strong statements about his commitment to end absolute poverty and, rather less plausibly, even claims to have found a 'passion' for this among the staff at the Bank (Boseley 2012b). Activists looking for evidence of the same radicalism in relation to health care will want to see a formal junking of the Bank's discredited 1993 strategy as a starting point – but could be excused for not wanting to hold their breath in anticipation.

The Bank's private wing: the IFC

The bulk of Bank activity on Africa and developing countries discussed in the pages above is carried out by two of the members of the World Bank Group: the International Bank for Reconstruction and Development (IBRD), which offers low-interest, long-term loans, and the International Development Association (IDA), launched in 1960, which is specifically focused on the lowest income countries and offers no-interest, long-term loans.

However, another arm of the Bank, the International Finance Corporation (IFC), has as its prime role the expansion and development of the private sector – including health care in Africa and in countries where the vast majority are unable to pay private fees or insurance premiums.

Established in 1956, the IFC describes itself as 'the private sector arm of the World Bank group': it is organisationally independent from other World Bank divisions, but declares that it 'shares its mission':

> To fight poverty with passion and professionalism for lasting results. To help people help themselves and their environment by providing resources, sharing knowledge, building capacity, and forging partnerships in the public and private sectors...
>
> (IFC 2009e: 1)

The IFC's actual work on health care seems consistently at variance with this proclaimed passion to fight poverty. Instead, the IFC in Africa and Asia has repeatedly targeted investment at already established, profitable companies, delivering health care for the wealthiest minority in the developing country concerned – and also boosting hospitals and multinational corporations which are offering comparatively cheap health care on a commercial basis for 'health tourists' from the US, Europe and other high-income countries where private medicine is more expensive.

The targeting of resources not at the poorest sections of society but at the already prosperous middle classes and wealthy is not a recent innovation in the IFC: it was explicitly adopted as a policy back in 2002. A confidential briefing paper which leaked out made it clear that, in order to ensure that it was investing in financially viable, profitable projects, the IFC would focus primarily on urban areas where the private market was already most 'mature'. The objective was to be:

increased involvement in private health insurance, to benefit the lower-middle and middle classes in countries without universal risk-pooling...

(IFC 2002, quoted in Lethbridge 2002a)

High-end treatment for higher returns

Interestingly, the IFC has now moved beyond this early focus on health insurance to sponsor the delivery of high-tech, high-cost treatment. This is in line with the detailed report researched for the IFC in 2007 by McKinsey that trumpeted the importance of the private sector in health-care provision in Africa (*The Business of Health in Africa: Partnering with the Private Sector to Improve People's Lives*). This argues that juicy profits that can be made by delivering health care to the wealthy elite in Sub-Saharan Africa:

High end clinics that target growing middle and upper-income populations in urban centers can deliver net profits of up to 30 per cent. These clinics provide the high-quality care that attracts patients and the well-equipped environment that attracts medical and nursing staff. An expected increase in the number of patients able to afford these services, as well as increasing acceptance of local treatment among patients, makes prospects for growth impressive.

(IFC 2007b: 40)

The report argues that half of the continent's current spending on health is already delivered through 'private enterprise' and that health spending is set to more than double to $35 billion by 2016, with the private-sector share expected to grow to 60 per cent – over $21 billion, offering profitable prospects for investors.

This appears to be the clear focus of IFC involvement in recent years. Indeed, the criteria for IFC financing seem to be at variance with the proclaimed commitment to equity: in order to be eligible, a project must not only be located in a developing country that is a member of the IFC, technically sound and in the private sector, but must also 'Have good prospects of being profitable'. If the project involves any kind of partnership with the government, it will only receive IFC support if 'the venture is run on a commercial basis' (IFC no date).

In the lowest income countries, where the majority of the population exists on $2 per day or less, there is clearly little or no prospect for a private medical facility to run at a profit unless it is either able to draw in government subsidies or deliberately targets the wealthiest few, largely ignoring the poor.

The commitment to profitability is certainly not a token gesture: the IFC makes the point that 'like other private-sector investors and commercial lenders', the IFC seeks profitable returns and 'prices its finance and services in line with the market'. The returns on IFC investment are considerable: IFC's Annual Portfolio Performance Review (FY09) show that its Equity Portfolio delivered an average 17.4 per cent annual return over the previous 17 years and that this level of profitability has been even higher in the years since 2000, averaging 22.7 per cent. In each case, the IFC's investments have outperformed the MSCI Emerging Markets Index.

Questions over private health in Africa

There is a major debate over the actual extent and character of private health care in the poorest countries, especially Africa. The McKinsey research claims that, of the $16.7 billion in total health expenditure in 2005, about half went to 'private providers'. Another 2007 report, from Merrill Lynch, also placed health care as one of the top-five most promising investment areas in Africa, on a par with African telecoms and infrastructure (*Economist* 2007). By contrast, McKinsey consultants, at an IFC conference, put Africa last on the list of profitable prospects, with the most lucrative potential in China, India, Asia in general, Latin America, the Middle East, Europe and the US (Kocher 2007).The IFC is nonetheless clearly convinced that private finance holds the key to improving the continent's health-care sector.

Oxfam and others have argued that the IFC depiction of private-sector provision vastly exaggerates the quality of what services are available on the ground and also gives a false impression of the preferences of African consumers. On closer analysis, the huge, profitable African 'private market' for health care includes unaffordable out-of-pocket payments that are bankrupting African families, plus a variety of health providers and services ranging from traditional 'healers' and non-profit charities and religious organisations, through to back-street shops selling pharmaceuticals over the counter which are near or beyond their expiry dates (Marriott 2009b).

Undeterred, Scott Featherston, senior investment officer at the IFC, has continued to insist that private investment is the way forward. He told journalist Susan Rundell that:

> Our role is to provide a stamp of approval and other investors can come in knowing the IFC has invested. Healthcare investment is on a par with infrastructure – offering long-term steady returns. The problem is that it is simply not known as an asset class. We hope that over time our fund will be a vehicle to show what is possible.
>
> (Rundell 2010)

One company in the IFC's sights is African Medical Investments, which provides specialised private health care via clinics and trauma centres for the wealthy and expatriates, and has opened a 35-bed private boutique hospital in the Mozambique capital, Maputo, with a trauma centre and Well Woman clinic. AMI already owned a 30-bed Dar es Salaam hospital and is still building an air ambulance service (AMI, no date). In March 2011, it opened a 22-bed boutique hospital in Harare with HDU and casualty services. Plans for future expansion after the replacement of its Chief Executive following 'financial irregularities' include Zambia, Uganda, Ghana and Nigeria. But the business has to cut costs by 25 per cent in a bid to turn a profit, after losses increased to $18.8 million on turnover which had doubled to $5.4 million (Lamberti 2011).

Insurance business

With at least half of Africa's health spending coming out of pocket – and much more in many developing countries – an expansion of health insurance is vital for any real expansion of the health-care market beyond the upper-income groups. Frost and Sullivan estimate that 80 per cent of Africa's private health-care providers' revenue comes from insurance (Rundell 2010). South Africa's Life Healthcare, backed by a $93 million investment from the IFC, which took a 5 per cent stake in the company (IFC 2010), has raised almost $700 million from investors to fund expansion plans across the continent.

But business has been less than booming for South Africa's Liberty Holdings, linked to Standard Bank, which had ambitious plans to sign up 1.5 million customers in three years through its medical health-insurance unit expanding into Africa (Rundell 2010). The health-insurance business has not yet proved to be the money-spinner that the company would like it to be: it has lost many of its core South African subscribers in the financial downturn and has yet to recruit the new customers it wants from the new markets it has been cultivating in the south and east of the continent. Liberty recorded a headline loss of R43 million for 2010 and lost a further R10 million in the first half of 2011 (Cairns 2012).

Other companies in this sector include Nigeria's health-insurance group, Hygeia Nigeria, which runs a non-profit community health-insurance scheme with 66,000 enrollees registered by family group. This scheme has annual premiums of about US$60 per person, per year in Lagos and US$27 per person, per year in Kwara State, mostly covered by external subsidies from donors including the World Bank (Centre for Market Innovations 2012), and a for-profit health maintenance organisation offering four levels of cover up to 'Hyprestige' level for the wealthy elite, costing just under £2,000 per year. The HMO now claims more than 200,000 enrollees from 250 corporate clients and contracts with 1,500 providers of health services (Hygeia Group 2012). However, not all of the relationships have been plain sailing and Hygeia drew some unwanted publicity early in 2012 when an SMS text message sent out to some customers, urging them not to resubscribe because they had made excessive use of their cover, was leaked to the press, forcing hasty apologies and not entirely convincing denials (Ahiuma-Young and Obinna 2012).

IFC's empty $1 billion promise

The publication of *The Business of Health in Africa* report was closely followed by huge IFC fanfares heralding the launch at the end of 2007 of a '$1 billion health-care strategy for Africa', including 'a new equity investment fund which could ultimately be worth up to $500m', plus provision to lend another 400 to 500 million dollars to help local banks lend to small and medium-sized enterprises in the health-care industry. The logic of this was puzzling: in the lowest income countries there is clearly little or no prospect for a private medical facility to run at a profit unless either it draws in government subsidies, or targets the wealthiest few. The *Economist* (2007) warned that private capital might 'only go into fancy facilities that serve the urban rich'.

Despite the IFC's ambitious plans, the sums of money raised have been much, much smaller than those suggested back in 2007 – and the amounts that have been spent have been even smaller. Two similarly named, relatively small equity funds, the Investment Fund for Health in Africa[5] and the Africa Health Fund, were subsequently established, raising far less than $1 billion.

Although all SMEs in Sub-Saharan African countries are eligible for financing, there are a number of target countries, including Nigeria, Ghana, Cote d'Ivoire, Senegal, Kenya, Tanzania, Uganda, Mozambique, Zambia, Angola, Rwanda, Burundi, DRC, South Africa and Ethiopia. If the limited pot of private capital were divided between all of these, it would leave so little for each as to make no real difference to anything. In practice, it is clear that the private sector is not by any means persuaded that health care can be profitably expanded in much of Africa, nor is it willing to take any risks: the limited funds that have been raised sit idle in bank accounts or have been invested with established businesses. The pattern set by the IFC's own limited investment in African health projects – just $12 million invested in the decade to 2009, a mere 2 per cent of IFC health investments (Akpofure 2009) – has not been changed.

Investment Fund for Health in Africa

The smaller of the two funds is the Investment Fund for Health in Africa, based in the Netherlands but also operated by 'a Mauritius-based company'.[6] This fund's investors include FMO; Goldman Sachs; the Social Investor Foundation for Africa (whose contributors include: ACHMEA, AEGON, Heineken, Shell, SNS-REAAL and Unilever); APG; Pfizer and the African Health System Management Company.[7] The fund had a target capitalisation of $50 million, up to $10 million of which was to be contributed by IFC. Its brief would be to invest with small and medium health-care providers. An additional €10 million was invested in the Fund by the African Development Bank, in a deal signed in Tunis in April 2010, but only a few small-scale investments have been announced: $8.8 million in Kenya's largest health insurer, $1.6 million in telemedicine in South Africa, an undisclosed amount in a Singapore company selling medical disposables in Africa, and other schemes.[8]

Africa Health Fund

In June 2009, a new, separate Fund was set up, the 'Africa Health Fund', as part of the ongoing Health in Africa initiative already begun with the Gates Foundation. The Africa Health Fund (AHF) comprises investments from the IFC, the African Development Bank, the Gates Foundation and the German development finance

---

5   http://www.ifhafund.com/index.php?page=investors
6   http://goo.gl/8al7y
7   http://www.ifhafund.com/index.php?page=investors
8   IFHA (2011) http://www.ifhafund.com

body DEG. Its initial target was to invest between $100 million and $120 million in two tranches, beginning with a first closing of $57 million.

Its first investment, of just $2.6 million, was in the Nairobi Women's Hospital, where even the most basic 'shortmat' maternity package is priced on the Nairobi Women's Hospital website at £280 – the equivalent of six months' wages for a Kenyan woman earning the average wage of £11.30 per week. This goes up by over £200 if an obstetrician is involved and by more again if a caesarean section is required. Additional, unspecified charges also apply for antenatal care medication and feeds or care for sick babies. More elaborate packages for maternity at Nairobi Women's Hospital range in cost from £420 to just over £1,000. A survey by the *Standard* newspaper in 2008 reported that an elective caesarean package at Nairobi Women's Hospital was going for SH99,000 (£866) with even a normal birth costing £393. These fees would be more easily affordable for those on professional wages, which (other than IT) average between £5,000 and £12,000 annually (Standard Digital 2008). But more than half the Kenyan population lives on $1 per day or less. More recently, TV news has shown a protest outside the Nairobi Women's Hospital by campaigners angry at the hospital's poor safety record, claiming two women a week are dying in childbirth (KTN Prime 2012).

It also seems that the sudden slight increase in private-equity involvement that has taken place in Kenya's health care may be linked to the recent expansion of Kenya's middle class on the back of economic growth, with spending on health services, much of it out of pocket, increasing by over 50 per cent from 2004 to 2008. But the inequalities are stark. The same survey by the *Standard* found that some women in Kenya were paying up to £3,500 (SH400,000) for maternity care in 2008 – while those on the lowest incomes in rural areas and city slums were spending little or nothing. Small wonder that only 42 per cent of women in Kenya (630,000) deliver their babies in hospital, leaving 870,000 every year to take their chances with little or no professional help, many in villages where there is not even a doctor. Thousands are obliged to depend on traditional birth attendants and, with no proper health care, maternal death rates are high, whilst infant and under-five mortality rates were worse in 2008 than in 1990.

However, the availability of extra cash in the private sector is not necessarily good news for improving access to health care in a country with such low incomes and such a small and under-developed health-care system. There are fears that the injection of a relatively small total of £4.4 million of private-equity funds into health care in Kenya in the last two years could trigger an increase in user fees, so as to ensure adequate profit margins can be delivered to shareholders and investors (Insurance News Net 2010). Kenyan statistics show that medical costs have risen at 20 per cent or more for each of the last three years, driven by a steep rise in doctors' fees and a corresponding increase in insurance premiums. Insurers have begun demanding co-payments in advance from patients, varying from under £1 to £7, as a way of reducing demand for treatment. A survey in 2009 comparing the impact of health costs on the poorest people in 18 low-income countries found that Kenyans already faced the greatest risk of 'hardship funding' – having to borrow money or sell assets to pay hospital and health bills (Kruk et al. 2009).

In other words, far from improving access to the poor, the first example of the

IFC policy of working through private-equity investment in Africa seems likely to help widen the affordability gap that separates the poorest Kenyans from even the most basic health care, and to benefit only the more prosperous middle class in urban areas.

Investing in successful companies

The pattern of investment has continued from this unpromising start: small amounts of money are invested in already-successful niche private hospitals and elite services in countries with vast unmet need for affordable health care for the poor. In July 2011, Aureos announced a $4.5 million investment in Ghanaian hospital C&J Medi-care, based in the capital, Accra. C&J specialise in delivering occupational health services to 100 companies, including multinationals such as Coca Cola. Its gesture towards the poor is to offer 'a regular programme of free-of-charge health screening drives' – which is a good way to drum up extra business from those whose screening shows health problems they might otherwise not have known about. More than $2 million of the Aureos investment will be spent on new radiology equipment for MRI and CT scans. The company plans 'in the longer term' to expand its services to other cities in Ghana (Private Equity Wire 2011).

In November came the announcement that Aureos was to invest $2.5 million in another Kenyan private hospital and health-insurance company, the Avenue Group, which already has a 70-bed hospital in Nairobi, seven clinics throughout Kenya and a range of services, again aimed at businesses, some of them relatively small scale. Avenue Group also see the value of offering 'non-profit' activities such as 'public health screening days' at its clinics as well as 'free medical camps' (African Capital Markets News 2011).

2012 began with the revelation that the IFC's chosen repository for private-equity funds was being taken over by a bigger private-equity manager, the Dubai-based Abraaj Capital, to create a company with $7.5 billion of capital under its manage-ment, of which the Africa Health Fund is only the smallest marginal component (Aureos Capital 2012a). In April 2012, Aureos continued the pattern of investment, pumping $5 million into one of the services the poor and sick millions in Sub-Saharan Africa have been crying out for: an IVF clinic. Therapia is run by Dr Richard Ajayi, described as 'a leading healthcare entrepreneur', and, not surpris-ingly, it is to be the first assisted reproductive centre in West Africa. The press release on the funding deal does not even pretend that any of this treatment will be available to the poor of Nigeria.

In July, just a couple of weeks before the final deal was done for the takeover of Aureos, another elite private hospital got lucky. This time, the $1.7 million handout went to Clinique Biasa in Togo, which describes itself, perhaps modestly, as 'one of Lomé's top three private hospitals'. The hospital is already established and running at full capacity: once again there is no attempt to suggest that the injection of donor funds to this company will benefit anyone but the wealthiest Togolese, who will no doubt enjoy the trebling of the hospital's bed capacity and the promised 'positive impact' on patient wellbeing (Aureos Capital 2012c, Altsassets Private Equity News 2012).

In fact, half of Togo's population of 6.6 million lives below the poverty line, with just 3.4 per cent of the population surviving to 65 or over and a life expectancy of 56. Private health insurance is almost non-existent, covering just 4 per cent of private health spending, while 76 per cent of all spending on health care comes out of pocket. The number of young women receiving contraception, at 17 per cent, is lower now than in 199, and there is just one doctor per 200,000 members of the population (Health Systems 20/20 2012).

Aureos itself once threatened to move its headquarters from London to Singapore to avoid EU regulation of hedge funds and, like the IFHA, it has been registered in the tax haven of Mauritius. The company is taking a hefty annual slice (2.25 per cent) from the investments as its 'management fees'. Save the Children has questioned whether the company has the necessary expertise for the extremely complex task of making the private health-care sector work equitably for the poor (Cometto and Brikci 2009). Now, although it will continue trading under the name Aureos (Aureos Capital 2012d), it has been taken over by a Dubai-based company. How much interest it now takes in the remaining Africa Health Fund is a question that will only be answered in the months ahead.

But five years of reliance on private equity to secure vital development in health care for some of the poorest populations on the planet have delivered nothing for any of the donors to be proud of. More money has been put into the pockets of already-profitable businesses, simply to help them maintain services that are unaffordable to those who most need them in their own country.

After all the IFC's big talk in 2007 of investing up to $1 billion, two funds totalling just over £100 million have eventually been established; and less than $20 million has been invested by Aureos in companies that didn't really need it, to treat patients already wealthy enough to pay their own way. Over this same period, more precious resources have also been spent on high level meetings, publicity and of course the management fees paid out to the two Mauritius-based companies controlling the Funds.

It almost seems as if the IFC has set out to disprove its own assertion that the private sector is the key to developing health care in Africa. Sadly, there are no signs that lessons are being leaned from this false start. It's clear that if any part of the World Bank apparatus is to be used as a conduit for effective use of donor funds, it should not be the IFC.

Egypt: IFC backs the existing winners – and boosts privatisation

While the going has been exceedingly slow for the process of equity-fund investment in Sub-Saharan Africa, the IFC has noted a 'boom' since 2007 in investment in the Middle East and North Africa (MENA). During 2007, the year in which the 'Investment Fund for Health in Africa' (IFHA) was launched, the IFC itself decided to invest $81.2 million in health-care companies in MENA countries, most notably in Egypt. $25 million was pumped into the Saudi Andalusia Group 'to increase access to private health care in Egypt', with the expansion of an existing private hospital and the construction of a new 100-bed hospital in Cairo. This investment that would benefit the most prosperous Egyptians and wealthy foreigners making use of the facilities was explained by the IFC's Health and Education Director, Guy Ellena, as a way of relieving pressure on public-sector hospitals:

> By expanding overall hospital capacity in Egypt, the project makes it possible for public hospitals to reduce overcrowding and waiting lists by referring patients to private facilities, thereby relieving the burden on the public health system.
>
> (IFC 2007a)

The IFC's Director for the Middle East and North Africa added with apparently no intended irony that the new facilities would 'increase employment opportunities for local professionals' – seeming to ignore the fact that professionals attracted to the new hospitals would not be delivering services in public hospitals for those unable to pay the fees demanded by Andalusia.

Indeed, with three hospitals and two specialised clinics in Saudi Arabia and Egypt, the Andalusia Group was no struggling small or medium-sized enterprise. It was already claiming to be 'the fastest-growing medical group in the Middle East', with 'a predominant position in both the Saudi and Egyptian markets' and seeking an even larger market share.

Another $4 million IFC investment was in Dar Al Fouad Hospital, another high-cost, high-tech hospital on the outskirts of Cairo: it is linked with the US Cleveland Clinic. The project was designed to expand the hospital's 'high margin/high growth tertiary care services': the IFC investment was specifically intended to 'further dilute public sector ownership'. The IFC argues that the extra money would help to expand and refurbish the Arab International Hospital in central Cairo and 'raise the quality of service in a highly populated and underserved area where there is an acute need for health care' (IFC 2007a). However, the Hospital makes the point on its website that it is 'located in the tourist area of the Sixth of October City' and boasts that it has been approved to deliver treatment to patients from the UK. Its charitable society 'helps those who are unable to afford the medical services that DAFH provides'. It raises charitable donations to pay for treatment for the poor, but delivered just 40 heart operations for children over a five-year period and has more recently 'partially funded a liver transplant' (Dar Al Fouad Hospital 2012).

The IFC involvement promoting private medicine in Egypt took place against a backdrop of growing popular anger uniting almost all opposition political parties and nearly every civil society organisation against attempts by President Hosni Mubarak's government to privatise the health-care system.

The political debate had raged since 2007 when, without any prior discussion or consultation with the Egyptian public, the Prime Minister issued declaration 637 which established a new 'Egyptian Holding Company for Health Care', a for-profit company to replace the non-profit, public-sector health-insurance organisation. The decree would have allowed the government to sell off the public-sector hospitals and other assets built up through years of subscriptions to the health-insurance system.

But it also restructured health-insurance cover, offering various packages according to people's means and excluding some treatments that were previously covered, such as kidney dialysis.

Co-payments equivalent to a third of the cost of treatment would also be introduced – including the cost of surgery, investigations, hospital accommodation and prescriptions – effectively negating the principle of health insurance and putting health care, especially specialist treatment, out of the reach of the poor. Campaigners against these plans pointed the finger of blame firmly at the World Bank and USAID, as well as the EU which also supported the change. USAID signed a Memorandum of Understanding in April 2007 as part of its effort to promote the reforms, committing to provide $1 million, to be matched by a similar sum from pharmaceutical companies which also favoured the plan (Shukrallah 2009, USAID 2007, People's Health Movement 2007).

The ruling National Democratic Party had argued for sweeping away the last vestiges of the old socialist-style public-sector health system and the establishment of a market-based system in which health-insurance funds would be used to contract with private health providers. Critics were concerned that the universal coverage promised by President Mubarak could be reduced to primary care, leaving heavy charges for hospital care (Bradley 2009). Even before the plans for co-payments, Egyptians were paying 56 per cent of health spending through out-of-pocket payments. Half the population was paying a subscription of between 60p and £1 per month for state health insurance, while a minority (30 per cent) were able to afford some form of private health insurance and 20 per cent of the population, living below the poverty line, could afford no health insurance at all. 44 per cent of Egyptians live on less than $2 a day. Another problem has been that most private-sector hospitals and clinics that can be used by those with health insurance are located in Cairo or Alexandria, giving little access to the rural poor in the north or south of the country (Shukrallah 2009).

There are 1,250 public hospitals with 116,000 beds, some running as low as 20 per cent occupancy for lack of adequate funding. By contrast, there are 1,200 mainly very small private hospitals with a total of 23,000 beds, averaging just 19 beds each. 84 per cent of hospital visits take place in public facilities. None of these problems was going to be remedied by further expanding the existing large, high-tech, high-cost private hospitals in Cairo. It is not clear how the IFC role of reinforcing the market dominance of a few large players in Egyptian and Middle Eastern health care complies with its commitment as part of the World Bank to fight poverty 'with passion and professionalism for lasting results'.[9]

In 2007, the IFC pumped $52 million into two other projects in MENA:

- Saudi German Hospitals, which was already running a network of five hospitals in

---

9   Despite the support for the government reforms, mass pressure and an appeal to Egypt's Administrative Court in 2008 forced a suspension of decree 637 (People's Health Movement 2008). A new proposed National Health Insurance Bill published in 2009 retreated from the establishment of the for-profit holding company, but still pressed for the establishment of separate insurance funds for catastrophic illness and for the poor, thus leaving the risk of breaking the principle of solidarity and universal entitlement (Egyptian Initiative for Personal Rights 2009). In the event, the new Bill was also dropped (Egyptian Initiative for Personal Rights 2010).

Saudi Arabia and was building a new hospital in Cairo. The hefty $37 million IFC investment carried minimal risk since the company was already established as a major player in the Saudi market, with a network including 1,600 hospital beds and employing over 5,000 staff (IFC 2007a).

- The Shefa Fund, a $100 million Shari'a-compliant health-care fund which invests in health-care providers and ancillary services in the Middle East and North Africa (MENA) region, with the objective of creating 'industry-dominant health groups with regional reach'. Shefa had been targeting the health-care industry through acquiring a majority stake in leading health-care providers in accordance with Islamic principles. The Shefa Healthcare Fund 'provides investors access to diverse markets in the MENA countries and offers them an opportunity to reduce risk by investing in a diversified portfolio of health-care providers.' The Fund aimed to raise the quality of regional health-care services to match global standards and transform the region into 'a high-standard health-care services hub' (IFC 2007a).

Exactly how supporting these projects assists in the development of equitable health services is not explained (IFC 2007a).

IFC and India: more health care for the rich at home and abroad

In India, the IFC has been investing in Apollo Hospital Enterprises, a high-tech, high-cost private hospital chain that is already the market leader in India and one of the leading proponents of medical tourism – while hundreds of millions of low-income local people lack access to affordable health care. India has a huge poor population, massive inequalities and, until recently, minimal levels of public health spending, at just one per cent of its GDP. As a result, a massive 80 per cent of health spending is 'private' – out-of-pocket payments at point of service. The private sector already runs 93 per cent of all hospitals, has 64 per cent of hospital beds and employs 80 per cent of all doctors, making India one of the countries most dependent on private provision and health spending (World Bank 2007a).

The private sector is already unhealthily large and dominant in Indian health care. So, as the Indian government seems belatedly to be recognising in 2012, the last thing India needs is a further expansion of private health care. UNICEF has also argued that it is *public* spending that needs to be increased in Asia and the Pacific: UNICEF has called for it to be increased by two per cent to improve access to care for the poor:

> As the world has moved past the half way mark and into the final laps towards the Millennium Development Goals' 2015 target line, what is needed now is political will and sound strategies to dramatically increase investment in public health services that specifically target the poorest and most marginalized.
>
> (UNICEF 2008)

Even the World Bank appears to agree, pointing out the ways in which the poor are failed by the existing private sector:

> India's heavy reliance on private health spending causes significant financial burdens for those who use it. For example, the average patient who enters a hospital spends over 58 percent of his or her annual income on private health services.
>
> More than 40 percent of inpatients borrow money to cover medical expenses, and at least 25 percent of them are forced into poverty by those expenses.
>
> India's reliance on private health spending also creates a 'two-track' system that discriminates against the poor by shunting them to inadequately funded public facilities.
>
> (World Bank 2007a: 33)

The Bank itself (IDA) has had dire problems from projects with various private companies in India. The report cited above, a two-volume internal World Bank report, commissioned in 2006 and completed at the end of 2007, revealed fraud and corruption running into tens of millions of dollars on five schemes with a total value of $569 million which were launched between 1997 and 2003. On one scheme, the $54 million 'Food and Drug Capacity Building Project', the investigation by the Bank's own Independent Evaluation Group (IEG) found fraud and corruption on a massive scale, in which almost $9 out of every $10 had been misspent. The 'Second National AIDS Control project' used defective test kit that delivered misleading or invalid results 'potentially resulting in further spread of the disease'. The $114 million 'Malaria Control Project' was found to have delivered poor quality bed nets. There were also strong criticisms over the $125 million 'Tuberculosis Control project' and the $82 million 'Orissa Health Systems development Project' – which was supposed to include work on 55 hospitals, but investigators found 'uninitiated and uncompleted work, severely leaking roofs, crumbling ceilings, mouldering walls, and non-functional water, sewage and/or electrical systems' (World Bank 2007a).

The fiasco and the scale of the subsequent revelations led the *Wall Street Journal* to comment:

> With the exception of Paul Volcker's investigation of the UN Oil for Food scandal, we can think of no comparable review of an international organisation that has brought such damaging facts to light, certainly not one that was internally conducted.
>
> (*Wall Street Journal* 2008)

However, none of these factors seem to have influenced the World Bank's private-sector arm, the International Finance Corporation (IFC), which has pursued a strategy in India which ignores the Bank's (and the IFC's own) proclaimed commitment to 'fight poverty with passion and professionalism for lasting results', instead focusing investment on further enhancing existing, highly profitable, high-tech private hospitals, whose fees are well beyond the reach of 90 per cent of the Indian population.

A 2010 report quotes Planning Commission estimates that private-sector outpatient services are 20–54 per cent more expensive than public-sector services in India, while inpatient care is 100–740 per cent more expensive, and notes the 'paradox' that health insurance is only affordable for those who could afford expensive health care – and 'beyond the means of those who are needy' (Sen 2010).

Just 11 per cent of the Indian population had any health insurance cover in 2007, with premiums rising rapidly. In 2008, the Indian central government launched a health-insurance scheme for 300 million people below the poverty line, for a premium of $0.80 per person per year, but offering a maximum coverage of $750 per family per year (Bhattachariya and Sapra 2008). The cost of care is a major factor in excluding the poor, with almost 38 per cent of the urban poor and 43 per cent of rural poor identifying financial hardship for not seeking even outpatient care (Yip and Mahal 2008).

On average, India has just 1.5 hospital beds per 1,000 people, but even at this minimal level there is a stark divide between the urban and rural areas, with urban centres having 1.8 beds per 1,000 people, roughly double the coverage in rural areas. Despite this desperate lack of facilities for its own population, which leaves India well down the league of the UN Human Development Index, some of its private hospitals have made the country one of the leading players in the new global market in 'health tourism'. They offer a range of specialist services, from cosmetic treatments and simple cataract operations through to open heart surgery and high-tech cancer care, using the latest equipment and offering luxurious accommodation for wealthy foreigners with money to pay, from the US, Europe and the Middle East.

Apollo, singled out for support by the IFC, is one of the market leaders in this field. Its website shows the range of rooms available to paying patients, ranging from the bog-standard 'air conditioned multibed unit' through 'semi-private', deluxe and the most extravagant 'Platinum/Suite', offering a separate bathroom as well as a sofa-bed for 'attendants', a lounge, a fridge, a pantry and 24-hour high-speed Internet. The company owns 26 hospitals and manages 17 more on a contractual basis in cities across India. Its total hospital capacity is 8,500 beds, with 4,500 beds in AHE's owned hospitals. According to Indian Stocks News, investors can be assured of a return on their money:

> The revenue per bed per day ranges from Rs 8,000 to Rs 17,000 (£119–£253), depending on the location of the hospital. The average length of stay has largely remained the same for the company at an average of 5.7 to 5.9 days across its various hospitals.
>
> (indianstocksnews.com 2009)

Operating in what is described as a 'recession-proof' sector, Apollo is also the market leader:

> Being the largest listed healthcare player, AHE commands a premium over its peers. It is currently trading at 25 times its earnings. Investors interested in steady

and predictable earnings growth can look at accumulating this stock with a long-term perspective.

Apollo treated 60,000 foreign patients in the five years to 2010 and emphasises its commitment to health tourism, making little reference on its main website to treating Indian residents and none at all to treating the poor. Websites and agencies such as Medical Tourism India help to keep a flow of wealthy patients coming, offering medical packages alongside tour packages (such as the 'Golden Triangle Tour', 'Rajasthan Cultural Tour', 'Kerala Backwater Tour' and 'Taj Mahal and Tiger Tour') and emphasising also that, in comparison with Western health care, 'you can get the treatment done in India at the lowest charges'.[10]

More recently, this leader in private health care has established its own two-tier service, opening a new chain of up to 250 'Apollo Reach' 150-bed hospitals in smaller towns and cities with the aim of drawing in income from a wider group of patients, at slightly lower prices than in Apollo's core prestige hospitals. This takes advantage of the availability of cheaper manpower and land, and the agreement with government that hospitals built outside the big metropolis areas will be free from taxes for their first five years.

Even at these reduced prices, only a small minority of Indians will be able to afford Apollo's services. Nonetheless, in this enterprise Apollo, which had already benefited from previous IFC investment, managed again to draw on IFC investment, with a $35 million loan and a further $15 million 'standby' loan to help fund the expansion plan for the first 25 new hospitals.

Just months after the loan agreement was agreed with the IFC, the real face of Apollo towards India's poor was underlined by a decision in the Delhi High Court to issue notice to Apollo Hospital for charging patients who should have been entitled to free treatment. On 30th November 2009, judges declared that 'It is completely unfair on the part of Apollo that they are not abiding by orders of giving free treatment to the poor.' International patients flown in to the Delhi Apollo Hospital pay 20–30 per cent above the bed charges for local patients, which have gone up almost three-fold since 2004 (Banrhia 2009).

The Indraprastha Medical Corporation, which owns the Apollo hospital site in Delhi, was established as a public–private partnership in 1994 and was given land at discounted rates by the Delhi government, with the lease making clear that the poor must receive free care. The government had also invested large sums in the hospital, seeking to secure the welfare of local people, with a requirement that 25 per cent of patients would be treated free. Earlier in the year, having heard that this requirement had been breached, the same court had ordered the Apollo Hospital to reserve a third of its beds for low-income patients and to treat them free of all charges, even for medical tests.

Apollo was just one of a number of private hospitals found by the Delhi court to have breached the agreements to set aside resources to treat patients on low incomes (defined in November 2007 as those with a family income of less than Rs4,000 ($85) per month). The World Bank estimates that 70 per cent of Indians live on less

10 http://www.medical-tourism-india.com

than the $2 per day required to live a decent life. Once again the Indian example shows the IFC using its resources not to help open up access for the poor to health care, or to sponsor small and medium-sized enterprises that might offer more afford-able treatment and fill in some of the gaps in India's threadbare health system; but rather to help entrench and expand a market leader in an exclusive system.

IFC helps bring privately financed hospitals to Africa

The hidden costs of Lesotho's new PPIP hospital[11]

The first major hospital built in Africa through a 'Public–Private Investment Part-nership' opened its doors on 1st October 2011: but the showpiece $120 million Queen 'Mamohato Memorial Hospital, a referral hospital in Lesotho's capital city, Maseru, was almost immediately the centre of controversy when it turned away an expectant 24-year-old woman, Metsana Rapotsane (*Lesotho Times* 2011).

The incident triggered an investigation by the Ministry of Health, amid public questions over arrangements for urgent care and emergencies at the new hospital, and the adequacy of the filter clinics.

According to the summary in *Handshake*, the quarterly journal of the World Bank's private-sector wing, the International Finance Corporation, the new hospital was to 'operate as the national referral hospital *as well as the district hospital for the greater Maseru area*' (IFC 2011: 27, emphasis added). A *Guardian* report on the dire state of health services, especially for Lesotho's rural poor, indicated the shortage of affordable health care and the much higher costs of private treatment and argued that the new is harder to access for many who were able to get treatment as outpa-tients at the QEII (*Guardian* Development Network 2011).

These controversies were a severe setback for a new hospital that had for several years been heralded as opening a new era for private-sector involvement in health care in Africa (GPOBA 2010, IFC 2009a, 2009b). The Global Partnership on Output-Based Aid (GPOBA), run by the World Bank, subsidised the new hospital by $6.25 million over three years and assisted the Government of Lesotho with contract management (GPOBA 2007). However, there are serious reasons for concern that the project will widen health inequalities and draw vital health-care resources away from patients with severe health needs in other parts of Lesotho.

The Project

The new 425-bed hospital (390 beds for the public sector and 35 which will be run separately as a private patient unit) is a long-overdue replacement for the 100-year-old Queen Elizabeth II Hospital, which was built back in colonial days by the British

---

11 An abbreviated version of this section has been published on the blog Global Health Check (http://www.globalhealthcheck.org/?p=481).

government and, with 450 beds averaging 83 per cent occupancy, was also far and away the country's biggest and most intensively utilised hospital (Lesotho Ministry of Health and Social Welfare (MHSW) 2008: 21).

The PPIP or 'Public Private Partnership' (PPP) was signed on 20th March 2009. It involved building the new hospital on a greenfield site on the edge of the city and the provision of clinical services for the 18-year lifetime of the contract, including the refurbishment, re-equipping and operation of three filter clinics (in Qoaling, Mabote and Likotsi in the greater Maseru area) and the training of health professionals. The contract stipulates that the hospital is to use the reduced number of 390 beds 'to treat all patients who present at the hospital, regardless of the type of condition' – up to 'a maximum of 20,000 in-patient admissions and 310,000 outpatient attendances annually, with very few clinical exceptions'.[12] In exchange, the Lesotho government pays an annual fixed service payment, which can rise only by inflation each year.

The lop-sided contract can be traced back to the managerial weakness of the Lesotho government and the failure of the IFC to give appropriate advice. A consultancy report establishing a 'Baseline study' for the PPP contract warned of such a problem in 2009, pointing out that:

> At present, sufficient expertise in hospital operations, financial oversight and analysis and systems analysis to manage the PPP contract in the interests of the Government and people of Lesotho does not exist…
>
> (Lesotho–Boston Health Alliance 2009: 72)

Nonetheless, the project carried on regardless. The same report argued (ibid.: 78) that the new hospital could not be adequately operated for less than 30 per cent of the MoHSW recurrent budget and that, as the cost crept up towards 40 per cent, there would be an increasingly adverse and severe impact on district health services. The report urged the Ministry to set an upper limit (40 per cent or less) to the amount of its recurrent budget to be devoted to the new hospital. This has not been done.

The consortium

The clinical services are delivered by South African private hospital corporation Netcare, which also heads up the consortium that collectively invested around 60 per cent of the capital cost of the new buildings. The consortium, Tsepong (Pty) Ltd, includes:

- Netcare Limited (40 per cent) – a large South African multinational health-care company
- Excel Health (20 per cent) – doctors and medical specialists from Lesotho who will jointly supply the hospital with specialist doctors

---

12 According to the IFC magazine *Handshake* (No. 3, p.28). Note that unless numbers of patients are reduced, 83 per cent occupancy of 450 beds would imply 95 per cent or higher occupancy of 390 beds.

- Afri'nnai (20 per cent) – doctors and medical specialists from South Africa – jointly responsible for supplying specialist doctors
- Women Investment Company (10 per cent) – an investment company for Basotho women – sub-contracting local security, gardening, linen and laundry
- D10 Investments (10 per cent) – the investment division of the local Chambers of Commerce – responsible for sub-contracting office facilities, vehicles and food for the hospital.

(Smith 2009: 9)

Capital costs

Supporters of the scheme claimed that it would be 'cost neutral' both to the government and to patients, whose fees for access have not been increased from the previous level. However, this is not a full picture of the situation. A very significant increase in spending and government investment had *already taken place*. According to the USAID-funded Health System Assessment for Lesotho (Mwase et al. 2010), the run-up to the PPP hospital project in Maseru was marked by a significant increase in spending on health, both by government and from other sources.

The Health Ministry had to raise a large share ($51 million) of the capital investment for the hospital. The Lesotho Ministry of Health and Social Welfare's total budget was just $100 million in 2007–8 ($39 million on capital and $61 million on recurrent expenditure). That figure itself represented a dramatic increase (169 per cent) on the previous year because it included an extra allocation of $24 million towards the new hospital (Lesotho MHSW 2008: 94). In 2005–6, the Ministry's combined recurrent and capital budget had been just $47 million. Constraints on government resources had blocked early plans for the Ministry to contribute almost 80 per cent of the capital required in order to keep its future payments lower.

Between 2006 and 2009, the cost of the PPIP scheme increased by more than 33 per cent above the original projection, which had projected an annual 'unitary charge' of $24.1 million for the hospital plus services (Stemmer 2008: 10–11). Mwase et al. (2010) identified a serious reduction in government income arising from a new treaty which has reduced the flow of revenue to Lesotho from the South African Customs Union. Indeed, overall resources available for health spending could even be further reduced, while the inflexible nature of PPP contracts means that payments for the new hospital would then consume a much larger share of a reduced budget – forcing cutbacks in other areas of health spending.

Revenue costs

The new hospital and its three primary-care feeder clinics are set to cost the Government of Lesotho (GoL) at least $32.6 million a year as a unitary charge for the core contract, index-linked to inflation, for 15.5 years, completing in March 2027 (Smith 2009: 14). Given that (according to the Health Minister) the annual budget for the QEII hospital and the filter clinics was less than $17 million in 2007–8, the new deal represents a near 100 per cent increase in costs and throws into doubt claims that the project is 'cost neutral'. Rates of inflation in Lesotho stood at 5.5 per cent in 2011 according to the Lesotho Bureau of Statistics:[13] if this were sustained, it would inflate the total cost over the lifetime of the contract from $489 million to $803 million, making it ever less affordable. These payments are on top of the government's own up-front investment of $62 million, including additional infrastructure costs of $11 million (Smith 2009: 10).

While the whole contract is shrouded in secrecy (like so many PPP deals), Matthew Smith's figures suggest that the consortium will make money in several different ways:

- A guaranteed profit on the capital investment
- A 10 per cent guaranteed return on its operating budget
- Full payment for any additional patients treated above the contract maximum
- And payment for those sent to South Africa for specialist treatment.

Hidden profits

By comparison with some health PFI and PPP deals, it appears that Netcare's likely direct profit is relatively modest. However, the $62 million capital investment by the Government of Lesotho and the ongoing unitary charge mean that public funds are not only paying for the beds open to citizens of Maseru and further afield – but also subsidising a brand new 35-bed private hospital, co-located with a full general hospital.

This private unit will be run by Netcare and have full access to the operating theatres, staff and other facilities in the main hospital; but it will only treat the minority who are wealthy enough to pay the full tariff fees for their treatment.

No details have been opened up to public scrutiny. However, it's clear that none of the profits from private treatment at the new hospital will be shared with the Lesotho government that helped finance it. As the largest operator of private hospitals in South Africa, Netcare will also be able to make additional money by sending patients to its hospital in Bloemfontein or elsewhere for specialist treatment not covered by the PPP contract (IFC 2008) – including organ transplants, advanced cardiac surgery and radiotherapy (IFC 2009d: 2). Lesotho patients will be referred to South African hospitals – with the GoL footing the bill for treatment. In 2006–7, it spent FY $24.8 million on 3,281 external referrals, of which 55 per cent were oncology cases (Mwase et al. 2010: 22).

A survey in 2011 showed Netcare charges of 2,000 Rand ($255) or more per night for bed only, in addition to consultant fees (timeslive 2011). If bills like this are potentially to be picked up by the Lesotho Ministry of Health, it gives no incentive for Netcare to reduce referrals. The company is still struggling to get free of the opprobrium from its involvement in the sale of kidneys transplanted, a number of them from children, to wealthy clients at the St Augustine's Hospital in

---

13 http://www.bos.gov.ls, accessed 16th October 2011

KwaZulu-Natal in 100 operations between 2001 and 2003. Only last November, Netcare was fined £700,000 after pleading guilty (Beattie 2011). In 2008, Netcare made profits in South Africa alone of R651 million on revenues of R4,907 million – a return of 13 per cent. Interim figures from March 2011 show a continued increases in revenue and profits.

Unequal access

But while the future looks rosy for Netcare, the GoL is committed by the contract to spend around 30 per cent of its health budget on a hospital whose main catchment area is Maseru, which has 350,000 inhabitants, just 16 per cent of the Lesotho population of over 2 million. Numbers to be treated at the hospital are capped at a relatively low level by the PPIP contract. Yet official figures show a hospitalisation rate of 3.2 per cent of the population each year (Mohapi 2011) – equivalent to 64,000 of the Lesotho population of 2 million.

The high rate of infection with HIV/AIDS also contributes to this pressure. Yet the new hospital, soaking up a third of the health budget, has a contract to provide for just 20,000 of them. To extend similar coverage to the rural areas would be unaffordable.

Figures from USAID's Health Systems 20/20 database show that the heavily impoverished population of just over 2 million, 58 per cent of whom live on less than a dollar a day, has an average life expectancy of just 45, with less than 5 per cent of the population aged over 65 in 2008. In part, this high level of mortality is driven by the level of infection with HIV, which has reached 24 per cent of the population. Along with high levels of infant and child mortality, maternal mortality was three times the average for other LMICs (lower-middle-income countries), at 960 per 100,000 births in 2005.

Tackling these health problems needs a good, affordable infrastructure of primary-care and small-scale local health facilities rather than one costly hospital in the capital, out of reach to many of those in greatest need. But Lesotho has a desperate shortage of hospital beds (with less than half the average in other LMICs) and doctors (one-fifth of the average in other LMICs). Nursing levels are also just half the LMIC average level of provision, leaving Lesotho short of 600 nurses and midwives, while those in post complain of low wages and excessive workload (IRIN 2006).

The plans for the new hospital claimed one advantage was that it would help improve the recruitment and retention of nursing and medical staff, but made no mention of how this is to be achieved, unless wages and conditions are improved and staffing levels are increased to match the workload. However, the problem is that implementing these policies in one hospital while leaving the rest of Lesotho's health workforce on the current levels will create another major distortion: staff would be attracted to the superior facilities and conditions in the new Maseru hospital, potentially leaving other areas even more desperately short-staffed.

There are more complexities and contradictions in the new hospital project than meet the eye. The PPIP scheme has already cost $62 million in capital investment from a ministry with extremely limited resources and pushed up the government's health budget. The new scheme has secured partial government funding for a deluxe private hospital unit on the main site, which will be unaffordable to all but a small wealthy elite in Lesotho and which will generate profits that will not be shared with the GoL.

While it makes perfectly good sense for Netcare as a private, profit-seeking company to take advantage of this situation to secure a foothold in Lesotho and establish facilities which will contribute to their growing profits, it is less clear that the project is consistent with the IFC's commitment to wider values of equity. A more useful contribution from the World Bank would have been to lend the money to build the new hospital at low interest directly to the Ministry of Health and to help ministers and civil servants negotiate a tight agreement to ensure prompt delivery on budget. This would have given the hospital management additional scope to negotiate as necessary with potential providers to deliver services without the long-term rigid constrictions of a PPIP which may soon turn out to be unaffordable.

Chapter five

Other organisations shaping health reforms

The number of significant players in global aid has risen and the issue of governance of the effort as a whole has become more complicated, with a growing proliferation of agencies, international donors, private and NGO organisations all playing a role in funding health provision in developing countries. The British government warned in 2007 that the involvement of 90 global health initiatives alongside more than 40 bilateral donors, 20 global and regional funds and 26 UN agencies was 'over complex' (McCoy et al. 2009: 414).

A major 2006 report for the World Bank and the Global Fund to Fight AIDS, Malaria and Tuberculosis pointedly reminds the Bank that the Global Fund was created in 2001 partly as a result of disappointing results from the Bank and UN agencies in responding to the AIDS crisis. But it warned of looming chaos from uncoordinated interventions:

> A multitude of international organizations providing HIV/AIDS services have been converging on countries with limited institutional, administrative and managerial public health capacities, creating what UNAIDS describes as 'an implementation crisis'. ... Recent studies of global health programs, while acknowledging their many contributions, conclude that 'their collective impact has created or exacerbated a series of problems at the country level' – including, for example, 'poor coordination and duplication, high transaction costs, variable degrees of country ownership, and lack of alignment with country systems. The cumulative effect of these problems is to risk undermining the sustainability of national development plans, distorting national priorities, diverting scarce human resources and/or establishing uncoordinated service delivery structures'.
>
> (Shakow 2006: 3).

Worse, the overall impact has been most negative in some of the most vulnerable countries:

> It is widely recognized that health delivery systems in Africa are now weaker and more fragmented than they were ten years ago, and yet the critical need for strengthening them has been further exacerbated as the Global Fund and other programs now promote universal access to treatment as well as for prevention of AIDS.
>
> (Shakow 2006: 36)

Each organisation brings its own transaction costs and there is already evidence of programs cutting across each other and becoming a burden on the countries they are setting out to assist.

Of course, there is a positive factor: there is more money in the system and more government-level engagement, even if few high-income countries have yet raised their aid contributions to the modest targets set. The sums seem very large: the combined volume of development assistance for health (DAH) from all sources doubled from 1990 to 2001, then doubled again in the six years from 2001 to 2007 to $21.8 billion – a quadrupling over 17 years (Ravishankar et al. 2009[1]). However, the sources of funding have shifted away from UN agencies (whose share of the total decreased from 32% to just 14% between 1990 and 2007), the World Bank and regional banks, and bilateral agencies (down from 47% in 1990 to 34% in 2001). This raises questions of control, accountability and coordination. By contrast, in the years immediately following the banking crash (2009–11) the 4% annual growth in aid for health to a total of $27.73 billion was largely driven by the World Bank's IBRD, whose contribution grew by 28% in 2009–10 and more than doubled (up by 128%) in 2010–11. Bilateral assistance fell back, growing just 4% over the two years, and the Global Fund announced it would make no new grants for the next two years because of inadequate funding (Leach-Kemon et al. 2012). US global health appropriations for 2012 were lower than 2011: 'the honeymoon is over' (Glassman and Duran 2012).

New funds

A growing share of DAH has come in recent years from specific funds, such as the Global Fund to Fight AIDS, Tuberculosis and Malaria (known as the Global Fund) and the GAVI Alliance (formerly the Global Alliance for Vaccines and Immunisation), and the Bill & Melinda Gates Foundation, established in 1994 (3.9% of DAH in 2007); along with NGOs (increasing from 13% of DAH in 1990 to 25% in 2006). Other significant donors in the final five years to 2007 have been governments, such as those of the UK, Japan, Germany, France, the Netherlands, Canada, Sweden, Norway and Italy.

Significantly absent is any substantial material support for initiatives to prevent and treat chronic disease in poor countries, where the cost and burden of noncommunicable chronic disease are rising. The lack of priority for this aspect of health care flies in the face of stark facts. In 2008, the WHO warned that chronic diseases are now the major cause of death and disability worldwide, accounting through cardiovascular diseases, diabetes, obesity, cancer and respiratory diseases for 59 per cent of the 57 million deaths annually and 46 per cent of the global burden of disease (Anderson 2009).

A World Bank report warns that what makes the challenge of these chronic

---

1   Curiously, Ravishankar and colleagues make no reference in their study to the US President's Emergency Plan for AIDS Relief (PEPFAR), established in 2003 by George W. Bush, which increased its spending from $2.3 billion in 2004 to $6.7 billion in 2009 and is a key component of the growing US share of DAH.

diseases especially difficult to deal with is that many developing countries are having to confront them now, while their economies are at a lower stage of development than their higher-income counterparts were when they had to deal with them. Noncommunicable diseases (NCDs) are also affecting populations at younger ages, bringing longer periods of ill health, greater loss of productivity, and premature deaths. Moreover, developing countries are often still having to deal with a heavy burden of communicable disease placing even heavier stress on over-stretched and under-resourced health-care systems (Baeza and Klingen 2011, Ollila 2005). Cardiovascular diseases (CVD) alone account for 35 per cent of deaths in Latin America and the Caribbean, compared with just 10 per cent for AIDS, TB, malaria and infectious diseases; and CVD is responsible for as many years of life lost as all communicable diseases put together (Anderson 2009).

There are fears that attempts to 'treat their way out' of the challenge of noncommunicable diseases will be 'too costly' for most middle- and low-income countries, obliging them to make 'often very difficult choices' and to place a strong emphasis on prevention measures (Baeza and Klingen 2011: 5).

Some of the preventive measures to reduce the incidence of these diseases are remarkably cheap and effective: they include promoting exercise, campaigns to reduce numbers smoking, campaigns to raise awareness of hypertension (one program in Brazil coming in at $1 per capita) and interventions to reduce hospitalisation for uncontrolled asthma (Anderson 2009: 204). In six middle-income countries the costs of a comprehensive prevention package, including one addressing individual health needs and several population-based interventions, ranged from $1.5 to $4.5 per capita (Baeza and Klingen 2011: 5).

Donors indifferent to NCDs

But the donors are not interested and so resources for these cost-effective measures are lacking. The four biggest donors of health-related aid – the World Bank, the US Government, the Bill & Melinda Gates Foundation and the Global Fund for HIV/AIDS, Tuberculosis and Malaria – between them contributed just 0.1 per cent of all health expenditures worldwide but, with the exception of the Bank, whose main investment has focused more strongly on prevention, they have a major impact on the shape of health-care systems and their priorities. This distortion means that $1,029 is spent for every person dying of HIV/AIDS, compared with just $3.21 per death from a noncommunicable disease (Sridhar and Batniji 2008). The missing elements that might otherwise attract the interest of the big bilateral and philanthrocapitalist donors to noncommunicable diseases seem to include the limited use of costly drugs or high-tech whizzy medical treatment; the lack of any high-paid CEO and board jobs on projects; and the public health focus resulting in few headline-grabbing stories (Wiist 2011).

The Gates Foundation is an important element in the growing contribution of 'private sources', which increased from 19 per cent to almost 27 per cent in the decade to 2007: other significant private sources include cash and 'in kind' contributions from pharmaceutical and other suppliers (Ravishankar et al. 2009).

But while the total resources may have increased rapidly, this proliferation of sources and the specific interests, 'pet priorities' and varied motivations of the various donors (Fan 2012a) do not necessarily make for an efficient, effective or coordinated delivery of the assistance. Each donor has their own distinctive structures, lines of accountability, focus on interest, methods of work and separate resources. The sheer volume of administration and organisation of dealing with so many schemes can be a real burden on governments and health-care systems in the developing countries:

> At one point Tanzania was producing about 2,400 reports annually to donors, and 8,000 audit reports just for multilateral development banks.
>
> (Health Poverty Action 2012)

Yet as far back as 2002, Danish aid workers were warning that Tanzania had just ten people in the whole country capable of dealing with the various international initiatives 'that are thrown at the country' (Muraskin 2004). It's not just paper work, either. An OECD report from 2008 highlighted the problems posed by 14,000 separate donor missions visiting 54 recipient countries in a single year, 'with Vietnam fielding an average of three per day' (McCoy et al. 2009: 415).

To make matters worse, many of the organisations clearly reflect the values and ideological aspirations of their leading donors, especially where these in turn are governments or big for-profit corporations. As a result, there is a tendency to focus on a few high-profile diseases to be treated according to medical models, and dramatic interventions through 'vertical programs' and costly drugs, or to rely on efforts to stimulate private-sector provision (which may or may not be affordable to the target population), rather than build a sustainable infrastructure of Alma Ata-style primary health care or invest in the longer-term training of doctors, nurses and other professionals to meet the gap in the global health workforce estimated by the WHO in 2006 at 2.4 million. Some organisations are based on an assumption that experts thousands of miles away know better what should be done in developing countries than health professionals on the ground (Muraskin 2004).

Even much of the training delivered by the Global Fund, GAVI and World Bank projects turns out to be short-term, in-service training of limited long-term value. There is little consideration of the longer-term sustainability of projects after the external projects are concluded: the Global Fund Round 10 guidelines failed to make any reference to sustainability in the evaluation criteria for bids (Vujicic et al. 2011). Concerns have been raised even by World Bank researchers that the proliferation of vertical programs could perversely result in disrupting and weakening local health-care systems rather than strengthening them, attracting local health professionals away to higher pay and new career options (Gottret and Schieber 2006: 135).

Development banks

The World Bank's favoured package of market-style health-system reforms is echoed on a very much smaller scale by the regional banks like the Asian Development Bank (ADB) and the Inter-American Development Bank (IDB). The IDB has in the past specifically endorsed a principle of fee-for-service payment for health care funded through its loans (IDB 1994) and a search of its lengthy statement on Public Health on its main website still yields no mention of 'equity' but a restatement of the principle that fees should be charged:

> Wherever possible a fee for services rendered principle should be applied. It is recognized, however, that in certain major instances, especially in the application of widespread measures for the control of diseases, the cost of such programs can be recaptured only through the general power of taxation. In those instances, however, in which services are rendered to income groups capable of payment, 'user' fees should be established.
>
> (IDB 2012)

The IDB's *Annual Report 2010* shows spending of $238 million in loans to five health projects out of a budget of $10.9 billion, so the priority attached to health issues at all is not great.

The Asian Development Bank (ADB) has stressed its commitment to expanding the private sector, although it has had false starts and mixed fortunes with experiments in Mongolia (Ulrich and Jigidsuren 2002). Its website states that health projects accounted for just 0.2 per cent of its loans in 2011, and again, clearly the main focus is on other issues.

USAID

A more significant global force in market-oriented economic reform has been the US Agency for International Development (USAID), which reported a budget of almost $6.5 billion for health development projects in 2011–12, up from $1.5 billion in 2003 (Michaud 2003).

Since its establishment as a subdivision of the State Department in 1961 – in the midst of the Cold War – USAID has been explicitly tied to the US administration of the day and its foreign policy objectives. Its *Strategy Document* (2004–9) proclaims as a core principle USAID's 'Loyalty: Commitment to the United States and the American people'.[2] The organisation and the work it sponsors are not primarily concerned with health but in its health work, as in all its policies, USAID demonstrates a consistent bias towards privatisation, economic liberalisation, private-sector involvement and socially conservative policies (Ollila 2005, USAID 2003a, 2003b). In the Philippines, a June 2005 USAID document stated that 'USAID is developing the private sector as an alternative source of health services.'

USAID's strong focus on privatisation can chime in with the pro-market inclinations of repressive and dictatorial governments: in Egypt prior to the dramatic Arab Spring upheavals that ousted President Mubarak, USAID played a key role in encouraging the regime's highly controversial drive to privatisation of health providers:

---

2 A major USAID policy document in 2002 is boldly titled 'Foreign Aid in the National Interest'.

> USAID has called for the implementation of so-called 'cost-recovery' mecha-
> nisms, a euphemism for transforming public health care and education into
> private, fee-based institutions. Indeed, USAID has spent nearly half of its health
> and education budgets – more than $100m per year – on privatisation measures.
>
> (Hickel 2011)

More recently USAID has launched the flagship SHOPS (Strengthening Health
Outcomes through the Private Sector) project to promote private-sector involvement in a variety of health-related projects in some of the world's poorest countries.
Among its initiatives was a joint project with the International Finance Corporation
to stage a jamboree of promotion for the private sector in Nigeria (SHOPS 2012).

USAID funding has underwritten projects and services, but also research and
consultancy work in many developing countries, much of it carried out via such
organisations as Abt Associates, which heads up the SHOPS project. This can cause
annoyance, such as resentment at the way in which USAID has been seen in Africa
as using much of its budget to pay consultants, mostly from the USA, instead of on
delivering treatment programs (Freeman and Boynton 2011).

Consultancies

Many of these consultancies are undertaken by private, for-profit firms which advise
on health-system reforms compatible with the US system and interests. On a worldwide scale, consultancy firms such as McKinsey also promote the drive towards
more private-sector and market-style policies, as indeed do the large-scale corporations involved in health care – the drug companies, US and other insurers and
private hospital chains and corporations such as South Africa's Netcare.

Much of the research and consultancy work procured by USAID is carried out
by Abt Associates Inc., one of the largest for-profit consultancies in the US. Abt
received a $42 million contract from USAID to supervise the reconstruction of
health-care services in Iraq from 2003 to 2004. However, this involved the imposition of a new system and structure much more akin to those of the US. During
that process, Abt convened meetings to agree on a policy document 'Iraq Healthy
and Free' which focused on breaking from Iraq's pre-invasion model of centralised, state-funded service that (prior to the prolonged UN sanctions) had once been
one of the best health systems in the Middle East (Library of Congress 2006).
The new 'Tenets for the Ministry of Health', published on the Internet, introduced
co-payments (with few exemptions), competition, provider autonomy, 'patient
choice' and the use of public funds to commission private-sector organisations. The
meetings to discuss the policy were reportedly attended by just 150 people in total
(Abt Associates 2003a, 2003b), so whether the proposals reflect any of the aspirations of Iraqi people is as yet unknown.

USAID also works with Abt and other consultancies through a variety of apparently wider formations in which generous funding for research and strong prospects
for publication draw in willing academics and researchers, such as the Data for
Decision Making Project, the Health Financing and Sustainability (HFS) Project,

Partnerships for Health Reform (PHR and PHRplus) and Management Sciences for Health (MSH). These generate academic papers, conferences, projects and debates which generally reflect USAID's underlying ideological assumptions and bias towards the private sector.

DFID

The British equivalent to USAID is the Department for International Development (DFID), which also has a network of academics drawn towards its considerable budget for commissioning research and sponsoring consultancy and projects, including the avid pro-market 'think tank', Adam Smith International (Corporate Watch 2005). It is accused by critics of spending a large share of its budget promoting privatisation (Monbiot 2004) and buying services from British-based companies (Provost 2012). As a result of this approach, DFID has been one of the international organisations accused in the past of attaching conditionality to the loans and assistance it gives to developing countries (Hilary 2005) and of evading, for many years, taking a clear policy line on user fees (Hutton 2004).

Even now, the doubt persists. In 2005, the British government issued a policy paper which focused on 'partnership' with governments in developing countries rather than conditionality. It pointed in particular to the pressures that had been put on developing countries to adopt policies of privatisation, often with embarrassing results for all involved with the policy (DFID 2005: 6).[3] The document also called for greater use of Poverty and Social Impact Analysis (PSIA) to anticipate and assess the likely intended and unintended consequences of policy changes. However, the problem was not entirely resolved by the new emphasis on 'partnership', which requires both donors and country governments to 'agree the purpose for which aid is given' (2005: 8) when the power relations between donor and country government are profoundly unequal. Nonetheless, in 2006 the British government did go as far as to threaten to withhold its contributions to the World Bank if it maintained its rigorous conditions of liberalisation and privatisation (Elliott 2006).

UK government policy developed at this time also discussed measures to ensure that money is spent in ways which do not jeopardise human rights, and which strengthen financial management and combat corruption. While the underlying intentions may be laudable, here too it seems that the conditionality of previous negotiations is simply translated into the less confrontational language of 'partnership'. A critique of the new policy commissioned by DFID from consultants Mokoro Ltd. found that neither the new conditions for accessing aid nor the milestones that countries are expected to reach were clearly enough defined. It also raised real doubts over the procedure where countries are perceived to have fallen short of a 'partnership deal' midway through a project (Mokoro 2005).

---

3   Interestingly, DFID itself was challenged in 2004 by members of Parliament over its 'privatisation' of its own research and consultancy work, handing over contracts for the conduct of projects worth a total of almost £38 million to the free-market neoliberals of the Adam Smith Institute.

Other development agencies

Both the UK and US seek to use economic levers in their control of aid policies to achieve policy change. This is different from equivalent programs from other countries. For example, Australia made only the most fleeting reference to the possible use of private providers in its 1998 document on health aid (Downer 1998) and continued to place little emphasis on this aspect of health reform (Barraclough 2005, AusAID 2006).

Denmark's government aid agency, Danida, explicitly criticised the impact of user fees (Danida 2005: 27). In an extensive document, the Danish agency accepted the need to encourage human rights but made no suggestion of conditionality or other political preconditions for the aid program (Danida 2003). A 2005 strategy paper on the fight against HIV/AIDS explicitly discusses in detail Denmark's eagerness to influence final outcomes, but never goes further than 'co-funding important programmes and participating actively in government-donor fora' (Tornaes 2005: 6). The programs for young people significantly make no US-style reference to religious calls for sexual 'abstinence' and the Danish definition of the 'private sector' is an extended one that includes trade unions.

Germany's equivalent organisation, the Deutsche Gesellschaft für Technische Zusammenarbeit (GTZ GmbH – the German Agency for Technical Cooperation), also follows a markedly different agenda from that of USAID. A major international conference it jointly organised in Berlin with the International Labour Organization (ILO) and the WHO was centred on the theme of social health insurance in developing countries. A central focus of the conference was on establishing universal coverage and solidarity-based financing schemes. The GTZ included a critique of the negative impacts of policies based on the Washington Consensus. The GTZ guidelines submitted to the conference stress the principles of 'universality, solidarity, social responsibility, subsidiarity, independent administration and pluralism, negotiation and consensus-building' (Schwefel et al. 2005: 6).

Emerging country donors

Other countries are beginning to play a role in funding and therefore potentially shaping health services in developing countries.

The biggest new player among these could even be India, which after decades as a recipient of international aid, in July 2011, announced the intent to establish its own aid agency, the Indian Agency for Partnership in Development (IAPD), overseeing $11.3 billion over the next five to seven years. It is not clear what proportion of this will be focused on health (*Economist* 2011a).

The new IAPD makes no secret of modelling itself and its strategy on USAID and of seeking to further Indian interests; but it has also served to highlight the contradictions of a country with massive unresolved health issues for its colossal poor population that is home simultaneously to a third of the world's malnourished children and to some of the world's richest men. The government has reserves of $300 billion (Basu 2011) and yet spends a minimal amount of its budget on health care. India's own government machine is so inadequate and places such low priority on the needs of its poorest citizens that, as the IAPD aid programme was unveiled, a staggering $22.6 billion of foreign aid to India was lying unused (Patel 2011).

It is this political weakness rather than any lack of potential resources that fuel doubts over the optimistic pronouncement by Nalini Saligram that 'Together the US and India have what it takes to tackle NCDs (Non Communicable Diseases)' (Saligram 2012). In neither country is there any lack of wealth, but in both a chronically dysfunctional political machine and health-care system make it very difficult to imagine coherent and coordinated policies emerging.

China

There is no clear consensus on the level of China's foreign aid, but most agree that it has grown – possibly by up to 30 per cent a year between 2004 and 2009. USAID suggests that, in total, China spent $38.54 billion in foreign assistance from 1950 to 2009, roughly the same amount the United States provided in 2010: 40 per cent through grants, the remainder as interest-free and concessional loans (USAID 2011). However, Freeman and Boynton (2011) estimate China's aid in 2009 at $3.1 billion, almost half of this going to Africa, and most of the spending focused on infrastructure rather than health: the *Economist* (2011a) quotes an official figure of $1.9 billion in 2009 (about level with Australia and Belgium).

China faces some of the same internal contradictions as India, with a still-low average gross national income, growing inequalities, problems with both infectious disease and with chronic diseases, and unresolved issues of access to health care for many on low incomes with minimal government investment in health care. However, despite this, and possibly with an eye to Africa's mineral wealth, China has focused its health effort in Africa since 2006 on building hospitals and clinics, training doctors, nurses and managers, and supplying medical equipment and anti-malaria materials. Chinese medical teams are now present in 40 African countries (Freeman and Boynton 2011).

Nor does the Chinese involvement have anything in common with the Maoist approach of equality, universalism and preventive health. Instead, in the 1990s China's projects in Africa echoed the World Bank's emphasis on charging fees for treatments and developing jointly run hospitals with the business sector (Huang 2011).

Even the funding level is far from generous. If the lower estimate of China's aid budget is accurate, it is eclipsed by that of Brazil, which has also been thinking about setting up its own aid agency and gives up to $4 billion per year (*Economist* 2011a).

Russia

There is similar debate over the actual aid spending of Russia: USAID (2011) argues that the Russian government spent 'more than $80 million' on global health programs in developing nations in 2010, mostly channelled through multilateral organisations. The *Economist* (2011a) has a much higher official finance ministry figure, suggesting an 'average of $422 million a year between 2007 and 2010'.

A remarkably vague analysis from the US Center for Strategic and International Studies fails to make the case for 'Russia's emerging global health leadership', although it does point out the ongoing health problems that beset much of the Russian population, which has one of the world's highest burdens of disease (Twigg 2012).

The big non-governmental donors

Global Fund

Launched in 2002, after decisions made at the 2000 G8 summit, the Global Fund has so far raised a total of $28.3 billion in pledges from the public sector, to be paid by 2015 (with 54 contributing governments), and another $1.6 billion (5 per cent) from the private sector and other initiatives. Up to 2012, $17.2 billion has been paid, the largest contributor being the United States, followed by France, Japan, Germany and the United Kingdom (Global Fund 2012).

Even these large sums of money fell well short of the goals that had initially been set:

> To bring all of sub-Saharan Africa up to the per capita spending of South Africa on health would require an annual expenditure of $72 billion, compared with total current government and donor funding of just $8.5 billion.
>
> (England 2004)[4]

One of the main arguments for a new fund to drive the fight to combat AIDS, TB and malaria was that the World Bank formula of extending loans was not delivering results:

> international assistance must be based on grants, not loans, for the poorest countries and be increased within the next 3 years to a minimum of $7.5 billion or more.
>
> (Attaran and Sachs 2001)

Despite this clear call for a change, for the first five years the Global Fund was headed by Richard Feachem (Donnelly 2002), a keen advocate of engagement with the private sector, who had formerly been in charge of the Health Nutrition and Population directorate of the World Bank, and had served as a Brundtland appointee as editor of the *Bulletin of the World Health Organization* in the period of Bank dominance (see above, Chapter 3).

---

4   In 2003, the Commission on Macroeconomics and Health confidently predicted that 'Assistance from developed nations should increase from the current levels of about US$ 6 billion per year globally to US$ 27 billion by 2007 and US$ 38 billion by 2015' (Global Fund website).

The Global Fund has remained more likely than the World Bank, and four times more likely than GAVI, to pay for health workers in the private sector (Vujicic et al. 2011). The Fund has also run into the generic problem of international projects setting up teams in developing countries with widespread poverty and low wages for health workers. With their generous funding and higher pay scales, Global Fund projects have been seen as potentially enticing vital health workers away from maternal and child health programs in Cambodia and, in Kyrgyszstan, drawing them into work on HIV, TB and malaria at the expense of other health care (Vujicic et al. 2011: 12) – a problem highlighted previously by Pfeiffer (2004).

However, the Fund has been hard hit by the global economic crisis following the banking crash of 2008. In May 2011, the Fund warned that it was short by \$1.3 billion of the amount needed to cover even minimum needs for 2011 through 2013. To make matters worse, revelations that \$25 million had been reported to be missing from community programs in four nations in Africa led to Sweden and Germany suspending their donations until an audit was completed, which in turn forced a pause in the Fund's operations (Hood 2011).

The change of General Manager has ushered in some fresh approaches, including the creation of a new Division for 'Strategic investment and Impact Evaluation' intended to shape investments 'by country and disease', in place of the previous 'one size fits all' approach, and new committees to monitor progress on each disease (AIDS, TB and malaria) (Fan 2012b).

The GAVI Alliance (formerly the Global Alliance for Vaccines and Immunisation)

The GAVI Alliance began in 1999 as a coalition of international health agencies, along with private industry, bilateral donors, philanthropic foundations and others. From the beginning, this alliance has marginalised the UN agencies, prioritising the private-sector partners (Ollila 2005) and leaving out the in-country fieldworkers from UN agencies and NGOs and governments in the target countries. As Muraskin argues, 'its vision came from leaders who were inadequately informed regarding fieldworkers' opinions about what could realistically be accomplished within a relatively short space of time.' Even governments of the target countries were left out of the frame: it was designed from the beginning '*for* the countries' good but not *by* the countries' (Muraskin 2004: 1,923).

As the name suggests, the organisation began with a single-minded focus on the issue of vaccination and immunisation which it has, at least until recently, retained. The GAVI sees this as the number one and indispensable route to improving health in developing countries.

Such an approach clearly has some strengths in focusing attention on diseases that can be prevented, but it also has the potential weakness of ignoring other crucial aspects of the development of sustainable health-care systems and primary health care, relating to the sensitivities and realities of different countries, their culture, concerns and priorities (Muraskin 2004).

The limitations of vaccination alone as a way to improve child health are underlined by performance figures for 2006:

2006 data, the most recent available, show a paradoxical relationship between GAVI funding in Africa and child mortality. Overall, child mortality improved more often in nations that received smaller than average GAVI grants per capita. In seven nations that received greater than average funding, child mortality rates worsened.

(Piller and Smith 2007)

Muraskin emphasises the lack of consensus behind the policy of vaccination as the single top priority for health systems in developing countries: neither field workers nor governments necessarily share the GAVI Alliance's view on this. Cochi too points to problems, not least 'competing health priorities, poor health system management, and inadequate monitoring and supervision':

The reasons for under vaccination and non-vaccination are multifaceted and often complex, and it is the most vulnerable populations in the low performing, low- and lower-middle income [LMIC] countries that are not receiving immunization services.

(Cochi 2012: 3)

Another flaw seen in the GAVI Alliance is its failure to achieve a balance between 'top-down' and 'bottom-up' relationships in its efforts to build projects in particular countries. And while some of the tensions that may result with governments and with health-care workers in the recipient countries can be eased by the availability of large sums of donor funding, many cannot (Muraskin 2004).

Cochi (2012: 4) argues that the GAVI proposal for an $800 million project for 'health systems strengthening' had 'poorly defined objectives, vague and ineffective links between investments and measurably improved vaccination results, and little in the way of tangible outcomes; it provides a cautionary example of what not to do.' The Alliance has now apparently agreed to devote 15–25% of its program resources to strengthening country-level health systems: hopefully, this will be done in conjunction with governments and with field workers on the ground.

In June 2011, the GAVI Alliance announced that it had overcome serious problems in raising sufficient resources and had successfully secured additional donor commitments of $4.3 billion to finance its work through to 2015, bringing its total resources to $7.6 billion (Cochi 2012).

However, there is a serious problem: GAVI support is only available to the low-income countries while the majority of unvaccinated and under-vaccinated children in the world will soon live in lower-middle-income countries (LMIC), which do not even qualify for the reduced prices that GAVI has been able to negotiate for the new and more expensive vaccines: these too are exclusively available to low-income countries. The cost of new vaccines is the largest cost driver for health services in low- and middle-income countries, making affordability a major issue for the future (Cochi 2012).

PEPFAR

In 2001, the Bush administration was apparently disconcerted to find the UN campaigning to raise $7 billion annually simply to fight AIDS in Africa, while the US had pledged just $200 million. As a *Time* magazine commentary at the time noted, 'To a problem that will kill more than 2 million Africans this year... the US contributed the annual budget of a Midwestern hospital' (Ramo 2001).

In response, Bush initiated the President's Emergency Plan for AIDS Relief (PEPFAR) with bipartisan support in 2003: funding through PEPFAR has risen since 2004 from $2.3 billion to $6.6 billion in 2012. Its website reports that, in fiscal year 2011, PEPFAR directly supported life-saving antiretroviral treatment for more than 3.9 million men, women and children worldwide; supported antiretroviral prophylaxis to prevent mother-to-child HIV transmission for more than 660,000 HIV-positive pregnant women; and three partnerships in more than 80 countries directly provided 13 million people with care and support, including nearly 4.1 million orphans and vulnerable children.

However, funding for 2013 is set to fall to $6.4 billion, having passed the peak of almost $6.9 billion in 2010. Up to 2012, 80 per cent of PEPFAR funding was directed through bilateral HIV and AIDS programs, 15 per cent through the Global Fund and 3 per cent through bilateral programs on tuberculosis (PEPFAR 2012a).

Among the bilateral arrangements are partnership frameworks in countries including Angola, Zambia, and Nigeria (where increased funding for public health care runs alongside collaboration with the private sector as the preferred way to reach primary-health-care clinics in hard-to-reach areas) (PEPFAR 2012b).

Interestingly PEPFAR appears to be more committed than some other funding agencies to the development of health systems and public health resources in partner countries: in Tanzania, the Global Fund acts as the purchaser of drugs while PEPFAR programs support test kits, training and the delivery of antiretroviral treatment to patients. In Namibia, PEPFAR and the US government have been working with the Ministry of health and social services to develop a transitional plan to ensure that health-care workers engaged in HIV/AIDS work are transferred to the public payroll (PEPFAR 2012b).

Under the Obama administration the focus has remained on strengthening health systems: a recent speech by Secretary of State Hillary Clinton emphasised the importance of improved health systems in reducing maternal mortality in China, Sri Lanka and Malaysia and stressed that when Zimbabwe's system began to crumble 'its maternal mortality rates shot up dramatically'.

She also focused on the challenge of integrating US efforts into coherent programs, learning form the mistakes at the beginning when PEPFAR set up a parallel network of clinics that were separately managed and paid for:

> We are trying to integrate our programs. And under our global health initiative each of our country teams now assessed how they fit within a comprehensive vision and program, based upon a health plan established by the country where

we are operating. And we have work with partners to develop these health plans in more than 40 countries.

(Clinton 2012)

However, it's clear that beneath this more collaborative and overtly public-sector focus, the private sector remains central to PEPFAR and is seen as 'contributing skills and results-based market-driven approaches'. In countries such as Namibia and Uganda, PEPFAR is promoting the notion of so-called 'low-cost private health insurance' (PEPFAR 2012b).

The Gates Foundation

The Bill & Melinda Gates Foundation, set up in 1994, has become a major player in the development of health-care programs for developing countries. Boosted by Warren Buffett's hefty $31 billion donation in 2006, and further multi-billion-dollar donations, almost 60 per cent of its spending has been allocated to global health projects.

While these very large donations from some of the world's wealthiest people are of course a positive development, opening up real possibilities for progress on various fronts, they take place in the context of a widening gulf between rich and poor on a global scale. So it does read rather strangely to see statements from multi-billionaire Bill Gates arguing that 'equity is the end goal' and that spending relatively small amounts of money to overcome the need for aid can 'continue writing the story of a steadily more equitable world' (Gates Foundation 2012c).

Far from being more equitable, critics have pointed out that some of the intended low-income beneficiaries of the Gates Foundation have actually suffered as a result of some of the activities of multinational corporations in which foundation money is invested. The Foundation has been split between those working on the front-line projects and those in a separate division handling the investment portfolio. Just 5 per cent of the total wealth of the Foundation is spent each year, while very much larger sums from the remaining 95 per cent are invested in search of profits to make the fund grow year by year. The ethical values applied in deciding these investments are not those of charity but those of big business, seeking maximum return regardless of the consequences.

Unsavoury investments

The result has been some investments in unsavoury enterprises that are undermining the Foundation's efforts. In 2007, a series of articles by Charles Piller and colleagues in the *Los Angeles Times* (Piller et al. 2007, Piller and Smith 2007) focused attention on some of these questionable investments by the Gates foundation. These included investments in:

- Oil companies responsible for massive pollution with serious health impacts on the population in the Niger Delta, including the Italian oil giant Eni, Royal Dutch Shell,

Exxon Mobil Corporation, Chevron and the French oil firm, Total. The oil industry is also blamed for clogging rivers, triggering water-borne diseases. The well-paid oil workers and the military forces that protect them bring rising levels of prostitution, resulting in teenage pregnancies and the spread of HIV (Piller et al. 2007).

- Sixty-nine of the worst polluting companies in the US (Democracy Now 2007).
- The big pharma companies whose unaffordable prices in developing countries are one of the main issues the charitable side of the Foundation seeks to address (Democracy Now 2007).
- Companies whose practices are in conflict with the Foundation's own charitable goals, including companies accused of forcing people to lose their homes, some using child labour and even some alleged to have neglected patients and defrauded people needing health care. Piller estimates that the Foundation has a total of up to $9 billion invested in such companies (Democracy Now 2007).

In 2010, a Seattle-based website criticised the Gates Foundation for increasing its investment in one of the corporations most notorious for promoting genetic modification, Monsanto (Vidal 2010). His Foundation's investments in global agribusiness corporation Cargill also stand in contradiction to Gates' professed wish to help 'poor farmers grow more food' and achieve 'self-sufficiency and overcome the need for aid' (Gates Foundation 2012c).

Other criticisms of the Gates approach focus on the limitations of the Foundation's fixed focus on vaccination and medical science to tackle specific diseases and failure to put resources into building up basic health-care systems. The issues raised include:

- That resources in many country programs are restricted to delivery of treatment against HIV/AIDS and do not cover basic equipment and infrastructure
- That the focus on advanced technology and recruiting professionals to deliver AIDS projects on higher rates of pay than other health workers can lure scarce professionals away from existing health-care systems, leaving crucial gaps in care
- That the vaccination on its own, without improving nutrition, without ensuring that transport is available for the poorest to access the services, can be ineffective: vaccinated children can die of hunger before even being at serious risk of diseases like hepatitis B, and health patients in Lesotho and Rolanda have described hunger so severe that they are unable to keep anti-AIDS pills down without vomiting.

(Piller and Smith 2007)

Botswana flop

Critics of the Gates approach cite the example of Botswana which, in 2000, the Gates Foundation and the drug firm Merck & Co. chose as a test case for a $100-million joint effort to prove that mass AIDS treatment and prevention could succeed in Africa. Deaths from AIDS fell sharply but AIDS prevention largely failed, despite a massive boost to health spending (by 2005 Botswana's health expenditure per capita, boosted by the Gates donations, was six times the average for Africa and 21 times the amount spent in Rwanda). The single focus on AIDS diverted attention and resources from other key health issues – including other MDGs: Botswana's rate of pregnancy-related maternal deaths nearly quadrupled and the child mortality rate rose dramatically in the same period of increased, but narrowly targeted health spending. Despite improvements in AIDS treatment, life expectancy in Botswana rose just marginally, from 41.1 years in 2000 to 41.5 years in 2005 (Piller and Smith 2007).

Indeed, just as the GAVI Alliance centres on an inflexible insistence that vaccination and immunisation is the one and only priority for health care in developing countries, and just as GAVI is driven from above by people with an inadequate understanding of the complexity and problems of implementing programs, the Gates Foundation formula centres very strongly on the medical model and makes little reference to the development of sustainable health-care systems or an infrastructure of primary health care. This weakness is reinforced by its first guiding principle, that 'This is a family foundation driven by the interests and passions of the Gates family' (Gates 2012). So there is little scope for broadening or varying the approach, and no democratic control over the Foundation at the top or in its programs around the world: big money calls the shots and the big money is still in the hands of a wealthy elite.

The sheer scale of the Gates Foundation resources (and its obligation to spend at least $1.5 billion each year in order to stay within the law as a charitable foundation) has led the *Economist* to brand it as an example of 'philanthrocapitalism' (*Economist* 2006). It points out the 'need for philanthropy to become more like the for-profit capitalist markets' and that today's mega-philanthropists 'need to behave more like investors':

> Mr Gates's big idea is to overcome the market failure afflicting poor consumers of healthcare by deploying his money on behalf of the poor to generate the supply of drugs and treatments they need. For instance, the money provides market incentives for drug companies to put some of their resources to work for the needy.

As such, the Gates Foundation has become a key partner for the big pharmaceutical corporations, which may well engage with charitable projects when it suits them, but always with their own distinct agenda: they are eager to establish favourable credentials and to retain their control of the development of new drug technology on a global scale.

Neglected diseases

This was illustrated in January 2012 when the Gates Foundation brought together the heads of 13 of the world's biggest drug companies in a project to tackle 10 of the many neglected tropical diseases that take a savage toll on hundreds of millions of people in some of the world's poorest countries (Boseley 2012a, Gates Foundation 2012a). Alongside a $363 million contribution from the Gates Foundation, the World Bank, USAID and the United Arab Emirates also put in cash and the 13 drug companies promised to donate an average of 1.4 billion treatments each year to those in need.

Among the companies getting positive headlines for the donations were Glaxo-SmithKline (which has just been fined a record $3 billion for the 'biggest healthcare fraud in US history' (Reuters 2012)), Astra Zeneca, Johnson & Johnson, Merck, Pfizer, Novartis and Sanofi. In some cases, there is a debate about the appropriateness of the drugs they are donating; in others, there are questions about the conditions under which they are donated or the real value of the donations.

The very principle of big pharma donations of drugs, however, is not uncontroversial, nor is it without its disadvantages – not least because the apparent generosity of wealthy corporations in donating drugs with ostensibly high market prices is not matched by any comparable donation of cash to assist in making use of them in the target countries. All of the costs of developing health-care systems therefore fall on low-income countries and other donors (Guilloux and Moon 2002).

Civil society organisations have repeatedly opposed drug donations to the Global Fund, arguing that they distort market incentives and have an adverse effect of therapeutic options. Large-scale donations of branded drugs can effectively block the development of potentially cheaper generic drugs by reducing the potential market for sales – since no company can compete against a free product (Baker and Ombaka 2009).

The impact on the development of generic drugs is especially important given the likely transition of a number of the countries currently defined as low income into lower-middle-income countries, a status which means that they will no longer be eligible to receive donated drugs, while they will not be able to afford the full price of the branded product. Industry forecasts suggest that the global market for prescription drugs is set to expand by $250 billion to $1.2 trillion a year by 2016, but predict that the bulk of this growth will be in generic drugs while the big pharmaceutical companies face reduced prospects for growth (Herper 2012). In this context, a strategic investment in donating drugs that can secure potential markets in developing countries – and prevent the emergence of potential rivals – could turn out to be a shrewd business move.

However, there are obvious contradictions and the motives are by no means necessarily all cynical – lives are potentially at stake: so while opposing all in-kind donations by drug companies, Baker and Ombaka also recognise the pressure on developing countries where many people with AIDS are still waiting for treatment to accept free products that would enable them to be treated straight away. But large-scale donations of drugs can also tie government treatment choices to particular so-called free drugs, thus delaying or undermining government motivation to select modified treatment guidelines.

From the company's point of view, this means donations of free products can result not only in product familiarity but even in the development of brand loyalty, influencing prescribers against later turning to generic equivalents or even to superior generic products. They can also enable corporations to enhance or even regain corporate goodwill through favourable publicity whilst at the same time obtaining tax advantages (Baker and Ombaka 2009).

Disease-specific donations

Other concerns centre on the implications of *disease-specific* donations of drugs by the pharma corporations. One problem is the geographical restriction of where the drug donations are available and which other developing countries are still required to pay the market price, even as it is supplied free of charge to people only slightly poorer elsewhere.

Some drugs are donated with a specific restriction that they must only be used for particular diseases and not for others, even where they can be effective: one example is Pfizer's Zithromax, which was donated for treatment of trachoma only, but can also be used to treat sexually transmitted diseases or acute respiratory infection (Guilloux and Moon 2002).

Time restrictions on drug donations raise the problem of how cash-strapped governments are expected to pick up the bill for what are still costly drugs once the donation program comes to an end. Critics also point to the upward pressure on costs (and the potentially harmful impact on longer-term health strategies) implicit in using some more sophisticated donated drugs when a less-advanced drug would be more appropriate:

> For example if the doctor has no first-line antibiotic available, but there is a donated third-generation antibiotic sitting on the shelf, rational drug use is very likely to be ignored. The wisdom of Glaxo Wellcome's donation of malarone – a second or third line treatment for drug-resistant malaria in sub-Saharan Africa – has been questioned with regard to resistance prevention.
>
> (Guilloux and Moon 2002: 192)

In-kind donations of drugs also obscure discussion of the actual value of the donation, since the marginal cost of production of the donated stock (a closely guarded secret) is clearly much, much less than the overt resale value of the drug at full price: Guilloux and Moon estimate that the marginal cost of production ranges from as little as one per cent to five per cent of the fair market value of a proprietary drug. Drug companies can also claim tax deductions on the basis of their donations, based on the cost of the goods, although not all do so.

The underlying issue is that 'companies may have motivations other than philanthropic ones for donating products including: improving public image, protecting patents, or responding to public pressure.' Drug donation programs cannot be considered a solution to the global access crisis (Guilloux and Moon 2002).

Another Gates Foundation initiative involves support for the Affordable Medicines Facility – malaria (AMFm), a scheme to subsidise the purchase of new antimalarial drugs in both public and private sectors. The starting point is that poor people cannot afford the new, highly effective artemisinin-based combination therapies (ACTs): unaffordable prices increase the risk that people will continue to use ineffective drugs against malaria or the slightly cheaper forms of artemisinin which are more likely to result in drug-resistant forms of malaria.

But if the objective is to maximise access to ACTs, it is difficult to see why the project is aimed only to deliver a 'high level subsidy' rather than to supply artemisinin free of charge to those who need it. The AMFm argues that an up-front co-payment by the project would 'ensure a stable demand for ACTs, encourage suppliers to invest in scaled up production of raw materials and lower the price of ACTs.' (Phumaphi 2009: 5)

But to make the drug available without charge would guarantee an even wider use of the drug and presumably allow even bigger economies of scale. The subsidised retail price of $0.10–$0.50 sounds eminently reasonable from a distance but could still prove unaffordable in practice for some patients in countries where the average income is below $0.50 per day. Strangely, the document actually discusses the problem that the program may benefit some who are 'not the very poorest':

> the policymaker needs to distinguish between absolute and relative poverty; people living on US $1 may be better off than those living on US $0.50 per day, but it is hardly sensible to try to exclude the former from the benefits of the AMFm.
>
> (Phumaphi 2009: 11)

This laborious attempt to distinguish between the poor and the ultra-poor seems especially bizarre in a paper for a project funded by one of the world's richest men, spending over $1.4 billion on this one project subsidising the purchase of drugs from one of the world's most profitable industrial sectors, the pharmaceutical industry.

This is a reminder that the capitalist system not only creates inequality and thrives on it, it distorts even charitable attempts to tackle the sharpest evidence of inequality. In a neoliberal world, charity, which taps into the decent instincts of countless millions the world over – and even billionaires – now needs to be planned around the vested interests of the big players: big Pharma, the insurance companies and profit-seeking consultancies. The Gates Foundation sets out not to supersede or supplant the market, but to preserve it: to 'overcome market failures' and to use market incentives to enlist the engagement of big pharma. In other words, the Foundation, no matter what its initial motivation, becomes another part of the ecology of the global marketplace, prolonging and embellishing the unequal system that generates the very problems it seeks to address.

In a capitalist system, donations are not what they seem – and even relieving the poverty of the poorest in the world can be exploited by some as a route to profits.

The policy-making elite

The system we have been discussing and the institutions shaping policies clearly need constant ideological reinforcement and some form of academic legitimacy; and, as always, the intellectuals are ready to follow the patron. In an increasingly austere and competitive environment, academics are drawn inexorably towards funding sources, finding more and varied ways to adapt their studies and their analysis to fit with the prevailing prejudices and nostrums of the funding bodies.

With big players like the World Bank, USAID, the Gates Foundation and others potentially keen to see research findings that support their policy initiatives, and hundreds of millions of dollars available to sponsor academic inquiry, it can hardly be surprising that the mainstream of academia has been so accommodating to market-style reforms and other policies, despite the lack of supporting evidence and the mounting evidence suggesting this is the wrong path for health reform.

Many of the most influential academics in the sphere of health policy and health economics are attached to universities and institutes in the richest G7 countries, especially the US and the UK. They constitute the core of a small and 'tightly integrated network of policy-makers, technical advisors and scholars' who have largely shaped and driven the policy reforms promoted by global bodies (Lee and Goodman 2002). Lee and Goodman argue that a small policy elite, an 'epistemic community', has effectively been imposing its view with the backing of the ideological – but also considerable financial and economic – weight of the World Bank, the International Monetary Fund and the WHO:

> Analysis of policy changes over time suggests that the process of policy initiation and formulation has been largely top-down, developed and supported through the Washington and London hubs.
>
> (Lee and Goodman 2002: 116)

This analysis follows the established critique of Walt (1994), which charts the rising influence of the World Bank on health issues since the early 1980s, enhanced by the powers of patronage flowing from its generous research budget.

In Britain, a network collaborating with the WHO emerged around the London School of Economics and the London School of Hygiene and Tropical Medicine. In the US, the lead was taken by USAID, which brought in consultants John Snow Inc and Abt Associates. By the mid-1990s the World Bank had moved to centre stage, promoting the importance of health economics and effectively eclipsing the WHO, which employed just one health economist.

Stone (2001: 352) also refers to epistemic communities and notes the role of a transnational network of 'élite, technical and scientific cliques' that have been able to effect change in policy and policy agendas and become 'entrenched in bodies such as the IMF, WTO, OECD and World Bank'. The influence can also work in other ways. Many of the main architects of the WHO's controversial *WHR 2000* were former or current employees of the Bank, some also involved in drawing up the Bank's *WDR 1993: Investing in Health*. Indeed, in addition to Bank employees, among those drafting *WHR 2000* only two were from health ministries of member states, but others came from health insurance companies, universities, the OECD and private health organisations (Ollila and Koivusalo 2002).

Bank's consensus

The Bank has successfully networked on a global level to establish 'a consensus across different institutions and national settings defining the "problem" of health care financing reform and potential solutions' (Lee and Goodman 2002: 116); but the 'consensus' often reaches no further than the elite community of policy-shapers themselves. Even PAHO has voiced criticisms of how narrow a circle of key people has had any voice in the formation of health policy affecting millions:

> It is simply unacceptable for health policy to be researched and conducted in small, closed circles of consultants and policy-makers... It is in the very definition of good governance that people have a right to a meaningful say in the decisions that govern their lives.
>
> (PAHO et al. 2001, Foreword)

It would be a mistake to see all such problems as simply flowing from the World Bank and the IMF. Market-style policies and ideological pressures flow also from adaptation to the global market itself and the prevailing ideas and policy frameworks elsewhere in the market system.

Seeking to re-enter the global market system, the Chinese government opted to implement policies, including privatisation of health care and user fees, without facing any explicit pressure from the Bank or IMF. The same is also true of South Africa. Other governments (such as Sri Lanka, Ghana, Thailand and Costa Rica) have withstood pressures and retained more progressive and equitable policies, delivering improved health outcomes for their population. Globalisation provides a context, but there is still a political choice in response.

Chapter six

The 'reform' agenda – market-driven (cost-cutting) reforms

There are many legitimate areas in which the right structural changes and an injection of sufficient resources could serve to enhance equity and access, accountability, professional skills, effectiveness and standards of treatment, and the empowerment of consumers. However, as this chapter will show, there is a serious mis-match between the objective problems faced by health-care systems and the policies put forward as solutions by the main groups and organisations proposing health-system reform.

The question arises: has the menu of policy prescriptions been formulated to meet the needs of the sick and the poor, or to maximise the profits of the rich and the private sector? This chapter works through the main 'menu' of the most commonly identified reforms, analysing the context in which they are being proposed and implemented, and discussing the evidence for success – or projections on their chances of success – in their proclaimed objectives. However, the evidence suggests that the reforms are driven not by concern for equity and efficiency, but by neoliberal values and the quest for profit.

The main elements of the reform agenda in the wealthier and poor countries can be categorised either as cost-saving ('market-driven') or as 'market-style' measures, although there are some which appear in different contexts under both headings.

Despite largely unsubstantiated claims that market-style reforms and private-sector involvement improve 'efficiency' (World Bank 2000, Fotaki and Boyd 2005, Maarse 2009a, Basu et al. 2012), cost-saving is at most a secondary consideration in market-style reforms, many of which are more expensive and less efficient than the systems they replace. It may therefore be deduced that market-style reforms are driven by ideological conviction rather than economic necessity and this overrides any questions arising from such reforms. The real questions should centre on their probable consequences – reshaping health-care systems around the principles of the market. For this reason, it is useful to differentiate between the two very different types of 'reform' if the underlying driving forces behind them are to be understood.

Overview: cost containment ('market-driven') reforms

As discussed above in Chapter 1, this study contends that market-*style* reforms involve attempts to restructure health-care systems to embody some or all of the features of a market (whether 'internal' within the public sector or, more commonly, a 'mixed economy' public–private market) in health services.

Market-*driven* (or *cost*-driven) reforms, on the other hand, date back long before the wave of market-style reforms and the nostrums of the New Public Management became fashionable in the 1990s:

> Cost containment has been driving health policy discussions in industrialised countries since the 1970s.
>
> (Mossialos et al. 2002: 1)

Market-*driven* reforms (in essence spending cuts, cost control) reflect the external pressures of the global market place and domestic capital on the government and the economy, and may include very basic measures designed to hold down corporate taxation by restricting expansion of the public sector – such as containing government spending on health-care services through imposing global cash limits or cutting public budgets for health care. There are many recent and ongoing examples as a result of the 2008 financial crash and the strains on the single currency in the European Union (McKee et al. 2012). As we have seen, this also dovetails neatly with the stock neoliberal policy agenda of 'small government' – and requiring individuals to cope without support from welfare or collective funds – so the two policies are by no means incompatible.

Most market-driven/cost-cutting reforms do not involve substantial restructuring of the health-care system. Services may be rationalised, rationed or restricted – leaving greater scope for private-sector provision – and subordinate elements of the service may be privatised in pursuit primarily of cost savings (regardless of quality): but the main driver is *cost* rather than *policy*. As a result, their organisational structure and the underlying funding system will generally remain unchanged (Collins et al. 1999), although very substantial erosion or pruning of public-sector support and intervention may eventually have the effect of changing the character of health provision, creating gaps which the private sector may profitably fill. In practice, the drive for market-style reforms can work most effectively if combined with moves to scale down public-sector provision, as happened in the controversial health-system reforms in England from 2010 (Lister 2012a).

The most dramatic and far-reaching market-driven changes are currently being implemented in Ireland, Iceland and Estonia – and more recently in Spain, Portugal and Greece – as a brutal continuation of the 2008 banking crisis,[1] and a raft of different measures have been introduced or attempted by other governments across Europe (Mladovsky et al. 2012, HOPE 2011). But however serious and long-lasting the damage done to health services and the health of the vulnerable population by these cutbacks, they do at least make no secret of being cash-driven and seeking

---

1   Cuts in government spending in Ireland reduced health spending by 7.6% in 2010, compared with an average yearly growth rate of 8.4% between 2000 and 2009. Health spending in Iceland fell by 7.5%, as part of a 9.3% reduction in public spending. In Estonia, both public and private spending on health fell: spending dropped by 7.3% in 2010. In Greece, total health spending fell by 6.5% in 2010 after a yearly growth rate averaging over 6% from 2000 (OECD 2012b).

first, foremost and solely to cut public spending to comply with the demands of the EU and the bankers for the so-called 'bail out' funds to repaid at the expense of the working class and the poor.

A contradiction of some market-driven policies is that by cutting public funding – or in many cases by seeking to squeeze the profits and force down the prices charged by the big pharmaceutical companies (Mladovsky et al. 2012) – they may restrict the potential development of the domestic market for health care and thus constrain the activities of private providers of health goods or services. Pharmaceutical companies in the USA, for example, normally strong advocates of neoliberal policies, have repeatedly lobbied Congress against legislation that would potentially achieve cost savings for Medicare and insurers of self-pay patients by opening up access to cheap imports of drugs currently sold at higher prices in the American market (McGregor 2003b). Their hugely expensive lobbying effort, which according to a report by the Center for Public Integrity, means that US Congressmen are outnumbered two to one by lobbyists for an industry that spends roughly $100 million a year in campaign contributions and lobbying expenses to protect its profits, has kept the cost of prescription drugs in the United States as the highest in the world (Singer 2007). In the US, at least the recession has also been good for health insurers, who have piled on profits because their policyholders have cut back on doctor visits because of tight finances and higher out-of-pocket costs such as co-payments (Stawicki 2012).

Market-driven policies involving substantial restrictions on government health spending have on occasion been forced upon some wealthier countries,[2] but in the past they were more frequently imposed upon developing countries (in various forms, including IMF Structural Adjustment Programmes). Now, interestingly, as Europe reels under the continued impact of the 2008 financial meltdown, with austerity cuts which undermine long-standing welfare provisions running alongside ideologically motivated 'reforms', the response to the financial pressures in many developing countries is the opposite. China, India, Indonesia and Philippines are among the major countries moving towards greater public spending to secure more equitable access to health services (*Economist* 2012). Mexico has responded to the downturn by a 10 per cent increase in spending on health and education. Low-income Sub-Saharan African countries, including those with IMF programmes, increased spending on health year by year from 2008 to 2010, and spending in 28 low-income countries was higher in 2010 than 2008. Other low- and middle-income countries to increase health funding were Honduras, Kenya, Peru, South Africa and Thailand (UNDESA 2011).

While the rhetoric employed by those politicians and managers who implement them at national and local level suggests that the focus of both market-driven and market-style reforms is the improvement of services and maximising their availability

---

2   Notably the British Labour government's 'IMF cuts', which resulted in cash limits on NHS spending from 1976: but also the more recent austerity policies in France and Germany designed to restrict spending on health, social security and pensions in order to keep the economy within the limits of the EU's 'Stability Pact' that underpins the single European currency. Latvia has had to take a World Bank loan to help get over the impact of the financial crash (HOPE 2011).

to the patient, some critics argue that the main underlying objective is the improvement of profitability and the expansion of market-opportunity for the private sector
(Vienonen et al. 1999).

The main elements of market-driven reforms are set out for clarity in the table
below, though experience has shown that while many countries are experimenting
with a number of these policies, until the full impact of the banking crisis hit Spain,
Portugal, Greece and Ireland, no governments embarking on health-system reforms
had been persuaded to implement all of these elements simultaneously.

> The reform agenda:
>
> Features of market-driven (cost-cutting) reforms
>> Cash limits
>> Rationalisation/bed cuts
>> Rationing and exclusions
>> Regulation of drug costs
>> User fees

An additional line of policy was advanced as justification for a further round of
rationalisation of hospitals and beds in the early 1990s in Britain: this was the notion
of substituting improved primary care services for hospital provision.

The myth of 'substitution'

The policy was always controversial and has frequently been opposed, not only
by hospital consultants but by some public health and primary care specialists
(Holland 2000, Edwards et al. 2000). Questions have been asked, especially over
the strong focus on reducing the numbers of accident and emergency departments
and attempting to divert as much as 60 per cent of their caseload to alternative
forms of treatment in primary care, community health services, so-called 'urgent
care centres' or similar, and self-care.[3] Perhaps the most stinging critique of the
assumptions underpinning these proposals came in *Primary Care and Emergency
Departments* by the Primary Care Foundation (Carson et al. 2010). The Foundation had been commissioned by the Department of Health with a specific brief to
'provide a viable estimate of the number of patients who attend emergency department with conditions that could be dealt with elsewhere in primary care' (ibid.: 4).
But it found that relatively few patients attending hospital accident and emergency
departments could be classified as needing only primary care – suggesting that NHS
London had drastically overstated the case for shifting work out of hospital A&E.
The 102-page report specifically took issue with 'widespread assumptions that up to
60% of patients could be diverted to GPs or primary care nurses' and argued that

---

3   Part of this focus can of course be explained by the steady and substantial year-on-year
    increases in the use of A&E services: but a starting point needs to be an understanding
    of why these increases are occurring and what weaknesses or gaps in other services are
    driving them.

the real figure is as low as 10–30 per cent (Carson et al. 2010: 5). The extensive study of patients in actual A&E departments also found no evidence that providing primary care in Emergency Departments 'could tackle rising costs or help to avoid unnecessary admissions.' The report authors argue that: 'Cost benefits may exist, but the evidence is weak' (Carson et al. 2010: 8).

The debate continues, animated once again above all by the perceived need to find ways to 'manage demand for secondary care' in order to reduce or contain costs (Edwards and Hensher 1998). In some cases this is attempted through the use of new 'referral management centres' (some of them run by private companies and many staffed by nurses and podiatrists rather than doctors) in order to reduce hospital referrals – at the expense of over-ruling patient 'choice' and GPs' clinical judgement (Duffin 2011, Davie 2011)

Even where the policy may be seen as increasing efficiency (cutting costs), questions have been raised over the impact on quality of care (Sibbald et al. 2007).

The planned reconfiguration of health services in London, as proposed in the 2007 report by Lord Darzi (Darzi 2007) and by a number of subsequent strategy documents covering the various areas of the city,[4] has pushed these issues back to the surface, with a concerted drive to reduce the numbers and size of hospitals. The Darzi plan, with its strong implications of private-sector involvement in funding and running a new network of 'polyclinics' (Beavers 2008) preceded the impact of the post-2008 austerity drive in the UK, which brought an end to ten successive years of increases in health spending, and seems set to hold spending down for anything up to 25 years (Appleby et al. 2009). But the drive towards downsizing and closing hospitals, not just in London but across the whole of England and in the devolved nations (Scotland and Wales, Northern Ireland) has been accelerated and exacerbated by the policy choices of the Conservative-led coalition government, which despite cynical pre-election promises to halt closures of A&E and maternity services, is driving through an unprecedented £20 billion in so called 'efficiency' savings over four years, alongside its market-style reorganisation of the NHS in a new, controversial Health & Social Care Act (DoH 2012, Lister 2012a).

Once the Bill had finally cleared its last parliamentary hurdles, a swift round of privatisation (especially in community health services) and fresh cutbacks were pushed through. The latter began with accident and emergency departments but also included jobs and the exclusion of a growing range of elective treatments from the NHS – forcing patients to 'choose' between going without treatment or going private. Neoliberals have been emboldened to raise publicly previously taboo topics,

---

4   NHS London's *Integrated Strategy* worked through a similar agenda and argued that five
    interventions could between them save up to £3.1 billion. Many of them consisted of deliv-
    ering less care or of seeking to bury the identifiable costs of delivering hospital services
    under a general heading of 'community' or primary care. The proposed interventions
    were: Reducing the cost of services delivered in the community; Providing more care in
    the community and less in hospitals; Stopping clinical interventions which 'have little or
    no benefit to those receiving them' – [including 'some joint replacements', although no
    more detail was offered]; Proactive care for people with long-term conditions, reducing
    the need for hospital admissions; 'Prevention to reduce the risk of ill health' (Healthcare
    for London 2010).

such as the introduction of 'top-up fees' that would undermine the key founding principle of the NHS – or even, from the cranky libertarian right, abolishing the NHS altogether (Ramesh 2012a, Moberly 2012a, Wellings 2012). Conservative cabinet minister Oliver Letwin is on record as having promised that this would be the result within one parliamentary term of the Tories taking office again after Labour (McSmith 2004).

Cutting services and artificially reducing access to services are both seen by the Conservative-led coalition as preferable to finding ways to get the wealthy and business communities to pay the estimated £120 billion per year of uncollected tax they owe, or raising taxes on big business and the banks which triggered the 2008 meltdown.

Switching a substantial volume of care from secondary to primary was seen as one way to contain the vast and growing costs of a new £400 million PFI-funded hospital project in Central Manchester (CMMH 2003), although concrete plans for achieving this objective have – as in so many other similar circumstances – been hard to find. This leaves the certainty of cutbacks and austerity, but only the vaguest hope of new, alternative services to take the place of the existing services as they are closed.

Market-driven reforms (spending cuts)

Cash limits (or 'global budgets')

Perhaps the crudest way of seeking cost containment in health care is simply to restrict the funds available, as a means of encouraging or compelling the providers themselves to seek ways to cut spending, increase efficiency and restrict (or 'manage') demand for more expensive services.

This type of policy has a long history: in theory Britain's NHS has always been cash-limited, although in its very first year it massively overspent the projected target (Lister 2008a). The IMF-inspired 'cash limits' imposed on the NHS from 1976 were made legally binding on health authorities by the Thatcher government in 1980 as part of its 'monetarist' policies (Mohan 1995). The imposition of global budgets is clearly a much simpler process in a Beveridge-style, centralised, tax-funded system, in which the government has effective discretion to fix the level of spending. However, it does carry a political price: even the Thatcher government in Britain felt obliged to ease its downward pressure on health-care spending, which had brought three successive years of negative growth in the mid-1980s, triggered a politically embarrassing series of winter bed shortages and sent hospital waiting lists soaring (Lister 2008a).

Imposing a limit on spending in Bismarck-style and other insurance-based systems, in which there is often a multiplicity of payers and providers, many or all of them acting at arm's length or even further removed from direct government control, can be much more difficult – as governments in France and Germany in particular have discovered (Mladovsky et al. 2012).

In general, the political scope for elected governments with developed and costly health services to squeeze spending downwards is restricted. High-spending health services generate high levels of popular expectation of prompt and appropriate treatment. Figures compiled by Dixon and Mossialos (2002a) comparing health-care spending in eight leading OECD countries[5] showed that only two (Sweden and Denmark) managed to reduce health-care spending as a share of GDP in the period 1988–99, while all eight *increased* actual real-terms expenditure per head by an average of over 50 per cent, with some governments far exceeding this increase[6] (Mossialos and Dixon 2002a: Table A1). Surveys of the impact of the post-2008 crisis on European health services also show that spending freezes and (sometimes drastically) reduced levels of growth in spending are far more common than outright cuts; and that many of the 'savings' measures have been focused on getting health workers to carry the main brunt of any reduction through job losses, vacancy freezes and reduced actual or real-terms salaries, rather than cut directly into front-line services (Mladovsky et al. 2012, HOPE 2011).

Levels of spending on health care also have to be viewed in the correct context. From the free market point of view, and the standpoint of for-profit health-care providers, the runaway expansion of *private* spending on health care in the USA or anywhere else is no problem at all – merely a reflection of the choices made by individuals and the play of market forces (Pauly 2003). However, the price inflation which continues to run through the US health-care system also leads to substantial increases in federal government spending – which potentially calls for tax increases, or reductions in other areas of social spending, if it is not to lead to a further widening of the US budget gap. Indeed the higher the cost of medical insurance, the greater the gap between this and the disposable income of the poorest sections of US society – and the more uninsured or inadequately insured people wind up reliant upon public funds (Hadley and Holahan 2003).

The escalation of insurance costs for the millions of Americans who are covered by workplace schemes also leads to divisions between the vested interests of different sections of employers – between those whose business is providing health care and those for whom health-insurance cover for their workforce is a substantial overhead cost, limiting their possible profits.[7] So while the wealthy see private payment systems and insurance as a way to purchase the health care they need, without constant contributions from them to the costs of treating others through income-related taxation (Evans 1997), there are political and economic reasons why important sections of US employers should be keen to see a more cost-effective system for delivering health-care services to their workforce. However, they are significantly less influential in pursuing this goal than the 'medical–industrial complex' has consistently been

---

5   Australia, Denmark, France, Germany, the Netherlands, New Zealand, Sweden and the United Kingdom

6   Deber (2000a) argues that measuring health care purely as a share of GDP leaves out any estimate of whether the economy is in recession: Canada has managed to reduce its share of GDP spent on health from 10.1 per cent in 1993 to 9.2 per cent in 1997 as it emerged from recession, though actual spending per capita had only dropped by around 5 per cent.

7   General Motors notoriously spends more on health insurance for its employees than it does on steel for the fabric of the vehicles it produces (Grant 2003, Mackintosh 2003).

in maintaining the system essentially unchanged – even ensuring that the Obama reforms have been designed around the health-insurance industry and preserve, even reinforce, the largely private financing model while bolstering it with more government funding and compelling people on low incomes to buy poor-value policies that do not fully insure them (Gibson and Singh 2012).

OECD countries have in general witnessed an upward curve of health-care spending since 1945: the imposition of austerity policies has until recent years been far more rigorously applied in low- and 'middle'-income countries, especially those under the disciplines of IMF Structural Adjustment Programmes. Health spending in Zimbabwe for example was reined sharply back following IMF and World Bank advice in 1988 – falling from 6.8 per cent of government spending in 1991 to just 2.7 per cent by 1994. The government also agreed in 1990 to introduce user fees – which eventually rose four-fold over the next five years (Kemkes et al. 1997). During the 1990s, the HIV/AIDS epidemic also had an especially brutal impact on Zimbabwe, with up to 20 per cent of the population (1.4 million people) infected with HIV by 1998, and 3,000 dying from AIDS each week in 2004 (Sapa-AFP 2004). The spending cuts brought shortages of medicines, a lack of functioning equipment and the closure of some rural hospitals: the user fees brought a sharp decline in hospitalisation, but also deterred poor people from seeking treatment for venereal diseases, thus contributing to the transmission of HIV.

Also in Africa, Ford and colleagues (2009) point to the dire consequences of cash-driven decisions to delay treatment for HIV/AIDS until a much later stage in the illness than in developed countries and to limit the poorest countries to using cheaper, sub-optimal antiretroviral drugs, which carry severe side-effects. Earlier intervention would reduce premature mortality and reduce the spread of TB and the HIV virus itself. It would also lead to the need for far less intensive treatment: the increased spending on this approach could reduce costs overall.

Of course, it's not only an issue in Africa: another example of the crude application of cash limits was the 'Country Assistance Strategy' for Ecuador, endorsed by the World Bank in 2000. This was a structural adjustment package which involved slashing health spending to *half* the 1995 level.[8] In countries where health-care spending is already well below the minimal targets ($35 per head per year) set by the World Bank and the WHO for a 'basic package' of primary and preventive health services, any cuts in spending are likely to have an exceptionally heavy impact on the services that remain and those who depend upon them.[9]

In fact, in many of the lowest-income countries, where there hasn't been much in the way of public spending to cut, the issue hasn't so much been the cutting of spending to match tough cash limits, but rather the identification of resources to

---

8   Ecuador spent just $71 per head per year on health care in 1995, against an OECD average of $1,827.

9   More recent estimates suggest that much more needs to be spent: a WHO Commission for Macroeconomics in Health report in 2002 suggested that a set of essential interventions would cost at least $34 per head per year in low-income countries, while the WHO's then director general argued in 2000 that countries spending less than '$60 or so per capita' would not be able to provide even a reasonable minimum of services (Labonté et al. 2004: 40).

raise spending towards the level of the WHO minimum requirement of $38 per person per year to deliver even the most basic package of health care.

Rationalisation: reductions in bed numbers

Hospital beds can be extremely expensive to run and consume the largest share of health spending, both in the wealthier countries (Hensher et al. 1999) and in many developing countries: in Sub-Saharan Africa, public hospitals absorb between 45 and 69 per cent of government health spending (Kirigia et al. 2002). Hospitals require not only revenue funding but sufficient qualified medical and professional staff – resources that are generally in extremely short supply. Market-driven reforms, aimed at capping spending, will therefore inevitably seek to reduce spending on excess numbers of hospital beds in the drive for 'efficiency', but also to reduce public hospital provision to ensure that the maximum numbers of patients with the money to pay privately do so.

Where it has been driven by advances in technique and medical science, this type of change has been inevitable. In much of Eastern Europe, it has been slow to take effect because the underlying model of care was hospital-centred, offering little in the way of outpatient, home care or community-based services, and the pace of technical change has been much slower (Kokko et al. 1998). In advanced health-care systems, the development of day surgery and minimally invasive techniques, together with improved anaesthetics and dressings, has enabled a substantial reduction in average lengths of stay for surgical treatment, reducing the need for surgical beds. Where these technical resources exist, this has given a sound basis for considerable reduction of surgical bed numbers over the last 20 years (Hensher et al. 1999). However, even in the more advanced systems, *medical* specialties have not achieved the same reductions in lengths of stay – for good reasons: most medical admissions are for emergency treatment, often for older patients.[10] In the UK since the mid-1990s, numbers of bed days for *medical* admissions have outstripped those for surgical procedures.[11] Nor have the promised improvements in primary and community health services always materialised or brought the expected reduction in demand for emergency medical admissions. This means that in any programme of bed reductions, a proper balance must be maintained between medical and surgical beds, if elective surgical work is not to be disrupted by emergency admissions of medical cases (Pollock and Dunnigan 2000).

For an accurate picture of current trends, it is also important to ensure that more recent changes are compared with those over a longer time frame. In England, large numbers of acute hospital beds closed in the 20 years from 1982: but the closures virtually ceased from 1994, when it became clear that hospital trusts could not cope with peaks in demand for emergency admissions without at least their existing complement of beds. This carried on until 2008, when ten years of annual rises

---

10 In Britain in 1992, 87 per cent of medical admissions were found by the Audit Commission to be emergencies (Audit Commission 1992: 57).

11 Hospital Episode Statistics for 2002–3 show 14.2 million bed days as a result of medical admissions, compared with 12.4 million for surgical (DoH 2004a).

in NHS spending began to come to an end (Lister 2008a). Indeed, a government-commissioned beds inquiry at the end of the 1990s found a substantial shortfall in available beds, not least for the delivery of more appropriate step-down and step-up provision in the community that could help reduce pressure on front-line acute hospital beds (DoH 2000a). By contrast, bed reductions in France began later and continued long after the generalised 'downsizing' of British acute hospital capacity had stopped (OECD 2012a). Hospitals in much of Eastern Europe are still facing the challenge of reducing capacity from the very large numbers of beds that were central to the Soviet style 'Semashko' system on which newly established health-care systems were based in the aftermath of the Second World War.

While political resistance to hospital closures – the loss of familiar and recognisable evidence of health services – has remained strong, one particular weakness in the plausibility of alternative proposals has been evident: they generally take shape under a financial pressure that prevents any serious attempt to set up alternative community-based systems before hospital beds are phased out. Plans for replacement services tend to be vacuous and unconvincing, pitched sometime in the future, in places which remain unspecified, often with no clear timetable or milestones to chart progress or plans to recruit and train staff: many such proposals are again being floated as part of the attempt to cut £20 billion in 'efficiency savings' from England's £100 billion budget (Lister 2012a).

Member state	Infrastructure	
	Hospital beds (per 10,000 population)	Radiotherapy units (per 1,000,000 population)
	2000–2009	2010
WHO region		
African Region	9	0.1
Region of the Americas	24	5.2
South-East Asia Region	11	0.3
European Region	62	3.9
Eastern Mediterranean Region	12	0.4
Western Pacific Region	47	1.5
Income group		
Low income	13	0.1
Lower-middle income	22	0.6
Upper-middle income	36	1.4
High income	59	7.3
Global	**29**	**1.8**

Table 1 (WHO Data 2012)

In the wealthier countries, the limited comparisons that can be made show that total acute bed provision over a 27-country OECD average has continued in general to fall – by around 10 per cent over ten years, from 5.4 per thousand population in 2000 to around 4.9 in 2009 (OECD 2012a). However, the average conceals some wide variations: bed numbers have been increasing in Korea, Turkey and Greece, while they have been squeezed down in most other countries. The largest proportional reductions in acute bed numbers were in France, Finland, the Slovak Republic, Estonia and Ireland.

In the low- and middle-income countries (table 2), the disparity in health provision compared with the OECD is stark. Progress in expanding services is slow and not necessarily helped by the focus of much external aid on vertical programs, which do not contribute to the development of health-care systems in the recipient countries. WHO figures show that on beds, high-income countries have four times the availability compared with low-income countries and almost three times as many as lower-middle income. Moreover, LIC and LMIC figures lump in poorly utilised private non-profit and a handful of for-profit beds, and most beds in high-income countries will be more productive. When it comes to delivering radiotherapy to treat the rising numbers of cancer sufferers in the developing countries, the contrast is even more glaring: high-income countries have 73 times the resources of LICs, the Americas 52 times as many and Europe 39 times.

The quest to increase throughput per bed

The proper objective of rationalisation is not simply to close surplus capacity but to ensure that the remaining beds are used more intensively and efficiently. This often requires additional investment in equipment and training of staff. OECD data on this aspect of the rationalisation process, although incomplete (in that comparisons cannot be made for all countries even back to 2000), show an enormous variation in the performance levels of hospitals and the extent to which throughput has increased in the last ten years.

The most intensive levels of activity per bed by a long way are in Israel (90 patients per bed per year), triggering angry complaints from Israeli doctors (IMA 2011a, 2011b). However, the rapid throughput of patients in Israeli hospitals goes back at least ten years and the rate of increase since 2000 is not the highest: the most intensive acceleration of hospital care has been in Norway, which increased throughput per bed by a massive 42 per cent from 2000, overtaking Mexico to become the second highest in the OECD with 70.4 patients per bed per year. Mexico is now the third most speedy at treating and discharging, averaging 63.2 patients per bed, followed by Turkey, which has pushed up throughput by an astonishing 52 per cent in ten years from 38.7 to 58.8 patients per bed, and the UK, up 34 per cent to 55 (OECD 2012a).

By contrast, despite a 27 per cent increase in throughput since 2000, Japan is still treating only 15.5 patients per bed, with the world's longest average length of stay: the hyper efficiency of Japanese productive industry has clearly not been translated into a hospital system, which raises questions over the comparability of the OECD figures.

Other countries are also making slow progress, given the advances in new anaesthetics, less-invasive operating techniques and continual experimentation with early discharge schemes. However, what these figures don't show is the extent to which the advent and spread of day surgery for many routine operations has changed the case mix of inpatient care, resulting in a more demanding cohort of patients in hospital beds, many of them with problems requiring medical rather than surgical intervention. Many of the innovations that have reduced length of stay have been focused on surgery (Lister 2008a).

Acute hospital performance: throughput			
	2000*	2010*	
Country			Increase %
Austria	43.7	53.6	23
Belgium	35.9	37.9	6
Canada	33.6	35.8	7
Chile	40.6	46.7	15
France	48.6	52.7	8
Germany	32.2	37.8	17
Hungary	37.7	39.5	5
Ireland	48.4	52.7	9
Israel	79.4	90.0	13
Italy	38.8	41.4	7
Japan	12.2	15.5	27
Mexico	56.7	63.2	11
Netherlands	27.4	34.0	24
Norway	49.6	70.4	42
Portugal	33.7	39.4	17
Slovak Republic	30.3	37.0	22
Slovenia	36.4	46.7	28
Spain	39.5	43.5	10
Switzerland	33.2	45.2	36
Turkey	38.7	58.8	52
United Kingdom	41.0	55.0	34
United States	40.1	43.6	9
Average number of patients treated per acute bed (*Nearest year or estimate) Source: OECD Health Data 2012			

Table 2

There is no obvious correlation between these measures of technical efficiency and the costly marketising reforms that are claimed to improve performance. The USA, with the most developed health-care market, lags well behind the leaders with just 43.6 patients per bed and a puny 9 per cent increase since 2000. British performance since 2000 appears high by international comparisons, but is not as dramatic as its 53 per cent increase between 1982 and 1992 – before any of the market-style reforms had been introduced (OECD Health Data 2012).

In Britain, the process of improving the productive use of hospital beds in these two very different ten-year periods can be seen as a complex and contradictory interaction between, on the one hand, the effects of cash limits and year-on-year reductions in real-terms resources for NHS hospital services in the mid-1980s and, on the other, rising productivity, a rapid expansion of day-case surgical treatment and the organisational changes facilitated through increased health spending and continual technical innovation since 2000.

The limited case mix of uncomplicated elective surgery delegated to the private sector in England and the heavy focus of private providers (including for-profit Independent Sector Treatment Centres delivering treatment on contract to the NHS) on day surgery ('ambulatory care') mean that increased use of private-sector providers has not really been a factor in these figures on inpatient treatment: the private sector handles none of the more complex and prolonged medical treatment that tends to involve longer-than-average lengths of stay (Lister 2008a).[12]

Rationalisation may be advocated for a variety of reasons. Centralising specialist services into fewer, larger units to improve the training of staff and focus skills may represent an advance in clinical terms: but it may also result in patients being treated in a larger, less familiar environment, often much further from their homes. Maynard and Bloor (2000), reporting research findings, conclude that the efficiencies of such changes may also be debateable: unit costs may well be higher in larger hospitals, while some medical conditions may be exacerbated by long journeys to hospital: the new hospital may even act as a monopoly, preventing any wider competition.

In 2006, the less than satisfactory experiences of hospital mergers in England were analysed by the UK Audit Commission, which found that:

> In the commercial sector many mergers do not achieve their intended aims for a number of years and it is common for costs and inefficiencies arising from the merger process to exceed any planned short-term savings. If this is the case where organisations come together for overtly financial reasons, and responsible boards demand full due diligence checks before proceeding, it is perhaps unsurprising that mergers in the NHS take a considerable period of time to settle, and do not always achieve their savings targets. NHS mergers can be embarked upon without any transparent published financial analysis in support of local reconfiguration plans. It is also unsurprising that mergers and reconfigurations, once under way, absorb a large amount of board directors' time.
>
> (Audit Commission 2006: 26)

---

12 It's also important to note that the 'UK' figures include results from a mix of diverging health-care systems in England (the biggest population and the focal point for marketising reforms since 2000), Wales and Scotland (where the direction of reform has been in the opposite direction), and Northern Ireland.

Interestingly, the USA has offered examples both of controversial cost-cutting rationalisation (with a particular pressure on health maintenance organisations to close 'surplus' and expensive Emergency Rooms) and of the proliferation of hospitals attempting high-tech (and high-cost) surgery despite small annual caseloads. Enthoven, arguing that the US faces continuing 'market failure' in health care, notes that California had 120 hospitals performing open heart surgery, 'half of them with annual volumes of fewer than 200 cases' (Enthoven 1997: 198).

Views on rationalisation are often sharply divided: different sections of the medical establishment in Britain have on occasion developed quite different policies and proposals for the future shape of services. Surgeons have been the most likely to favour the concentration of services in fewer, larger units; physicians have been the least likely – with support for centralisation strongest among super-specialists dealing with a small minority of major complex cases, rather than generalists or GPs. The latter have, however, been strangely reluctant to address the logical consequences that flow from centralisation: the creation of extremely large and very costly buildings required to take the caseload from a number of smaller ones and the inevitable loss of senior medical posts along with local access (RCS 1997: 6). But the existence of even a paragraph of medical endorsement for a controversial closure is certain to be exploited by politicians and health-service management searching for protection against public anger (Lister 1998b, 2008).[13]

Rationalisation in developing countries

As with cash limits, the scope for substantial rationalisation of hospital services in many poorer countries is restricted, both by the inadequate infrastructure of hospital and primary care and by the lack of technology and sufficient suitably skilled staff.

In many cases, the problem is not to centralise resources: too many resources are already concentrated in huge, costly, showpiece teaching hospitals, generally in the capital or in large urban areas (such as Kenya's Kenyatta National Hospital and Ghana's Korle Bu and Komfo Anokye hospitals), and too few located accessibly for poor rural populations. The new PPP-funded referral hospital in Lesotho's capital is accessible only to a minority of the country's impoverished rural population. The problem in these countries is not that there are not too many beds, but too few – and too little money and too few staff to utilise them fully or facilitate their use by those with the greatest health needs. Medical expertise – hugely scarce in many of the least developed countries (see Table 3) – tends to gravitate to these big centres rather than reaching outwards.

---

13 In England in the 1990s, the medical Royal Colleges and the BMA called for a greater concentration of specialist services in a few 'super hospitals' covering very large catchment populations, in order to facilitate the training of junior doctors and the expansion of consultant numbers. However, there was never any indication that the government intended to build any hospitals large enough to meet the needs of this wider catchment (RCS 1997, BMA 1997).

Health workforce	Physicians		Nursing and midwifery personnel	
	Number	Density (per 10,000 population)	Number	Density (per 10,000 population)
WHO region:				
African Region	173,677	2.3	805,575	10.9
Region of the Americas	1,930,909	22.5	5,259,128	61.5
South-East Asia Region	903,408	5.4	2,224,133	13.3
European Region	2,950,761	33.3	6,620,725	74.7
Eastern Mediterranean Region	626,923	11.0	870,490	15.4
Western Pacific Region	2,586,199	14.5	3,599,720	20.3
Income group:				
Low income	215,761	2.8	522,425	6.7
Lower middle income	3,742,065	10.1	6,208,439	16.8
Upper middle income	2,189,890	22.4	4,333,111	44.5
High income	3,024,161	28.6	8,315,796	78.6
Global	**9,171,877**	**14.0**	**19,379,771**	**29.7**

Table 3
Figures from WHO Health Data 2012

Rationing services: exclusion as a cost-saving measure

One relatively unsophisticated way of reining in public spending on health care is to ration care by drawing up a list of treatments or drugs that will be excluded from coverage. This process is politically easier if it is possible to create an argument that the treatment or drug is somehow ineffective or potentially dangerous – though ineffective or dangerous drugs should probably be barred from use by *any* patients, not just those covered by public funding or insurance schemes (New 1999).

In 2009, the British government commissioned a report from McKinsey, preparing the ground for measures to bridge the 'gap' that would open up between frozen health spending and the mounting demand for health care after the ten years of large budget increases came to an end in 2010. Among many other proposals, this suggested 'decommissioning' treatments which the management consultancy insisted were of 'limited clinical benefit' to save up to £700 million in England: the treatments included hernia operations and hip and knee replacements (McKinsey 2009: 51–2). Since then, local health commissioners in England have drawn up varying lists of treatments now unavailable on the NHS in their area. This policy has continued after the change of government, spreading to over 90 per cent of primary care trusts, despite denials from ministers that any exclusions or rationing are taking effect. One survey of 101 PCTs found that 91 per cent had measures in place to limit GP referrals on some procedures, including cataract surgery and bariatric surgery: 59 per cent were imposing limits on joint surgery (Moberly 2012a).

Explicit exclusions in publicly funded health-care services are politically sensitive, since the implication is that the excluded services – previously available to all – will be available only on a private basis to those who can afford to pay (Drache and Sullivan 1999). In Britain, there had previously been various attempts at this, beginning with the Thatcher government's 1987 legislation to exclude eye tests and most provision of spectacles and lenses from the NHS, along with dental check-ups and a big increase in co-payment charges for dental treatment (Lister 2008a). The issue remained on the agenda of cash-strapped British health authorities during the 1990s (Klein 2000, Lister 1998a) and has now resurfaced in the current economic crisis.

A wider debate on rationing developed during the mid-1990s, partly in response to the perceived levels of under-funding of the British NHS but also encouraged by American and other advocates of private medical insurance, either as a 'top-up' or as a substitute to publicly funded health care (Marmor 1999). The starting point of claims that 'rationing is inevitable' (Ham 1997, Ham and Honigsbaum 1998, Smith R 1996b) is that health-care demand (or, more properly, the *need* for health care) is infinite – a 'bottomless pit' (Light 1997) – whereas health-care resources are of necessity finite. With only so much money and human resources to go round, the argument goes, 'hard choices' have to be made (Lenaghan 1997).

This view was challenged by Light, who argued that levels of health spending were politically determined rather than geared to measures of need (or demand) for health care. He pointed prophetically to the German health-care system as one example where resources had *matched* demand and yet demand had conspicuously failed to increase to 'infinite' levels.[14] Health care is unlike most other commodities under capitalism, in the sense that the demand for it is closely linked to need – and that demand is self-limiting. Few people wish to prolong treatment beyond the point where drugs, surgery or other therapy have taken effect. Frankel and colleagues (2000) have challenged what they describe as a 'pessimistic' thesis of the 'infinite demand' for health care.

The German experience offers a definitive answer to the 'bottomless pit' pundits (who almost invariably want us to conclude that the state should abandon the quest for universal and comprehensive health care and instead revert to some regressive form of private insurance or system of 'top-up' fees). Costing around 11.6 per cent of GDP in 2010, the German health-care system is one of the most costly in the world (OECD 2012a), despite more than two decades of attempts at cost-containment (MSI Healthcare 2000, Busse et al. 2002: 54). But with Germany's waiting lists completely eliminated, and amid revelations that 20 per cent of German hospital beds were empty, hospitals seeking to ride out the squeeze on prices from the sickness funds and utilise their spare capacity began searching for private patients from

---

14 Germany, then spending up to 10 per cent of its GDP on health care, was by 1997 heading towards the surplus of beds and patient care facilities which led in 2002 to German health-care providers seeking to market spare capacity to other European health-care purchasers.

Europe and beyond. A private company GerMedic visited Ireland, Denmark and Sweden offering 'package deal' operations in a network of 80 hospitals and clinics (Payne 2001). The German example suggests that, far from being 'infinite', the cost of providing a comprehensive health-care system could be somewhere below the 11 per cent figure which produced a surplus of facilities and a shortage of patients in Germany – even with the costly and complex system of insurance funds that remain features of the Bismarck system (Lister 2008a).

Alternatives to explicit rationing

Four different approaches offer a less overt alternative to explicit rationing by exclusion: the first is the establishment of an 'approved' register for new drugs and treatments. In Britain, the National Institute for Clinical Excellence (NICE) was established in 1999 by New Labour as an impartial body that would assess the cost effectiveness and appropriate use of new drugs and treatments, and advise the government. Of course, such a body only solves part of the dilemma since 'cost effectiveness' is a composite measure embodying the contradictions of use value and exchange value, leaving the question of which aspect of the treatment is to be uppermost in the decisions of NICE – the *cost* of a drug or its effectiveness? A decision by NICE to recommend that a treatment should be made available, and funded by the NHS, can open up a fresh dilemma in the context of cash limits (Boseley 2003c, Revill 2003).

The second alternative is to establish an 'approved list' of treatments which will be funded. This was the underlying method behind the so-called 'Oregon experiment' which began in the late 1980s as a reform to the Medicaid scheme. The US state of Oregon passed legislation in 1989 which offered to increase access to health insurance for some of its poorest residents, but imposed restrictions on the range of health-care services that would be financed. The most controversial element of the plan was implicitly excluding the poorest people in the state from receiving treatments that were not on a list of 'priorities'. The priority list was drawn up by an 11-strong health services commission, which received professional advice, research evidence, and the findings of public hearings and focus groups involving the local community. Despite fears that this would lead to a distortion of medical priorities reflecting popular prejudices over 'deserving' and 'non-deserving' patients (Dixon and Welch 1991), this process resulted in a list of 696 treatments – of which, 565 were initially deemed to be priorities that should be funded. According to Ham (1998: 1,966) the main exclusions were treatments for 'self-limiting conditions and conditions where no effective interventions were available.'

Ham's assessment of the exercise concluded equivocally:

> Whether the outcome looks like a glass half full or a glass half empty depends on your perspective.
>
> (Ham 1998: 1,969)

For those who see rationing as the way forward, Oregon offers not so much proof of success as vindication that it does not have to lead to the horrors of populist shroud-waving and large-scale exclusions of the vulnerable. Similar efforts in the Netherlands and New Zealand to define packages of care that would be funded, effectively excluding the remainder, have also proved unsuccessful (New 1997: 81). The spread of rationing has been limited by these negative experiences and by strong disagreements even among advocates of rationing as to how it should be carried out (New 1996, Maynard and Sheldon 2001, Coulter and Ham 2000). Saltman (2002) concluded rather optimistically from his survey of evidence that there has been 'no explicit rationing' of publicly financed or publicly controlled health services in Western Europe.

The third alternative approach is a form of implicit rationing of the kind that prevails in health services that levy charges for care, such as the US, or that tolerate sometimes hefty, illicit 'informal' payments to health-care staff in systems where resource constraints have eroded the morale of professionals – and that is the restriction of demand by price. This is facilitated by the lack of any affordable health-insurance policy offering unlimited cover – and the very high co-payments and deductibles which are built into apparently 'affordable' health insurance for those on low incomes in the US (Cohn 2011, Hancock 2012). The pricing mechanism, the most crude of all the market-driven devices to manage demand, clearly takes no account of ability to pay and has its most severe impact on the poor, exempting only those wealthy enough to be able to afford treatment.

The fourth and final alternative is also a form of implicit rationing: the limitation of resources (money, staff, facilities) available to deliver publicly funded health care, through caps on spending, global health budgets or other formulae with similar effects. In the USA, most rationing is entirely achieved in this way, with people on low incomes deciding what policy they can afford or how much they can raise through loans and the sale of assets to pay for their own health care (though this is coupled with administrative staff in insurance companies ruling on whether their customers are covered for particular treatments, as discussed brilliantly in Michael Moore's film *Sicko*). When the imbalance is especially severe, the result is waiting lists, queues and shortages – or in the US case, large gaps in care for those whose means do not cover the costs of treatment. In this sense, America's poor share a similar experience with the chronic sick and poor of developing countries; except that in the USA, the economic exclusion from services takes place cheek by jowl with the most expensive and extravagant high-tech health-care provision in the world.

One further form of exclusion which has been more widely adopted, leading to a substantial shift of the funding burden from governments to individuals and their families, has been in the area of long-term care, especially for older people. Continuing care for older patients in nursing homes, frequently now simply described as 'social care' (Mossialos et al. 2002), has been widely seen as an appropriate area for the expansion of private enterprise, even at the heart of what have until now been predominantly publicly financed health-care systems in the more advanced economies. Systems of care for older people in much of Europe have up to now been converging on a model in which a relatively low level of state-funded (often privately provided) provision of continuing care is supplemented by low-cost care, mainly delivered by unpaid family members. This is discussed in more detail in Chapter 8 below.

Regulating the costs of drugs and medical goods

At least 26 European countries have turned to this avenue for economies in the aftermath of the 2008 meltdown, using measures such as generic substitution, price negotiations, claw-back mechanisms and changes in prescribing (Mladovksy et al. 2012). The question of the regulation of medical devices was thrown into the spotlight by the scandal at the end of 2011 over faulty silicone breast implants made by a collapsed French company (Adams 2012a).

'Market failure in both supply and demand' is blamed by Mossialos and Mrazek (2002: 149) for the widespread intervention and regulation that governments have applied to the pharmaceutical market. They argue that part of this market failure arises from the so-called 'moral hazard' in many insurance-based systems, under which the consumer/patient does not have to pay, or is reimbursed, the cost of the drugs they consume, so 'neither they nor the physicians have any incentive to economise'.

The drug companies have been quite happy with this. According to Fortune 500, the world's top ten pharmaceutical companies had average revenues of $35 billion (the largest, Johnson & Johnson, with $63 billion) and average profits of more than $7 billion. Even as the cost of drugs came under scrutiny, a chirpy and optimistic forecast from the IMS Institute for Healthcare research predicted a resumption in the rise in spending to create a $1.2 trillion market for medicines by 2016, although located not so much in the traditional markets of the developed economies as in the 'pharmerging markets', centred more around generics than branded products (PharmiWeb.com 2012). These wider markets can offer an extra mark-up to companies wanting to keep profits high – a 2010 study of the availability and affordability of cardiovascular medicines in 36 developing countries found they were much more readily accessible through private hospitals than public health services, and that patient prices were generally well above international reference costs: 'chronic treatment with anti-hypertensive medication cost more than one day's wages in many cases. In particular where monotherapy is insufficient treatment became unaffordable' (van Mourik et al. 2010). An earlier study had come to similar conclusions, stressing that as a result of these inflated costs, spending on drugs consumes 20–60 per cent of health spending in developing and transitional economies, compared with an average 18 per cent in the OECD (Cameron et al. 2008).

A large share of the profits of US pharmaceutical companies depends upon the continuation of large-scale public spending to subsidise medicines for the poor and elderly: big pharma has certainly been hit by the drastic austerity drives that have sought to squeeze down the price of patented drugs and force greater use of cheaper generic medicines in Europe, especially in Portugal, Greece, Spain and Hungary (*Economist* Intelligence Unit 2011a, 2011d). The quest for economies is also shaking up drug sales in Italy and Ireland: even big-spenders France and Germany are trying to rein in drug price inflation and maximise the use of generics (InPharm 2012, *Economist* Intelligence Unit 2011b). The political power of these corporations is one reason why, until the desperate crisis forced governments into seeking even bigger savings, measures to restrict spending on pharmaceuticals had previously concentrated more on deterring demand and forcing patients to cover a larger share of the cost rather than on forcing down the prices of the drugs themselves.

There has also been a long-running battle over the protection of patent rights and the use of branded rather than cheaper, generic drugs when patents have expired. In Britain, growing pressure on GPs to prescribe generic drugs for their patients has continued since the 1980s (Rivett 1998). The British 'internal market' reforms in the 1990s meant that non-fund-holding GP practices were strictly monitored for their adherence to generic prescribing guidelines, while fund-holders, subject to cash-limited prescribing budgets, were given the financial incentive of retaining any unspent surpluses: as a result, fund-holders made greater use of generic medicines (Mossialos and Mrazek 2002: 158–9). New Labour's introduction of cash limits throughout primary care has resulted in a high profile for GP prescribing budgets in local financial reports, and pressure has continued on 'high-spending' practices to conform to the prescribing patterns of the majority and regard the drug budget as a target for savings (McKinsey 2009: 32–5).

The contradictions of a world market in which different prices are charged for the same drug in different countries has spawned a curious trade in 'parallel imports' of drugs from low-cost to high-cost countries and a new layer of management within the US 'managed care' industry – 'pharmacy benefit managers', whose role is to secure low-cost supplies of drugs (Gryta 2011). Physicians are told to prescribe the cheapest alternative from a restricted list, while pharmacists make a higher margin every time they switch to a cheaper prescribed drug.

Other mechanisms, such as the use of co-payments related to the costs of the drugs prescribed, have sought to enlist consumerism as a means to scale down prescribing costs and exclude unauthorised products: in Germany and the Netherlands, patients receiving drugs above the standard 'reference cost' pay the full difference in price in addition to the standard prescription charge of 4–5 euro. However, the price of some generic drugs which were originally below the reference price have been found to rise to the reference price level (Dixon and Mossialos 2002a, Mossialos and Mrazek 2002).

France and New Zealand give no reimbursement for any drugs that are not included on the Pharmaceutical Scale (Dixon and Mossialos 2002a). Other attempts to control drug prices include the establishment of a 'cost-effectiveness price' for medicines sold in Australia, Canada and Finland. In Britain, the government each year negotiates a target rate of return (17–21 per cent) with each pharmaceutical company, but allows the companies to set their prices within this margin (Mossialos and Mrazek 2002).

Elsewhere, New Zealand (which has no resident drug multinationals to worry about) has led the way and Belgium has experimented with the 'Kiwi model' for forcing down drug prices: drug producers are encouraged to underbid each other in proposing the lowest price for the same treatment. Whoever wins the tender is compensated for having the lowest price by becoming eligible for a preferential 75 per cent reimbursement rate, with patients paying just 25 per cent of the cost, while all other existing versions of the same drug are reimbursed at just 50 per cent.

The pharmaceutical companies jealously guard their role in the research of new drugs but resist any attempt to steer them towards particular areas of research. In fact, numbers of new 'chemical entities' registered each year have fallen dramatically, from 100 in 1963 to just 37 in 1998. Almost half the drugs approved for sale in the USA in the 15 years to 1990 were for cardiovascular conditions or antibiotics (Mossialos and Mrazek 2002). In 2010, only 29 new drugs were registered (Graul and Cruces 2011). Drugs such as Viagra to combat erectile dysfunction are proliferating alongside 'me too' equivalents Cialis and Levitra (Angell 2005), while large-scale killer diseases which haunt the African continent are all but ignored.

Drug companies make no secret of the fact that they are run for profit: but this means that they allocate little or no research work to diseases and conditions which largely affect low- and middle-income countries, while the drugs they develop for other diseases are often inaccessible or unaffordable in the poorer countries. This is despite near-unanimity among the various advisory agencies on the priorities for drug research (GFHR 2002: 92–5).

While inflated drug costs are a problem in the established health services of the wealthier countries, they are literally a matter of life and death in the poorest countries, especially in those facing an HIV/AIDS epidemic. This is the arena in which the case for generic medicines and against the exorbitant prices charged for patented drugs has been most hotly fought.

Washington has tried its best to fulfil its cast-iron guarantees that any concessions made on behalf of big pharma to the very poorest countries, in the limited WTO agreements, will not translate into the mass production of much cheaper generic drugs in India and Brazil (Chandrasekhar and Ghosh 2003).[15] However, the Indian government has now changed the game with a bold new policy. It has announced its own scheme, spending up to $5.5 billion a year to supply free generic medicines to the poor who access care in public health facilities: under the plan, doctors will be limited to a generics-only drug list and face punishment for prescribing branded medicines. A health ministry spokesperson stressed that generics are 'much, much cheaper'. While private patients will still have to pay for drugs and may be supplied with patented rather than generic medicine, the new policy is a major blow for pharmaceutical giants in one of the world's fastest-growing drug markets, at a time when some of the high-income countries are also squeezing their profits (Foy 2012).

Market-driven user fees

Robinson (2002), examining user charges in the context of East and West Europe, argues that user fees can be viewed as:

> different positions on a continuum ranging from full third-party payment (zero cost-sharing) to full user charges (costs met completely by out of pocket payments).
>
> (Ibid.: 162)

---

15 There are also fears that the focus on procuring drugs to treat AIDS has diverted attention from the need to develop specialist expertise in using the drugs to ensure that patients benefit and that drug-resistant forms of the virus do not result (Kumar 2004).

Noting that the main claim that user fees help to improve 'efficiency' revolves around their effectiveness in discouraging 'unnecessary' demand or, in some cases, in generating additional revenue for funding health care when alternative funds are not available, Robinson points out that such a policy has little to do with efficiency: it is more accurately seen as 'public sector cost containment' – in other words, a market-driven, cost-cutting measure.

Summarising surveys conducted in 1998 and 1999, and including Russia, Central Eastern Europe and the former Soviet Union republics of Central Asia, Robinson notes that user fees are widely used by most countries in the form of co-payments for pharmaceuticals – covering as much as 35 per cent of the drug cost in Hungary. Nine EU countries imposed charges for general-practitioner consultations and most EU countries impose co-payments for specialist consultations. Sweden levies extensive user charges, including charges for children's outpatient services. However, only Greece, Italy and Portugal relied upon user charges to raise more than 20 per cent of health-care funding (Robinson 2002: 174).

Portugal and Italy have each had to increase charges or introduce new ones, Portugal having more than doubled charges for seeing a doctor and increased other charges for hospital care and treatment. As part of EU-imposed austerity measures, Greece has had to make brutal cuts to reduce government spending on health, resulting in soaring costs for prescriptions and cancer, and in other patients going without drugs they cannot afford (McKee et al. 2012, Frayer 2012, Tagaris 2012, Athens News 2012).

In the USA, where inflated costs for the private provision of both insurance and health care mean that co-payments and deductibles have long been a feature of the health-care system, an unpleasant and under-discussed side-effect of President Obama's 'Affordable Care Act' has been to compel those on low incomes to buy subsidised health-insurance policies which carry potentially huge co-payments and deductibles. So large are these additional charges that they effectively negate any advantage of the insurance policy for those too poor to be able to afford any more generous cover (Hancock 2012).

Robinson argued that a number of countries in Central and Eastern Europe and the former Soviet Union were levying user charges as part of new health-insurance schemes. Yet the evidence of limited research shows that total revenue from user charges rarely exceeded 5 per cent of total health revenue, while the charges had strongly reduced utilisation and thus worsened equity of provision, having a heavier impact upon the poor. There was some evidence that charges had an adverse effect on health outcomes – and that they carried hidden costs in managerial and administrative effort (Schieber and Maeda 1997, cited in Robinson 2002: 177).

A wider survey of OECD countries by Docteur and Oxley (2003) found a varying pattern, with just over half the OECD countries levying some form of charge (sometimes relatively small) for hospital in-patient treatment and a similar number charging for consultations with a general practitioner or, for a slightly more imposing charge, a specialist. While supplementary private insurance schemes may cover some or all of these charges in some countries (notably France), in Australia private insurance is *prohibited* from covering fees for outpatient treatment – suggesting that this functions very much as a cost-containment/demand-limitation measure: indeed, the Australian government has no powers to intervene to control the level of fees charged for health care (OECD 2012c: 74–5).

In the UK, even while national governments in Wales, Scotland and Northern Ireland have abolished prescription charges (which still apply in England), a team of Nuffield Trust and other academics has been working on systems to enable the NHS in England to introduce 'person based resource accounting', in which the basic health costs of individuals can be calculated as a way to decide precise budget allocations to GP practices and local commissioning groups. This would break down the national risk-pooling of the NHS (Dixon et al. 2011). But the same calculations could also form the basis for cash-limited allocations of health services per person, leaving individuals to 'top up' from their own pocket or from health insurance if they need additional treatment.

'Personal budgets' which work on the same basis are already being rolled out for more and more mental health patients and frail elderly people (despite the reservations of the NHS Confederation's Mental Health Network) – tacitly posing the issue of top-up payments where the budgets are too small to meet needs (Davies 2012: 80, Mental Health Network 2011).

In July 2012, the Nuffield Trust published a report by the Institute of Fiscal Studies which predicted that the NHS will be charging for treatment within ten years and suggested a 'review' of the range of services that the NHS should continue to offer 'free at point of use'. Soon after this, the *Health Service Journal* launched an open discussion on top-up fees (Girach and Irwin 2012).

'Top-up charges' is a misnomer: they are simply charges. They would require payment for health treatment, with each patient's access to services decided not on clinical need but on their ability to pay. In the UK, where such charges have not been seen since 1948, their implementation would be a massive change that would create a two-tier health service, fly in the face of equity and undermine the NHS as a universal service. It would limit or reduce demand while making no impact on health needs. The most widespread charge already levied in the NHS is the £7.65 per item prescription charge: the only reason this regressive charge has survived in England is because of truly massive exemptions, with something in excess of 85 per cent of prescriptions issued free. Even so, charges raise hardly any money (£400 million, a mere 0.4 per cent of an NHS budget that is in excess of £100 billion) but they do deter low-paid workers from accessing proper treatment.

Of course, the introduction of charges can both save money, by reducing the numbers treated, and act as a market-style measure to drive people who can afford it, and want to avoid the risk of charges, towards private health insurance – especially if the charges are large and difficult to deal with. This would create a defensive 'market' of people seeking protection from unacceptable costs rather than a market gratefully embraced or emerging in any organic fashion from public demand. Far from demonstrating any positive impact of 'patient choice', the experience of low-waged patients in the areas of care where 'top-up' fees and private provision have been established in the UK since the 1980s has been grim: dental services, opticians and 'social care' services have been dismantled and quality largely abandoned, while charges have continued to increase.

While user fees may have an inequitable impact in the wealthier countries, in the poorest countries, where the poor have even less income and resources at their disposal, the impact is more severe. The imposition of user fees, according to Newbrander and colleagues, 'is a strategy that places much of the burden of financing health care on the individual patient' (Newbrander et al. 2000: 12). Creese argues that user fees shift the burden away from risk sharing towards payments by individuals and households:

> The higher the proportion of user payments in the total mix of financing for health, the greater the relative share of the financing burden falling on poor people.
>
> (Creese 1997)

Among the techniques proposed for the introduction of fees in previously free health services is that of bringing in the charges at a very low ('minimal') level and then increasing them, 'to avoid creating public reaction':

> If there is public and political sensitivity to introducing new fees, it may be best to have a wide range of exemptions and relatively easy access to poverty waivers in the beginning and to reduce them gradually.
>
> (Newbrander et al. 2000: 104)

Another device to soften the negative political impact of user fees is the use of a different phrase to describe the charges which patients must pay for treatment. According to MSH, the Kenyan government was reluctant to announce that it was instituting a system of user fees, so:

> It chose the term 'cost sharing' to emphasise its continued commitment to providing high quality services to its population.
>
> (Management Sciences for Health 2001)

Presumably, any Kenyans who had failed to spot the significance of 'cost sharing' would soon have worked out that money was to change hands when they saw the networked cash registers installed as part of the MSH initiative. Indeed, user fees are a blunt instrument. As the WHO (2000) has argued, payment of charges at point of use restricts services to those who can afford to pay, irrespective of the level of *need* for treatment.

After a vote by the US Congress to oppose the imposition of user fees for health by either the IMF or the World Bank, there was an apparent rethink on the issue. Moreover, evidence emerged that user fees not only deter the poorest but also discriminate heavily against women (Nanda 2002). Despite this, user fees appear to be one of the policies most deeply ingrained in the thinking of those responsible for shaping policy in developing countries. A 2006 survey of 30 African countries found 27 still imposing fees (Oxfam 2006) and the Bank's *WDR 2004* actually argued that 'paying for services confers power'. It claimed that:

modest co-payments can also provide an entry ticket to clinical services for poor people by reducing capture of supposedly free services by richer groups.

(World Bank 2003b: 143)[16]

Any illusions that patients might be 'empowered' by fees should be dispelled by reports from Burundi where, following the introduction of a 'cost recovery' system in 2002 to make the system more 'financially efficient', patients were forcibly detained for weeks or months for failure to pay hospital bills (Human Rights Watch 2006). Similar confrontations have also been reported in Ghana, where new-born babies have been held in hospital in a bid to force mothers to pay maternity bills (Amanfo 2006, UN Office for the Coordination of Humanitarian Affairs 2005, 2006).

Although they deter poor people from accessing care and cause real problems to those struggling to pay, fees don't bring in significant income: health-care cost recovery experiences in African countries show that average fees yield only around 5 per cent of operating costs, meaning that the net yields are lower – or even negative – when collection costs are factored in. A Harvard University study in Tanzania found that the administration of the user-fee programme cost more than the user fees brought in (Kessler 2003). Similar experiences apply elsewhere: in Honduras, despite minimal exemptions, the fees raised less than 2 per cent of the Ministry of Health's income, but two-thirds of the funds collected were used to administer the fee system itself (Flores 2006). In Uganda, the abolition of fees resulted in a loss of $3.4 million per year for the health system, but generated $9 million worth of economic gains because of reductions in work time lost through illness (Morestin and Ridde 2009).

Many of the user fees imposed largely through World Bank pressure in the 1990s remain in place, although there have been some 'astounding' successes where they have subsequently been abolished – notably in Uganda (Hutton 2004). Another 2004 study of 24 priority countries supported by DFID revealed that 20 of them had user fees at primary-care level and that two-thirds of health spending in developing countries comes from out-of-pocket payments rather than governments (Save the Children 2005). The fact that Save the Children, Health Poverty Action and Oxfam have continued to feel the need to publish research arguing the case against user fees also underlines the fact that such fees remain a pervasive and enduring feature of health systems in many developing countries and in the independent states of the former Soviet Union (Emmett 2006, Edwards 2010, Hovhannisyan 2012, Marriott 2012a).

Schieber (1997) claimed that cost sharing is a means to combat 'moral hazard' and Wang'ombe claims that only 'frivolous demand' is affected (Wang'ombe 199b7: 151). However, there is little evidence of 'frivolous demand' in developing countries

---

16 A 2001 DFID manual, discussing the objectives of introducing user fees, does not even mention the most common motivation and impact of the policy – effecting an immediate reduction in demand – but suggests euphemistically that it 'encourages more efficient use of resources' and 'creates greater accountability to the consumer'! It goes on to claim that the 'almost universally negative' effects of fees on the poor are almost always due to a technical glitch – 'the result of poor design, planning and implementation' (Bennett and Gilson 2001: 1, 11).

– or in other contexts of health care (Deber 2000a) – and reducing 'demand' does nothing to reduce the need for health care. Those most likely to be deterred from accessing health care are the poorest – and especially women: in fact this effect is the most consistent and predictable result from any cost-recovery programme (Creese and Kutzin 1995).

The fees can be very substantial, regardless of ability to pay: poor people in Peru are expected to buy their own drugs and medical inputs, which are charged to the user at full cost plus a mark-up; fewer than one in five of the poor are exempt from payments (Cotlear 2000). Research from Nigeria indicates that when poor users are deterred, they are replaced by wealthier sections of the population who can afford to pay – a backward step for equity (Blas 2004: 19).

All of the empirical evidence confirms the initial assumption that the imposition of charges will above all reduce the utilisation of services (Lagarde and Palmer 2008, Steinhardt et al. 2011): the scale of the reductions observed ranges from 52 per cent in Kenya (Mwabu et al. 1995) to 64 per cent in Zambia (Kahenya and Lake 1994). Other countries where the same effect has been observed include Ghana and Zaire. High levels of user fees 'which exclude the poor' have been seen by donor groups as a problem in Mozambique (Brown 2000a) and Uganda (Brown 2000b). The UN Research Institute for Social Development has concluded that 'Of all measures proposed for raising revenue for local people, this [user fees] is probably the most ill-advised' (UNRISD 2000, cited in Whitehead et al. 2001). The abolition of fees invariably results in increased use of services: in African countries the increases have varied from 17 per cent in Madagascar to 84 per cent in Uganda. By contrast, the removal of fees in public-sector health care can bring dramatic reductions in the use of private health care (in Kenya the consultations dropped by 32 per cent) (Morestin and Ridde 2009).

The Bamako Initiative is a variant model of user fees, largely restricted to countries of Francophone West Africa, in which the fees go into community-owned 'revolving funds', to be spent and controlled locally. This model is still running in Benin, Mali and Guinea, and the World Bank (2003b: 76–7) claims that it has contributed to improved health outcomes, dramatic improvements in immunisation rates, a narrowing of the gap between rich and poor, and a tenfold increase in the use of health services by children. However, on closer examination it becomes clear that immunisation is provided free of charge and, even though user fees had been held down below the price of alternative, traditional healers, 'a large proportion of the poor still do not use key health services in all three countries'. In some instances, Bamako Initiative health centres have become a service for the affluent (Blas 2004).[17]

After twelve years, government subsidies to the BI system in Guinea were still benefiting richer groups rather than the poorest and there is still an unresolved question of how to subsidise and protect the poor. Ridde, pressing for a simple abolition of user fees, argues that:

---

17 A similar phenomenon has been reported in Peru, where user fees led to reduced use of hospital services by the lowest-income and also the middle-income groups, while higher-income group usage increased by around 50 per cent (cited in Flores 2006).

> Little progress toward equity has been made in the context of the Bamako Initiative over the past 20 years.
>
> (Ridde 2011: 179)

The exclusions always hit the weakest among the poor. Among the poorest social groups, those most likely to be excluded from treatment by user fees are women, children and the elderly. Nanda (2002) explored the additional barriers which limit women from accessing the funds to pay for care, and the additional informal and hidden costs faced by women.

User fees have nothing to do with equity. Even defenders of the policy admit that almost all of the 31 African countries that were persuaded by the World Bank and other advisors to implement user fees were simply seeking to raise money: only four claimed that either 'efficiency' or 'equity' was an objective (Leighton and Wouters 1995).[18]

However, the abolition of fees would carry significant additional costs in the short and medium term because a large body of pent-up demand would potentially be released (Gilson and McIntyre 2005, Meessen et al. 2009). There are real dangers that if this is not properly prepared and resourced (with appropriate increases in staffing, equipment and other supplies) the result could be the inundation of local services, as the Zambian example in 2006 shows (McPake et al. 2011).

The serious contemplation of such a change of policy in the poorest developing countries, therefore, requires serious preparation (SCUK 2008). More commitment from the Bank and other donors would be needed, in terms of policy guidance and also practical, material and financial support, than the general statement that there is 'no blanket policy' on user fees.

There is at last evidence of sustained activity directed towards lifting fees in Afghanistan (Steinhardt et al. 2011) and in six Sub-Saharan African countries (Hercot et al. 2011), and a wider discussion on lessons that can be learned from early attempts to avoid potential pitfalls (McPake et al. 2011).

---

18 A finding echoed in a separate study of user fees by Russell and Gilson (1997).

Chapter seven

The 'reform' agenda – market-style (ideologically driven) reforms

Introduction: reforms, the underlying agenda and the New Public Management

Market-style reforms, reflecting the dominant neoliberal ideological approach, make constant reference to what they claim to be the values and merits of a competitive market system: but it would be a big mistake to take this at face value. As Evans (1997) sums up:

> In practice advocates have never wanted a truly competitive market, but rather one managed by and for particular private interests.

He goes on to stress what has become increasingly evident: that the advocates of using market forces do not really believe that this can be applied without extensive regulation:

> International experience over the last forty years has demonstrated that greater reliance on the market is associated with inferior system performance – inequity, inefficiency, high cost and public dissatisfaction. The United States is the leading example. So why is this issue back again? Because market mechanisms yield distributional advantages for particular influential groups.

Evans points to the advantages of higher prices for suppliers and service providers, and the advantages of inequitable systems for the wealthy who want the freedom to buy what they see as better quality care for themselves while contributing little or nothing to the health care of the poor. He concludes:

> Analytic arguments for the potential superiority of hypothetical competitive markets are simply one of the rhetorical forms through which this permanent conflict of economic interest is expressed in political debate.
>
> (Evans 1997: 427)

The pitiless drive for ever-deeper cuts in public health spending in the aftermath of the 2008 financial crash continues to lay waste publicly funded health-care services, notably in Greece, Spain, Portugal and Italy, in what McKee and colleagues (2012) have described as a 'failed experiment'. As this continues, it is clear that the weight of the crisis has been deliberately loaded onto the working and middle classes, leaving the interests of the ruling rich largely intact. As Klein (2008) argues, the crisis also showed that governments can act decisively and mobilise very large resources to solve problems when the system itself is seen to be at risk. If billions can be spent to bail out banks and billions more created in the US and elsewhere as 'stimulus' to restart flagging economies, why could not much smaller sums be used more constructively to preserve and enhance health-care systems?

Of course, in the current context, in which the ideological climate has moved firmly against the welfarist consensus of the past, the cuts and 'reforms' have never been simply a question of saving money or ensuring fiscal correctness: they have been targeted in a specific way, with an underlying intention to undermine public-sector provision so as to ensure that increasing numbers of the middle classes will begin to question the value of the services they get for their taxes.

As McKee and Stuckler (2011) argue, this can open up a situation in which 'public services will become like public hospitals in the United States, a service for the poor'. Drechsler and Jütting (2007) note the case of Chile, where public health care was consciously downgraded and, as a result, abandoned by the rich, who opted for private health care – making public provision 'de facto an insurance of last resort'. Systematically undermining confidence and public support can in time open up a possibility of further withdrawing public funding for health and other welfare services, leaving the lower and middle classes to fend for themselves as best they can – a policy which can benefit only 'the very rich, who no longer have to pay for services they never used anyway' (McKee and Stuckler 2011).

So the 'reforms' proposed for health care and presented under the general guise of reducing costs (with the IMF, entering the arena of health reform, even creating new jargon to describe 'Excess Cost Growth' (Clements et al. 2012)) turn out to have a consistent ideological thrust and not to prioritise cost-cutting at all.

In fact, on closer examination, the main 'reform' menu promoted by the IMF, the OECD and the World Bank (and obediently echoed by many academics eager for their generous research grants) are not centred on costs at all or on any real evidence of effectiveness. Instead, ignoring all the negative experience of recent decades, they continue to promote the 'zombie' policy prescriptions of New Public Management. Evans (1997: 432) points out 'the advocates of private markets tend to make arguments as if the last forty years had never occurred' while McIntyre and colleagues (2007) state that 'many of the assumptions underpinning the health sector reforms initiated since the 1980s have been shown to be invalid' and call for 'more rigorous evidence to support health sector policymaking'. Whitehead, Dahlgren and McIntyre sum up by asking:

> Do we have an 'evidence-free zone' around the health sector reforms that have been taking place over the last few decades?
>
> (2007: 354)

Given the dominant role of public sector and social insurance systems in health care across much of the OECD, neoliberal values have in many cases been translated into health-sector reforms through the combination of theories which has become collectively known as 'New Public Management' (NPM). The NPM approach aims to model public services on (initially US) private-sector assumptions, theories and practices, and to make public services feel and operate like private businesses (Hood 1991, Osborne and Gaebler 1992, Newman 2000, Preker and Harding 2003). The 'key levers' of reform have been itemised as:

- Privatisation of functions 'better performed by businesses operating in competitive markets'
- Uncoupling steering and rowing [separating purchasers/commissioners from providers]
- Performance measurement and performance contracts
- Decentralisation of authority
- Public–private competition
- Accountability to customers through choice, customer service standards and customer redress.

(Osborne and Plastrik 1998: 36)

There is a substantial and growing literature on both the NPM and its application to health care, which will not be detailed here. However, it is clear that within the literature there are critics as well as enthusiasts for NPM and its applicability to health care in particular. Pollitt (2000, 2003) is one of several who have emphasised how partial have been the attempts to evaluate NPM policies and methods where they have been introduced and the severe limitations of the studies that have been attempted (Pollitt 2000: 187). Simonet (2011), in an otherwise terribly confused article, asks why NPM has remained so popular despite 'relative failure and little success'. He points out that it has been differently interpreted in different countries, although it began 'with its emphasis on health care as a private consumer good, on outsourcing, on quasi-market competition': in some contexts, by contrast, it has been:

superseded by a public health model that aims for public values (e.g. equity, access to care) and population-based outcomes.

(Simonet 2011: 824)

In other words, NPM has been most acceptable where its main principles have not been applied and opposing values have been embraced instead.

The pro-market assumptions of the NPM approach often sit uneasily in policy documents alongside professions of concern for 'equity' and maximum access to services for the poor, and there is little to support the assumption that NPM delivers compensating economies or increased efficiencies in the operation of the public sector (Pollitt 2000, Manning 2000). The Australian experience of NPM in nursing has been that nurse managers found their ability to manage services and provide professional and clinical leadership was 'seriously diminished', along with job satis-faction and confidence in future services (Newman and Lawler 2009).

In the twenty-first century, some of the hype and jargon of NPM may have been dropped but the ideological consequences linger on as an expensive burden on health care. It remains a vehicle for the introduction of the neoliberal project.

As Connell and colleagues point out, the neoliberal/NPM approach opens up space for an expansion of private providers:

> Under neoliberalism private, and specifically the corporate part of the health sector, is allowed to grow, fuelled by demand from the affluent, subsidies from government, and the profit logic of insurance firms – which themselves are being transformed from mutuals [a kind of cooperative] into profit-seeking corpora-tions. Under this regime private care becomes normative, and public health care becomes a residual system, the second best choice for those who can't afford the real thing.
>
> (Connell et al. 2009: 332)

The expansion of private-sector providers, driven by government subsidy and feeding from public and social insurance budgets in the absence of any organic growth of a genuine competitive market, has become a major feature of the changes in health-care systems in many OECD countries; and it is clearly becoming a model for export to middle- and low-income countries as well.

For the purposes of this investigation, it is useful to note that the shotgun marriage of NPM with health systems outside the USA has brought a steadily increasing series of measures making reference to such stock NPM shibboleths as:

- **Competition** ('managed' or otherwise) – but with little discussion of the surplus of capacity that needs to be in place to enable unfettered patient choice, or the poten-tial cost of so much additional (under-used) capacity. Advocates of the merits of competition often seem unable to grapple with the actual issues and contradictions of existing systems in the real world.

- **Contracting out** – increasingly of clinical as well as non-clinical services. This is often linked to various forms of privatisation but always to increased fragmentation and complexity of systems, with a question mark over quality and local and wider accountability.

- **Various forms of increased local autonomy** for hospitals – encouraging public-sector hospitals to break from their public service ethos and behave as businesses.

- **Decentralisation** – although the extent of the loss of central control is often in question.

- **Public–private partnerships**, few of which attempt any examination of the poten-tial conflict of interest between public and private sectors – such as the vexed issue of developing and retaining appropriately skilled human resources.

- **User choice and user empowerment** – concepts which could fit more appro-priately into an agenda for a collaborative, cooperative system than one in which policy decisions of purchasers and providers are shaped by market pressures and competition.

- The introduction of **internal or quasi-markets**, separating purchasers ('steering, not rowing') from providers, again with little debate over the potentially inflated overhead and administrative costs involved or the resultant lost opportunity for local, regional or national government to plan the efficient and equitable allocation of resources according to social and health needs.

- And seeking ways to draw in **private insurers**, initially to offer supplementary cover but in many cases seeing a key role for private health insurance, regardless of the many well-attested risks and market failures that can make such policies expensive and inequitable.

The neoliberal/NPM policy package is of dubious value even for the wealthier countries but it can be even more wasteful and disruptive in the context of resource-poor developing countries. As early as 1998, one of the most eager advocates of NPM, Allen Schick, learning from bitter experience, was urging low-income countries not to attempt reforms based on NPM (Schick 1998).

Overview: limits to the health-care market

Within a free-market system, the main drivers are competition and private and corporate gain. In private-sector enterprises, these gains generally take the form of profits and shareholder dividends: but where market-style competition is introduced within a public-sector framework, the gains may take the form of increased revenues for providers. This results in surpluses and the possibility of enhanced rewards for executives and other sections of staff – at the expense of the less-successful providers, which may face loss of contracts, budget reductions, redundancies or even closure. Interestingly, as Lenin pointed out in his detailed critique of the emerging global capitalist system at the beginning of the twentieth century, the end product of competition is the opposite – *monopoly*, the dominance of a few massive global players controlling markets and making it close to impossible for rivals to emerge and gain access to significant shares of those markets.[1] There is plenty of evidence that this has taken place on a large scale in the pharmaceutical industry and in other sectors relevant to health, especially in the USA, although this aspect of competition is prudently never referred to by those who see it as a driver to force down prices and force up efficiency and quality.

While there may be a by-product of heightened prestige for the most successful public-sector providers, it is clear that the introduction of a market mechanism focuses much more strongly, if not exclusively, on the exchange-value (money) element of health care as a business, rather than on the use values delivered by health

---

1   'Capitalism in its imperialist stage leads right up to the most comprehensive socialisation of production: it, so to speak, drags the capitalists, against their will and consciousness, into some sort of new social order, a transitional one from complete free competition to complete socialisation. Production becomes social, but appropriation remains private. The social means of production remain the private property of the few. The general framework of formally recognised fee competition remains, but the yoke of a few monopolists on the rest of the population becomes a hundred times heavier, more burdensome and intolerable.' (Lenin 1917)

care as a service and public good: health care is effectively commodified through market measures.

Unregulated markets make no reference to equity and represent a direct opposite to centralised planning: however, despite claims that competition necessarily leads to lower prices and improved efficiency and cost-effectiveness,[2] the opposite is often true. In health care, markets which are less than perfect (in other words all actually existing competitive markets) create and encourage many perverse incentives – as can be seen in the USA.

This is one of the reasons why, even in many otherwise-neoliberal proposals for health-care system reform, it is generally accepted that the outright privatisation of existing health-care systems, to replicate the dominance of private provision in the US model, is not desirable (Maynard and Bloor 2000). As Evans (1997) points out, there is no health system anywhere in the world that relies exclusively upon competition and market mechanisms. The US system itself evolved some time ago away from a largely unrestricted free market in health care, exhibiting what Enthoven (1997) describes as 'profound and multifaceted market failure', towards more regulated regimes of 'managed care' (Marmor 1998, Enthoven 1997). Hence the limited objectives of the Obama reforms to reorganise the system around the rooted vested interests of the private providers and private insurance industry.

In fact, while it is possible to envisage a publicly provided health-care system with no private-sector involvement, the private sector remains in many ways dependent upon the existence of a public-sector infrastructure and government intervention. Only with the involvement of public or collective health budgets is it possible for the majority of the population (and therefore most of the 'market' for services) to afford access to health care, which they otherwise could not pay for. In more and more instances, the private sector benefits from this, picking up profitable contracts to treat patients paid for by public health budgets and filling otherwise-surplus private beds and facilities with patients they would not otherwise have.

In almost every OECD country, public-sector hospitals are the largest facilities and the only ones able to offer a full range of services, with multi-disciplinary teams and the resources to treat the chronic sick, complex cases and high-risk patients without first considering the balance sheet. As such, they provide a dumping ground for the private sector, not only taking the poor but also providing a safety net for patients receiving elective treatment in private hospitals who may develop complications and need emergency care.

Private health providers also depend on a vast hidden subsidy from the public sector, which, through educational services and public-sector hospitals, community and primary care services, trains the overwhelming majority of health professionals. Many of these doctors, nurses, therapists, technicians and other specialist staff are

---

2   The OECD's recent major study on competition begins by arguing that: 'The introduction of competition has mainly been motivated by increasing healthcare expenditures. ... Attempts to control costs by regulatory means, such as reducing fees paid to health-care providers and rationing user access, have typically only been temporarily successful. Market-oriented approaches have been introduced to foster productivity with the objective of cutting costs without reducing quality or entitlements' (OECD 2012c: 9).

then 'poached' to work in small private-sector services which provide no training themselves and do not contribute towards its costs.

Another hidden subsidy comes in the form of public-sector research: much of the work that opens the way for the 'innovative' techniques which are later trumpeted and exploited for profit by the private sector is conducted in public-sector hospitals and institutions, funded or subsidised through public or collective health budgets.

And of course, the private sector needs government to take an active role to regulate and maintain standards in the health-care marketplace, to limit the frequency, scale and visibility of multiple market failures, and to allow private medicine to appear much more socially acceptable than would otherwise be the case. As Gupta et al. point out:

> If a country is willing to let healthcare be rationed among its citizens by price and ability to pay, then it can delegate most of the functions to be performed by the health system to market forces, and use regulation to make private markets function honestly and efficiently. If a country aspires to a roughly egalitarian health system, in which the quality of healthcare is to be roughly the same for everyone regardless of socioeconomic status, then government inevitably needs to step in, as well as strictly monitor and regulate the private sector.
>
> (Gupta et al. 2012: 11)

It is the 'managed care' devices developed in the US intended to *regulate* the market, rather than the extravagant, fraud-ridden, bureaucratic and socially exclusive US system itself, which governments elsewhere have sought to emulate, especially as a result of the efforts of Enthoven and others (Enthoven 1985).

Over and above seeking to avoid the high and escalating costs and problems of a US-style system, most World Bank policy documents since the mid-1990s have also tended to accept that some form of collective risk-sharing and public-sector provision is necessary in developing countries. This is often only to provide subsidies to private insurers and the most basic infrastructure of primary care and preventive services, leaving more expensive hospital and specialist services as the prerogatives of the private sector (World Bank 1993). As a result, there has been a certain convergence between the Bank and the WHO at the level of the 'essential package' of care (Buse and Walt 2000a).

Many of the health-system reforms that have been implemented in the last 15 years have *begun* with neoliberal ideology – of 'small government', low taxes, decentralisation, competition, privatisation and consumer power. Yet ironically, in many cases – perhaps all – the end result of such reforms has been *increased* state spending, massively inflated costs, more bureaucracy and colossal waste (Hay 2001, Leys 2001, Leys and Player 2011, Fox 2009)[3] – and of course, the ultimate dependence

---

3   It is estimated that these changes increased NHS overhead costs, from 8 per cent in 1991–2 to 11 per cent in 1995–6 and increased administrative staff by 15 per cent and general and senior managers by 133 per cent. Between 1995 and 2008, Department of Health statistics show that numbers of (whole time equivalent) senior staff rose by another 91 per cent, more than double the 35 per cent increase in the total of doctors and nurses.

of the banks upon national governments to bail them out of the financial crisis their reckless actions triggered in 2007–8.

The 1989, British health-care reforms – pushed through by the Thatcher government despite popular and professional opposition – were widely quoted as a model for reforms to restructure similarly centralised systems along market lines (Busse et al. 2002). However, amid doubts over the extent to which these and subsequent market-style reforms have delivered their promised improvements in efficiency or effectiveness, relatively few wealthier countries tried to follow Thatcher's route of imposing unpopular policies in one 'big bang' reform package (Maynard and Bloor 2000: 6, Smith 2000: 4, Danzon 2002).

Desperately seeking evidence – the OECD and market-style reforms

In October 2010, health ministers from 30 of the world's richest countries, the member states of the Organisation for Economic Cooperation and Development (OECD), met in Paris to discuss 'Health system priorities in the aftermath of the crisis'. This came six years after the first-ever meeting of OECD health ministers in 2004 had effectively backed away from embracing some of the more radical pro-market 'reforms' that were then being driven through by countries such as the United Kingdom (England) and Portugal.

In the aftermath of the 2008 banking crisis, ministers were looking for 'tough choices' in order to improve health-system performance in the context of a long-term squeeze on public-sector budgets as the recession took hold. In most countries up to this point, the health system had been one part of the economy not particularly affected by the crisis and the subsequent recession. However, public-sector deficits were unsustainably high in many countries and nobody wanted to raise additional funds by taxing the wealthy, the banks or corporations and so, as a result, some countries had already been forced to make sharp cuts in public expenditure.

The urgent need to find ways to control spending whilst maximising the efficiency and effectiveness of health care may be greater than before; but there is still little or no evidence that market-style reforms and the use of private-sector providers can deliver either efficiency or economy. The OECD country with the most notoriously expensive, the least inclusive and the most inequitable health-care system is the one with the greatest reliance on 'market' forces and competing providers – the USA.

Back in 2004, OECD researchers drafting the ambitiously titled report *Towards High-performing Health Systems* for health ministers had struggled to find good arguments in favour of many market-style reforms (OECD 2004). A central issue was seen to be the appropriate role and methods of regulating the private sector, which

---

Senior management numbers peaked at almost 45,000 in 2009, but after two years of reductions the total was still 82 per cent higher in 2011 than in 1995 (Health and Social Care Information Centre 2012). So this is hardly a reduction in cost or an exercise in small government.

was implicitly assumed to play a valuable role, although no satisfactory means of regulation had been discovered.

The final chapter of the 2004 report looked at 'increasing value for money in health systems' – but was forced to dismiss as unproven many of the stock policies proposed by pro-marketeers, such as cost sharing; the purchaser–provider split; decentralisation; payment by results (activity-based systems of payment); and competition between providers. All these policies, widely touted by pro-market academics and policy-makers, were found wanting, while contracting out (i.e. privatisation) of support services was given only the most fleeting and uncritical attention.

The section on private insurance and efficiency underlined the concern that although, in theory, private insurance schemes could employ market power to secure cost-effective health-care delivery, in practice most of the evidence, especially from the US, suggests that they do not and will not reliably do so. US-style 'managed care' schemes may have delivered short-term efficiencies through selective contracting with providers (Colombo 2007) but they have since tended to break down under pressure from providers and consumers, in the relentless rise in US health spending that has mushroomed from just $75 billion in 1970 ($356 per person) to $2.6 trillion ($8,402 per person) in 2010 (KFF 2012).

In any event, the report concluded, genuine competition in health-insurance markets was limited in OECD countries – and where it did occur, it offered no guaranteed improvements in cost-efficiency.

Dissatisfied but still not deterred, the ministerial meeting immediately mandated a further round of research and discussion, with increased resources allocated from a range of sources including individual member states. As a result of all these efforts, a new booklet was published five years later titled *Achieving Better Value for Money in Health Care* (OECD 2009).

But despite deploying the combined research resources of the world's wealthiest countries and generous funding from the European Union, the OECD had still failed to come up with any convincing – or even up-to-date – evidence to support a call for market-style reforms. The new booklet embodied papers from a 2008 one-day conference, many of which were in turn simply a rehash of material dating back to 2006. One aim of the 2008 conference had been to 'identify a checklist of policies or good practices worthy of consideration by national administrations': but virtually none of the ideas discussed stood up to any objective scrutiny and it was clear that the evidence cupboard was bare. Many examples harked back 15 years or more to the controversial 'internal market' experiment carried out by the British Conservative government in the 1990s, while others were simply assertions, not backed by any references or examples. The argument peters out after the sad phrase:

> Finally, the evidence base for setting policy in this domain remains feeble and there is a pressing need for more and better research.
>
> (Ibid.: 72)

Two decades or more of agitation from the neoliberal right for governments to adopt market-style reforms in health care had yielded no significant hard evidence to support their argument. This of course has not been enough to deter the neoliberals, whose policies have always been based on ideology rather than pragmatism or evidence. In 2012, the OECD researchers came up with an even bigger volume of material, *Competition in Hospital Services*: but the larger number of words did not result in a qualitatively stronger analysis. Indeed, one overwhelming theme is that regulation and government involvement, rather than competition, are the key to prevent the private sector from amassing profits, widening inequities and ignoring and excluding the poor:

> Competition is a difficult concept. Difficulties are exacerbated by different associations with the concept. In the health care literature competition is often associated with privatisation and 'laissez faire'. It is likewise equated with compromised public health objectives and deteriorating health outcomes.
>
> (OECD 2012c: 26)

Competition on price is especially suspect, tending to lead to reduced quality of services:

> It is clear that a well-functioning competitive process will drive firms to lower their costs in order to improve their competitive situation. In hospital markets with fixed prices and asymmetric information for example, competition may result in suboptimal levels of quality being provided. While this does not affect the competitive process and is indeed only a manifestation of a functioning competitive process, it is typically not associated with positive outcomes.
>
> (Ibid.: 27)

Interestingly, OECD researchers contest the notion that this loss of quality is a 'market failure': rather, they argue it is a result of the market working successfully – but delivering undesirable consequences!

The main burden of demonstrating a positive value to competition in the latest OECD volume falls upon the 'expert' analysis of two papers supplied by Zack Cooper from the London School of Economics, based on his team's curious analysis of data from the UK NHS. Both papers have been hotly and consistently challenged by other academics for their flawed methodology (Pollock et al. 2011a, 2011b), while this author would suggest that the premise of seeking to measure the effectiveness of competition by measuring death rates – using old figures – on specific services where competition does not apply tends, if anything, to underline the desperate lack of solid evidence available to back the claims of the pro-marketeers.

Meanwhile, another weighty tome, this time from the IMF, has also taken up the struggle to find evidence for the neoliberal menu of market-style reforms (Clements et al. 2012). This also faces the limitations and limited objectives of the reforms, admitting that the main focus is not cost saving:

> Recent healthcare reforms in most countries are unlikely to alter long-term public health spending trends.
>
> (Ibid.: 10)

Although the implicit presumption of the IMF approach is that there must be a way in which the private sector and market forces can somehow play a constructive role in improving the efficiency and quality of health care, the evident problems with this view and the lack of evidence to support it mean that a more balanced approach has to be taken. Cheng and Reinhardt warn that the idea that all or most social problems can be solved through a competitive free market approach is 'like a religious belief that need not be questioned' among some policy analysts and management consultants (2012: 78).

While, hypothetically, markets can be regulated and contradictions and perverse incentives can be contained, in practice the weaknesses are hard to tackle:

> The role of the private sector is constrained by market imperfections such as asymmetric information, lack of transparency in pricing, and monopoly power.
>
> (Clements et al. 2012: 11)

> Private payers are also associated with higher administrative costs, which increase overall expenses.
>
> (Kanzler and Ng 2012: 62)

Nor are the problems merely theoretical: while the researchers struggle to shape evidence to suit their foregone conclusions, in the real world of people and politics, governments that have tried more recently to drive through far-reaching reforms and restructuring, such as those of Bulgaria and Romania, have run into serious popular opposition (Stoiciu 2012, Ilie 2012). Even the British Conservative-led coalition government faced stiff opposition and took 16 months to force their highly controversial market-style reforms through parliament (Lister 2012a, Lister 2012b). In recent years only the government of the Netherlands appears to have managed to carry through a similar radical restructuring of its health-care system without facing severe political problems – and some of the consequences of these policies are now becoming more obvious, meaning that 'the jury is still out' (van de Ven and Schut 2008, Maarse 2012).

Wherever in middle- and low-income countries attempts have been made – almost always at the instigation of external global agencies – to implement market-style reforms, the political and practical obstacles have centred on the hard fact that, in societies polarised by class division between rich and poor, the main burdens of ill health and illness are directly related to poverty – and poor people cannot afford market prices for health care. As Hsiao and Heller have argued, in low-income countries 'the average cost of a hospitalization typically exceeds the annual median household income' (2007: 6–7).

As a commodity with an exchange value which is likely to be least affordable to those for whom its use value is greatest, health care is not readily suited to a competitive market. In a sector like this with no organic market based on conventional supply and demand, the effectiveness and usefulness of market forces are plainly limited – if not completely irrelevant. Those most needing health care tend to be the very old (who are systematically ignored by the MDGs) and the very young. Both of these groups tend to be among the poorest groups: so the vast potential 'market' for health-care services in the developing world is largely composed of individuals and countries least able to pay for them. Health care in many poorer countries and poorer areas is correspondingly less likely to attract sustained investment by hospital corporations or by drug companies that follow purely market criteria. Indeed, even its most avid proponents have to admit that private health insurance tends to be most developed in low- and middle-income countries, where the levels of inequality are the highest, and to focus on the highest-income groups, leaving the poor to whatever public health care might be available:

> Private for-profit health insurance does benefit from an unequal distribution of wealth, because the rich are more likely than others to buy coverage, even if it is provided through other channels.
>
> (Drechsler and Jütting 2007: 40)

Noting that market reforms are based on ideology and not evidence, the remainder of this chapter will explore the results of some of the market-style measures that have been brought forward as part of the international reform agenda.

Features of market-style (ideologically driven, restructuring) reforms
- Competition
- Contracting
- Provider-payment reform
- Decentralisation
- Provider autonomy/entrepreneurialism
- Public services purchase care from private sector
- Privatisation
- User fees as market-style reform to expand private insurance
- Managerial control over medical professionals
- Patient's choice/consumerism
- PFI and Public Private Partnerships
- Managed care
- Medical savings accounts

Competition

The triumph of hope over experience is neatly expressed in the latest offering on health reform from the IMF, where Gupta and colleagues rehash an old, evidence-free mantra:

> Among micro-level reforms, strengthening market mechanisms – increasing patient choice of insurers, allowing greater competition between insurance,

relying on the greater degree of private provision and allowing local competition between providers – are particularly effective in containing costs.

(Gupta et al. 2012: 12)

The evidence for this assertion? Not experience from any health-care system in the real world but a 'simulation analysis' by Tyson and colleagues (2012: 101–24), which on closer examination is even less convincing. By contrast, the previous chapter of the same IMF volume, by Cheng and Reinhardt, stresses a different picture:

Given these shortfalls from the competitive ideal – asymmetry of information, lack of user-friendly information on quality and prices, and monopoly power on the supply side – it would take an enormous regulatory effort to move healthcare markets closer to the competitive ideal. Indeed one invariably sees attempts to move the health system closer to 'more market' accompanied with a whole host of government regulations, including price regulation, that belie the move to a free market. We see this clearly in the Dutch, German and Swiss systems.

(Cheng and Reinhardt 2012: 80)

Indeed, the Dutch system presents problems for those who argue that competition can contain prices: ever since the 'bold experiment' of the Netherlands government in 2006 to abandon mandatory social insurance in favour of a system based on competing private insurance companies and 'managed competition', health spending has been rising rapidly (Okma et al. 2011, cited by Cheng and Reinhardt 2012). Moreover, 'managed competition' has to be highly regulated by the government, setting global budgets, caps on cost-sharing, fees for specialists and general practitioners, and the prices of hospital services. In other words, it's not really a market at all. Indeed, after a flurry of activity in 2006, the numbers of people switching policies under the new system rapidly fell back to the numbers who had done so before and almost all of these turned out to have been motivated by the price of the policy rather than any issues of quality of care (Brabers et al. 2012).

In addition to the Netherlands, some other OECD countries (Czech Republic, Germany, the Slovak Republic and Switzerland) have strengthened competition between insurers since the early 1990s; but a 2010 study for the OECD shows that in 'most OECD countries, competition is virtually inexistent, as citizens have no choice among insurers for basic coverage (e.g. NHS countries and countries with a unique social insurance system)' (Joumard et al. 2010). The German competitive experiment has been hedged with imposed ceilings on premiums (Lisac et al. 2009).

Brekke and colleagues (2010) drew attention to the 'almost unanimous' academic view that *in theory* competition with fixed prices could lead to improvements in quality, while empirical findings are 'more ambiguous': but there seems to be no real evidence that competition can reduce costs without damaging quality.

Indeed, in the case of insurance funds, it seems from the US experience that if various competing insurers cover a population and negotiate prices separately with health providers, the divided strength of the insurers can result in 'rapid inflation in health care prices' (Cheng and Reinhardt 2012: 82): so competition can force prices up as well as down.

Despite the problems involved in trying to make it work, competition is central to the full operation of the various market-style reforms, since it represents the greatest break from traditional public service notions of planning and centralised state provision and control.[4]

Some continue to argue that competition 'empowers patients' (Bevan and Skellern 2011), although even these authors admit that there are questions to be answered about the cost-effectiveness of competition, about its impact on clinical outcomes[5] and about the problems of relying upon competition as a lever when in many parts of a country there is little meaningful choice of provider and therefore no prospect of competitive pressures.

Some – especially those with a vested interest as major figures from the private sector such as UnitedHealth's Simon Stevens – argue, largely from theory and generalities, that competition can set health providers free, break up bureaucracy, 'raise standards, unleash productivity and improve equity' (Stevens 2011). Others from a more independent point of view are much more sceptical of the minuscule improvement in quality allegedly delivered as a result of competition in the National Health Service, at a time when it was only at a rudimentary level and in a sector to which competition did and does not apply (Mays 2011).

To create conditions for competition – and thus open up the possibility of patient choice – centralised systems must be broken up and decentralised. The policy options for those seeking to introduce competitive systems include almost the full repertoire of market reforms identified at the start of this chapter:

- The restructuring of centralised systems to separate purchasers from providers
- The enhancement of public-sector providers' autonomy and the encouragement of 'entrepreneurialism' and competition between them
- The deregulation of public purchasers (or the adoption of other measures to permit, encourage or compel them to buy services from private rather than public-sector providers)
- The privatisation of publicly run services.

In the English National Health Service, the move to open up a centralised and publicly provided service to competition has required a dramatic investment since 2000 in bureaucracy and management. A complex new system of 'payment by results' has been introduced, establishing a system of cost-per-case funding with fixed prices for NHS providers to replace block contracts and allow the NHS budget to be divided between a variety of public and private for-profit and not-for-profit providers. This has gone along with a subsidised expansion of higher-cost, private-sector provision of elective care for NHS-funded patients, in the form of 'Independent Sector Treatment Centres', initially under the guise of delivering additional capacity to reduce waiting times but later specifically to create 'contestability' and destabilise existing public-sector providers.

---

4   Conspicuously, the promotion of competition comes as the first of the ten principles of the New Public Management as outlined by Osborne and Gaebler (1992).

5   Further questions also need to be asked as to whether the 'empowerment of patients' would result in any improvement – or even potential worsening – of clinical outcomes: would they make evidence-based choices? Harold Shipman, the mass-murderer, was the 'patients' choice' as an ostensibly attentive GP.

The most successful hospital and other provider trusts were encouraged to break from NHS management systems and control to become autonomous 'foundation trusts', accountable no longer to the Secretary of State, local commissioners or strategic health authorities, but to a new independent regulator, Monitor, many of whose staff and senior figures come from McKinsey and other private-sector consultancies (Lister 2008a). Community health services were separated off from the primary care trust bodies that had managed them and opened up for competition, inviting bids from 'third-sector' non-profit organisations and private for-profit organisations like Virgin and Serco.

To police this process of fragmentation of public-sector providers, a new, blatantly biased 'Cooperation and Competition Panel' was established by the Labour government. The Panel was headed by a former boss of a private hospital chain and filled with city accountants and lawyers, with a brief to keep cooperation to a minimum (it was branded 'collusion') and to promote competition at all costs. The Panel has remained as a court of appeal for aggrieved private-sector operators seeking a slice of the NHS budget (Lister 2012a). The extent to which competition needs to be ruthlessly imposed by legal threat was underlined early in 2012 when the Dutch Association of General Practitioners was fined €7.72 million for contravening competition law that protects the free-market principles underpinning Dutch health care. Its alleged crime was unlawfully advising its members that they could restrict the freedom of new GPs to set up practice (Sheldon 2012).

Behind these English-style reforms is a mounting drive by neoliberals within the EU to open up the lucrative $1-trillion-plus European health-care market to a private sector hungry for profit. The market reforms driven through by the UK's right-wing coalition government since 2010 are intended to complete the process of transformation from a public service to a competitive market, and the pressure of EU competition law helps ensure that as each new sector is opened up to competition and private providers move in, it becomes ever more complicated and difficult to reverse the process (Lister 2012a). EU laws, with power over member-state governments and backed up by the WTO, have created what appears to be a one-way valve driving the process towards privatisation but blocking any return to planned systems, or towards democratic control and accountability over services and providers.

Of course, competition brings with it new overheads in the form of regulation and transaction costs. Modern health-care systems are complex and the requirement to formulate precise specifications and standards, then to administer and monitor the resulting contract, means that any efficiency savings that may be generated through competition have to be offset against the overall cost increases. These are among the factors that help push the costs of administering the US health-care system to over 30 per cent of its spending (Light 2003).

Since 1993, the World Bank has seen competitive market systems as a general 'one size fits all' formula, applying to all countries and circumstances. Yet the possibilities for establishing genuine competition between health-care providers, or even 'managed competition' between rival health funds, are largely restricted to the wealthier countries, where budgets are sufficiently large to allow the possibility of surplus capacity and where there are a sufficient number of properly resourced competitors to create the semblance of a 'market'.

Even where a degree of competition exists, it by no means guarantees a positive long-term outcome for health-care services to the poor. One USAID-funded study of Tanzania illustrating this point noted with approval that the public sector is now obliged to compete with private providers on an unusually wide front, whether in curative services at all levels of care in hospitals or even 'in providing preventive and other high-priority public health services.' (Munishi 1995: xvii) Yet the same report also noted the profoundly unequal provision of competitive for-profit private health care in the rural areas. Private provision is concentrated in Dar es Salaam and it is clear that if the private sector emerges as the 'winner' in this type of competition, the end result will be to leave the public sector shouldering the costs of care for the poorest and the rural population – with resulting negative implications for equity.

The same pattern has been noted time and again in low- and middle-income countries around the world. Such competition as there is focuses on the provision of lucrative elective treatment to the middle classes and the wealthy in the cities. In the poorer and rural areas, there is no competition and no interest in private provision (McIntyre et al. 2007).

> Citizens in poor countries and poor-country governments often do not have a choice of health provider. In many instances they are lucky if they have one at all. This means that competition, the main engine for efficiency in the market, is absent. ...
>
> Without a guaranteed minimum standard of health care accessible to all, competition to attract low-income, poorly educated patients will continue to drive a race to the bottom amongst private providers in both price and quality.
>
> (Marriott 2009b: 15, 36)

Indeed, a crucial factor in making competition a positive force in developing countries is a strong, high-quality public sector that can give a real choice to those on low incomes and even force down the prices charged by some private-sector providers (Marriott 2009b: 37).

Not much has changed since the World Health Organization (WHO) concluded from an extensive literature review on contractual efficiency that:

> the conditions necessary for competition, and even contestability, are generally absent from most areas of most low and middle-income countries.
>
> (WHO 1998)

The issue is equally difficult in middle-income countries. Waitzkin (1997) notes the failure of 'managed care' and competition to hold down costs or ensure universal coverage in the USA and warns that attempts to extend these into Latin America, with the prospect of competition between large private companies, are likely to replicate similar problems.

Hsiao and Heller (2007: 18) sum up the reservations of those who are focused on how the policy will work out in practice rather than the fundamentalist zeal of the pro-market theorists:

A blanket policy to allow the health sector to operate fully on a free market basis will not yield efficient outcomes. Market competition can be used only selectively for the benefit of a country's health and welfare.

Contracts between purchasers and providers

For market mechanisms to come into play, a market has to be created through the separation – where they have been linked in a common centralised system – of purchasers and providers. Once the chain of command of a centralised system has been broken in this way, a new system of contracts must be put in place in order to establish the responsibilities and accountability of service providers. The role of government and public agencies is changed from the provision of services to the commissioning and monitoring (sometimes called 'stewardship') of services. The result, a more complex system, is likely to include sharply increased management and administrative costs.

Contracting out services ('steering, not rowing') is part of the economic and 'New Public Management' philosophy dominating much global policy discourse, which aims for a minimal public sector and maximum private involvement. It has been a feature of health policy in the OECD countries since the 1980s but the pace-setter in this, as in many other aspects of the NPM agenda, has been the British government.

The Thatcher government required health authorities to put hospital non-clinical support services[6] out to competitive tender from early 1983 (with competition based on price) – long before hospitals were given local autonomy as trusts or the introduction of the internal market (Lister 2008a). The consequences were severe in terms of the fragmentation of the hospital ward teams and virtual casualisation of the support staff, which also helped to exacerbate a sharp decline in hygiene standards and was in turn followed by a proliferation of hospital-acquired infections: in 2002, an international study established the links between cleaning and hospital-acquired infections (Lethbridge 2012).

A similar process driven by the Victoria Government in Australia in the 1990s had similar effects in terms of a tail-off in quality of support services, the disruption and break-up of ward teams and the willingness of senior managers to gamble with long-term risks in exchange for short-term gains (Young 2008).

While devolved governments in Scotland, and especially in Wales, have subsequently worked to bring support services back 'in-house', there have been only partial and localised attempts to roll back the process in England where it always had its biggest impact. Instead, there has been a continued fragmentation of formerly unified services, coupled with a process of monopolisation of 'competitive' contracts by a handful of powerful multinational corporations (Lister 2008a, Leys and Player 2011).

Since the early heyday of the small, unreliable, low-wage, low-standard private cleaning companies, things have moved on: now the recipients of profitable contracts

---

6 Initially defined as catering, cleaning and laundry services.

are increasingly likely to be large-scale multinational corporations or their subsidiaries. Generalist companies like Serco and Sodexo tender far and wide for a wide range of services both inside and outside the health sector, bringing economic clout, managerial structures and economies of scale – but little or no specific expertise in delivering health-care services. This helps to ensure that the contracts, which are drafted in terms of cash, inputs and outputs, represent a first step away from notions of public service and social solidarity, towards the establishment of health care as a commodity to be bought and sold – and towards a market in which these transactions can take place (Leys 2001).

The replacement of an internal process (of budget allocation and matching resources to needs) with the development of a formal contract between the public purchasing agency and a range of providers – over which the agency has only the indirect control of a customer – also opens up the possibility of contacting *out* (or in more recent jargon 'outsourcing') purchasing services from the private sector in place of publicly owned and run services. Such a culture may also be encouraged at much more local level, sometimes as a precursor to wider-reaching market-style reforms.

In England, the early experiments, in which the goalposts of competitive tendering were successively shifted by government in the mid-1980s to minimise the chances of a successful 'in-house' bid and maximise the prospect of it ending in privatisation, have now been followed up by measures to oblige local commissioners to contract out an ever-wider range of clinical services. This began with the Labour government as part of its 2000 NHS Plan working to bring in private companies on contracts to deliver diagnostic and treatment services, notably CT and MRI scanning (some of which resulted in scans and images being reported by consultants in South Africa), and then elective surgery, to be delivered initially by overseas doctors and professional staff in new for-profit 'Independent Sector Treatment Centres' (Lister 2008a).

The contracts negotiated centrally in the English NHS with the for-profit companies that were brought in to set up new ISTCs to deliver uncomplicated elective surgery, paid for by the public purse, are among the most generous contracts that have been signed. Preferential five-year deals, at rates well above the standard tariff rate within the NHS, and with a guaranteed volume, regardless of how few operations were actually required, were seen by Tony Blair's government as the way to stimulate the growth of a new private sector, creating a competitive pressure on the existing public service. But the contracts were also one-sided: only the private sector could apply, restricting the 'competition' to one between mainly overseas for-profit companies (Player and Leys 2008, Lister 2008a, Leys and Player 2011).

Contracting has now reached well beyond the boundaries of the hospitals. In primary care, having made a major change in GP (family doctor) contracts in 2002, allowing them cheaply to buy their way out of their previous commitment to provide round the clock care for patients on their list, the government followed up with moves to contract out the out-of-hours (OOH) services. One of these contracts, with jack-of-all-trades contractor Serco to provide out-of-hours GP services in the large rural county of Cornwall, has proved a continual source of complaint and controversy: in July 2012, the company was found by the Care Quality Commission to be failing to supply adequate staffing to meet its legal requirements in four areas – and manipulating its daily performance reports. Serco was given 14 days to put things right: but as this study is written, the local hospital trust has complained that, following Serco's introduction of a telephone triage system staffed by people without medical training, the number of emergency cases arriving at accident and emergency departments has risen significantly (Lawrence 2012).

The contracting out of GP services was not restricted to OOH: in 2005, the first APMS (alternative provider of medical services) contracts were opened up for private provision of regular primary care services. A few were controversially awarded to the new UK subsidiary of the US giant multinational UnitedHealth, despite the company at that point lacking any staff or track record of provision of primary care: its only strength appeared to be having employed Simon Stevens, a former health advisor to Tony Blair and architect of many of the Labour government's more far-reaching experiments in market-style reforms (Lister 2008a). Other contracts were awarded to French multinational Atos (which has since become much more notorious in Britain for its role in delivering assessment services designed to reduce sharply the number of disabled people deemed eligible for disability living allowance) and to various new organisations formed by 'entrepreneurial' GPs to cash in on the new openings. By July 2010, nine companies had ten or more contracts and 227 GP surgeries and health centres had been effectively privatised, run for profit by commercial companies paid for through the NHS: they were attracted by the opportunity to gain a toe-hold in a growing market, but also by the prospect of gaining a voice over the allocation of much larger local commissioning budgets (Leys and Player 2011).

Another major area for private-sector involvement and contracting in England has been community health services. From 2006, concerted moves began to split these services away, putting them 'at arm's length' as separate units from the commissioning bodies (primary care trusts) that had been providing them, preparing the ground for them to be offered out for tender, either as a single package of services or split up to make them more attractive to smaller companies.

The Labour government promoted this approach as 'Transforming Community Services', pointing to examples where some of these neglected and under-funded services were of poor quality and implying that almost any new management or ownership would result in improved services. However, some of the first community services to face changes were among those already described as of high quality or 'excellent' – and there is no way to guarantee that contracting out these services, especially in the current tight financial circumstances, could bring any improvement even where quality is poor (Lister 2012c).

Since 2010, the Conservative-led coalition government has cranked up the pace and required a minimum number of local community health services in every area of England to be contracted out to 'any qualified provider' by September 2012. Large-scale community contracts have already been won by Virgin and by Serco which, along with some other private companies, have their eyes on a greater share of the £11 billion community health-care budget (Davies 2012). The controversial Health and Social Care Bill was amended during its lengthy parliamentary process to change the wording from 'any willing provider' (the original formulation used when community services were first opened up to tender under Labour) to 'any qualified provider'. Yet no requisite 'qualification' is stipulated: the list of 'qualified' providers will be drawn up by Monitor – the regulator, with an expanded role from 2013 – with a guiding brief to maximise competition and apply only a 'light touch'.

The fragmentation and privatisation of community health services, following on from the previous ISTC contracts, mark a watershed because, until this point, at least in theory, contracting out could have resulting in a contract going either to a public-sector (in-house or a rival provider) or private-sector provider. This was excluded for ISTCs and is no longer an option with many community services, where existing in-house management teams have concentrated all of their energies on breaking away from the NHS – dragging their staff with them – and forming some form of 'social enterprise'. The bias throughout has been consistently towards breaking up public-sector providers and bringing in the private sector, whether this be for-profit corporations and companies, charities or 'social enterprises'.

Other varieties of contracting out, or 'outsourcing', have emerged in the neoliberal forcing house of the English NHS since 2000: there have been experiments, not all of them very successful, with outsourcing the transcription and typing work of medical secretaries – in some case to call centres and other enterprises in India or the Philippines (*HSJ* Local 2012). Some hospital pathology services and sterile-supplies services have been outsourced, others are being assessed: similar moves have also been proposed for hospital labs in Sweden and family doctor diagnostic lab testing in Ireland (Healthcare Europa 2012).

There have been various moves in England since 2010 to outsource work in the highly sensitive blood transfusion service, whether this be the storage, collection and delivery of blood supplies (Beckford 2011) or, more recently, the bringing in of the investment bankers Lazard to investigate ways of injecting private capital to enable state-owned Plasma Resources UK to 'compete in a global market' (Handal 2012).

Moreover, learning nothing from a hugely unsuccessful experiment in outsourcing the management of Good Hope hospital in the West Midlands, which had to be brought to a premature conclusion by buying out the contractor (Lister 2008b), Labour ministers, followed by the right-wing coalition government, embarked on the contracting out of the management of a small, financially challenged district general hospital, Hinchingbrooke in Cambridgeshire.

The private company, Circle Health, is a provider of small, bijou and high-cost private hospitals and a vehicle for private equity and other investors. But after all the boasts, less than two years on from the contract, the company is struggling, its share price is falling and it is resorting to old-style cuts in staff and services in an attempt to balance the books and deliver a profit (Lister 2013). Nonetheless, there are persistent rumours that up to 21 financially struggling hospital trusts could be handed over to private management – and furtive preliminary discussions have taken place with the German private hospital giant Helios (Clover 2012).

Nor is the British government alone in seeking private solutions to public-sector debts: in Greece, it seems likely that the all-powerful troika of the IMF, the European Central Bank and the EU may force the government to hand over the country's underperforming public hospitals to private-sector management. In Poland, health reforms passed by the right-wing government in 2011 put the responsibility for debt-laden local hospitals in the hands of local authorities, which have the option to convert them into commercial enterprises (Healthcare Europa 2012).

The Labour government was also eager to encourage the use of external contractors – in the form of management consultants – to advise and effectively steer much of the commissioning work of the NHS local commissioning bodies, the primary care trusts, which have assumed responsibility for the spending of 80 per cent of the NHS budget in England. So in 2007 it established an approved list of 14 companies, mainly major US and UK health insurers or city management consultancies and accountants, to provide 'support' in what was termed the Framework for Procuring External Support for Commissioners (FESC) – resulting in the prospect of the process of privatisation itself being privatised and steered by private companies (Lister 2008a, Leys and Player 2011). The proliferation of consultancy work from companies such as McKinsey, Ernst & Young, PricewaterhouseCoopers and KPMG has followed, effectively marginalising many of the senior public-sector management teams which had previously been expected to carry out this work.

Wherever contracting takes place, contracts may be enforced either positively, through incentives for providers to meet targets, or (less frequently) negatively through the imposition of sanctions in the case of failure. In many cases (including in England), the early 'contracts' are better described as planning agreements since they did not have the legal force of a normal commercial contract and the purchasers lacked any effective sanction in the case of failure, other than to seek an alternative provider (Palmer 2000).[7]

However, the 'contract culture' that emerged from the 'new managerialism' of the 1980s leaves a number of unresolved problems, notably that of:

> how to be sure that when an organisation or individual is recruited to pursue the interests of the purchaser, they do not use it as an opportunity to pursue their own interests. Contracts always have 'gaps', performance indicators can always be manipulated or used perversely, and even worse, as 'contract culture' takes over from trust and good will, everyone looks to exploit these opportunities more forcefully.
>
> (Ling 2000: 99)

Another perennial difficulty with contracts is that they require expertise in drawing up precise specifications and constant monitoring if they are to be upheld. In Romania, for example, where a system of contracts including an age-weighted capitation fee for each doctor's list was used to improve primary care services from 1994, purchasing authorities were found to have insufficient capacity and experience:

> Policymakers had to strike a balance to avoid under- or over-specifying service requirements, to set workable and monitorable performance targets, to allow the flexibility to respond to demand, and to protect the funding system against abuse and budget blowouts.
>
> (Vladescu and Radulescu 2002)

---

7   In Britain, new regulations making contracts between hospital trusts and primary care trusts legally binding began in the spring of 2004, amid warnings that the new system would 'throw up even bigger risks and challenges' (Plumridge and Kemp 2004).

Another difficulty with contracts revolves around fixing the length of the agreement: too short a period can serve to deter providers from any longer-term investment in capacity, whereas too long a contract can remove any incentive to innovate and effectively neutralise competitive pressures (Palmer 2000).

The level of expertise and the challenge of regulating the quality and contract compliance of external providers is a serious challenge in the OECD countries and has had mixed results: but it is an even bigger challenge in the developing countries and low-income countries where management expertise is at a premium, providers are thin on the ground and resources are limited.

Palmer notes that:

> It is unlikely that any approach to contracting can be comprehensively transposed from developed country markets for health, which in turn are not functioning entirely as envisaged, to the different environments of a range of low- and middle-income countries.
>
> (Palmer 2000: 826)

Even a pro-contracting enthusiast like the World Bank's Maureen Lewis has to accept that:

> Where government oversight is weak, there are limited private and NGO options, or where shifts in government administration lead to changes in contracting arrangements, the use of contractors can be problematic. Managing a poorly performing contractor can be costly in both time and money. While contracting out can work, it is not a panacea.
>
> (Lewis 2008)

While the ideological commitment to market-style measures may be strong and the market-driven pressures on health-care systems may press in the direction of tighter contracts, the progress has not been even. Abrantes (2003) points to the varying levels of progress towards contract-based service provision in the Southern Cone countries of Latin America, while Slack and Savedoff (2001) identify a large variety of types of contract in Latin America and the Caribbean countries.

Nor is the mere existence of a contract sufficient to ensure control and the delivery of targets. Slack and Savedoff, examining the working of these systems, identified a number of issues that show a need for more precision and monitoring if the contract is to deliver the intended results. Examples singled out show that:

- Fee-for-service contracts with no volume restriction carry no incentive to keep costs down: Slack and Savedoff noted that in Uruguay high-tech services from private facilities were 20–25 per cent more expensive than those from public units.
- Fee-for-service contracts with volume restrictions give an incentive to claim for treatments not delivered: in Brazil in 1995, an estimated 28 per cent of hospital inpatient services that were claimed for were not delivered.
- A fee-for-service contract with volume restrictions that was not properly monitored led to increasing numbers of treatments and an overspend of more than $1 billion in Colombia in 1998 (Slack and Savedoff 2001: 20).

Nonetheless, USAID, the British Department for International Development (DFID) and the Asian Development Bank have spent millions of dollars funding large-scale programmes to contract out service delivery to the private sector in countries such as Afghanistan, Bangladesh and Cambodia (Marriott 2011).

According to a literature review by Liu and colleagues (2007), contracting out has been most successful where publicly provided services have been irregular or unavailable but only a minority of schemes have assessed the issues of equity, quality or efficiency. They suggest that more evidence is needed on the 'programme effects' of contracting out, not least 'assessments that incorporate a more comprehensive treatment of the costs of contracting out (from the perspectives of the purchaser, the provider and the household)' and hidden costs, such as the fact that:

> introducing contracting in areas with existing public service delivery may result in further fragmentation of health care systems, and linking payment to specified services may lead to gaming of the system and, as a result, reduced availability and quality of non-focal services.
>
> (Liu et al. 2007: 12)

In the WHO's Eastern Mediterranean Region (which reaches as far east as Afghanistan and Pakistan), Siddiqi and colleagues found that Afghanistan, Egypt, the Islamic Republic of Iran and Pakistan had experience with outsourcing of primary care services; Jordan, Lebanon and Tunisia extensively contracted out hospital and ambulatory care services; while Bahrain, Morocco and the Syrian Arab Republic outsourced mainly non-clinical services (WHO Eastern Mediterranean Regional Office 2012). Although drawing generally positive conclusions, the authors emphasise the distinctive interests of the contractors, whose central objective was to secure a regular source of revenue and (in the case of NGOs) gain enhanced recognition and credibility.

Interestingly, the sample of ten projects reviewed by the most gung-ho advocates of contracting turn out to be focused on primary care and nutrition services, many of them funded by external donors and all of them delivered by non-profit organisations. They admit that there is little experience in developing countries of contracting with for-profit providers: yet they go on to recommend not only contracting but maximising the amount of autonomy given to contractors (Loevinsohn and Harding 2005). In a later, larger sample of 14 evaluated contracts, as part of a 'Toolkit' to encourage more contracting out, only two of the contractors were for-profit providers, underlining the limited and untypical experience of contracting (Loevinsohn 2008).

The omission is important: in a review of contracting for health, only five studies were found that attempted to compare operating costs between public and private providers (Marriott 2011). Two of the studies (for Bangladesh and Cambodia) found private providers were either less efficient or up to 61 per cent more costly than their public counterparts and two produced inconclusive results (Bloom et al. 2006).

Marriott (2011) also points out that in the case of Cambodia – where the evaluations are considered the most rigorous of all contracting studies and the results widely used by the World Bank and others, and where contracted INGOs achieved improvements in access, equity and quality indicators:

successful outcomes were automatically taken to be a result of contracting out, and other, arguably far more important, factors were played down. These included: salary increases of five to eight times that paid by government; improved staff management including agreements to cease private practice; and drastic reductions or wholesale removal of user fees supported by increases in financing of nearly two and half times that spent in government-run districts.

(Marriott 2011: 18)

Marriott also emphasises the sometimes forgotten increases in costs of management and administration, reaching 13–17 per cent of the budget for nutrition services in Senegal and Madagascar and up to 20 per cent for private management of public hospitals in Chile and Argentina (Ibid.: 18). This extra cost is not necessarily leading to improved quality. Among many examples:

In Lesotho, only 37 per cent of sexually transmitted infection cases were treated correctly by contracted providers compared with 57 per cent and 96 per cent of cases treated in 'large' and 'small' public health facilities respectively.

(Ibid.: 21).

Privatisation

While contracting could involve public-sector providers, possibly in a more commercialised arrangement delivering services to other public-sector organisations, the logical next step is to move towards more substantial privatisation, the private provision of services. As another facet of the New Public Management it comes from the same neoliberal school of policy.

There is a qualitative jump from any form of public provision to privatisation. However tenuous the level of accountability between a public service and the local public, there is no similar accountability in the case of a private provider, who is not bound to serve the public interest and is unlikely to deliver any more than is required under a formal contract. Any arrangement with a private contractor is a substantial step beyond the 'new contractualism' that Schick (1998) detects as the essence of the management reforms implemented by the New Zealand government.

Kay and Thompson (1986), analysing the wholesale sell-offs of major public-sector utilities by the Thatcher government in Britain, famously summed up privatisation as 'a policy in search of a rationale': they pointed to the Treasury's interest in realising the proceeds of such sales, the implicit Thatcherite objective of undermining and disciplining the public-sector trade unions – and 'the promotion of a kind of popular capitalism through wider share ownership'. This latter point underlines the very different tactics and strategy that have been applied by successive governments and in general by governments seeking to open up public and socially funded health-care systems to the private sector: far from a big-bang, high-profile sell off of entire health systems, discrete services and particular sectors have effectively been salami-sliced with as little overt discussion as possible.

Only in Germany, 'the world champion of hospital privatisation', has there been an extensive privatisation of substantially sized full-service and teaching hospitals – and even there it has been controversial, with some schemes abandoned under public pressure (Böhlke et al. 2011, Tiemann et al. 2011).

Since new legislation in May 2007, Swedish counties can sign over the management of entire hospitals or certain services to private companies, although the medical care would still remain tax funded and regulated by contracts with the supervising authority (HOPE 2009).

In Spain, the 'concession' (concesión) system allows a private company to manage a public hospital on a contractual basis – in 2001, for example, management of the biggest public hospital in Madrid was turned over to a private structure. An autonomous community can also draw up a contract with a private health establishment to provide a public health service, along the lines of the 'Concordat' drawn up with private hospitals in England by the UK government in 2000 (Lister 2008a). The Spanish agreement, known as a 'concierto', is also primarily to help shorten waiting lists by allowing the private sector to handle cases for the public health service. In Catalonia, this type of contract represented more than 44 per cent of its health budget in 2005 (HOPE 2009).

In Portugal, half of the country's formerly public hospitals, including the biggest hospitals in Lisbon and Oporto, have been transformed into limited companies, known as 'Hospitais SA', with the state as the sole stakeholder, as a result of legislation in 2003. However, while the private-sector rules still apply to these new bodies, the government had to convert the legal status of the 'Hospitais SA' to public undertakings, so-called 'Hospitais EPE', to allay fears of a privatisation of public hospitals brought on by the new status. These hospitals are now governed by commercial law and enjoy financial and administrative autonomy, although the government remains responsible for providing capital (HOPE 2009).

As the sensitivity over the Portuguese changes shows, privatisation of health and social care is controversial in Europe and generally not seen as popular (Stolt and Winblad 2009): the motives come from neoliberal ideology rather than populism. In 2008, the UK Office for Public Management investigated outsourcing and found that it was 'primarily driven by dogma rather than evidence-based practice' and that there was little evidence that it offered any improved value for money.

The international organisation of public-sector trade unions distinguishes between a number of levels and forms of privatisation:

- Privatisation of ownership – of health facilities and service units
- Privatisation of responsibility – management of public services privatised or state provision withdrawn in favour of private sector
- Privatisation of provision – health-care services contracted out, or even publicly owned facilities leased, to the private sector
- Privatisation of finance – the use of Public Private Partnerships, Public Finance Initiatives, borrowing private capital for public health schemes, charging higher fees for health-care treatment and services, or shifting from public funding of health care to private health insurance

- Privatisation through markets – creating conditions where the private sector can compete with the public sector for government or social insurance scheme funds, where necessary splitting purchasers and providers.

(Public Service International 1999: 9)

Maarse (2006) further distinguishes between privatisation that is 'policy-driven', the result of purposive government action, and that which is driven by other factors. He also distinguishes between privatisation and liberalisation, making the point that many services have been privatised without being fully exposed to the competitive market, allowing the new public provider to enjoy a monopoly position (Maarse 2006: 988).

There is also a distinction to be made between for-profit private providers and not-for profits, certainly in the initial motivation and values of the organisations involved, although the distinction can turn out to be largely theoretical and irrelevant:

In the hospital and nursing home sector, for example, the not-for-profit institutions are thought to seek high quality, high occupancy, and merely 'satisfactory' profits, while for-profit hospitals and nursing homes are thought to maximize the singular goal of profits. In practice, however, both forms of ownership tend to pursue mainly profits and behave similarly, especially in highly competitive markets with some excess capacity.

For-profit enterprises seek profits to enhance the wealth of owners. Not for profits seek 'excess of revenue over expenses' – their delicate term for 'profits' – to announce the power and prestige of the institution by reinvesting these funds in the enterprise for the growth and more prestige.

(Cheng and Reinhardt 2012: 71)

These authors sensibly conclude that it's best to think of 'private sector' as a synonym for 'commercial sector'. The World Bank and IFC come to a similar conclusion for different reasons, lumping the broad mix of non-profits in developing countries together – NGOs, charities, religious organisations, untrained small shopkeepers that informally sell drugs, traditional faith healers and so forth – especially where they are trying to make the case for the vital role of the private sector and the IFC's attempt to kick-start the development of health care in Africa by purely funding the private sector (IFC 2007a, Marriott 2011).

In fact the convergence between non-profit and for-profit is far from theoretical: the contracting out of services to non-profits tends to be part of a market-style restructuring of services that effectively forces the non-profit to compete as a business with the for-profits, including large-scale multinational corporations. In this tough, competitive environment, the non-profits either have to behave like for-profits or lose out to them in future competitive tenders: this has already happened in England with the failure of the first, largest and best-publicised community health social enterprise to win a second contract, losing out expensively to the multinational Virgin group's health-care subsidiary in a £500 million contract over five years. For many critics, this underlined concerns that social enterprise and non-profit businesses are simply a staging post to full-scale privatisation by for-profits (Thiel 2012).

In 2009, a report prepared for PricewaterhouseCoopers revealed the uneven spread of privatisation through health-care systems in Europe (Wootton 2009), identifying Germany as the leader with 26 deals and a thin spread of privatisation across other countries: but the pace has now increased. At the same time, some governments are keen to dump any responsibility for resolving debts in struggling hospitals and are therefore willing to contemplate privatisation of management or outright privatisation (Germany), regardless of the resulting efficiency or value for money (Tiemann et al. 2011). But the overall pattern is an uneven one of numerous piecemeal and partial shifts towards the private sector.

In the past there have been attempts to press home a more thoroughgoing privatised model, especially in middle- and low-income countries. The model aspired to by many neoliberals was the situation in Chile, in which wholesale privatisation of the economy was driven through by the extreme right-wing Pinochet junta after the 1973 coup, with advice from neoliberal guru Milton Friedman and his 'Chicago Boys'. The Pinochet regime did drastically cut health care spending, slashing per capita health spending by more than a third by 1979 and to 34 per cent of its 1974 level by 1990 (Taylor M 2003). The proportion of private beds increased from 10 per cent to 25 per cent between 1981 and 1992.

But such policies could only be sustained under a military dictatorship: the new government from 1990 was obliged to implement substantial increases in government spending on health care, which more than doubled in seven years in the mid-1990s. This increased spending did not reverse Pinochet's expansion of the private sector, which by 2000 collected two-thirds of Chile's health-insurance contributions and 46 per cent of total health spending, but covered just 23 per cent of the population, maintaining a rigorous system of risk-adjusted contributions and excluding those most likely to require health treatment. The system also imposed substantial co-payments for the public-sector service, with some subsidy for the poorest. Yet even at its peak of 'authoritarian neoliberalism', Pinochet's regime pulled back from privatising the entire system and left 75 per cent of hospital beds in the public sector (Taylor M 2003).

Most Latin American countries have had difficulties implementing the neoliberal reform package and most have only implemented aspects of it, such as decentralisation or some form of privatisation. The privatisation of hospitals has led to large investments in improving financial information, estimating costs and developing contract and payment systems, but there is no evidence of an improvement in quality of care (Homedes and Ugalde 2005b).

Developing countries can face pressure from global bodies and from powerful donors (notably the World Bank and USAID) which are ideologically committed to privatisation and the expansion of the private sector (World Bank 1987, 1993, Skaar 1998, Mudyarabikwa 2000, IFC 2002). USAID launched new initiatives (notably Private Sector Partnerships) aimed at expanding the level of private-sector provision in developing countries. The USAID PSP website notes with approval the changes in Indonesia which it claims had:

successfully shifted market share from predominant reliance on the public sector to reliance on the private sector. The Indonesian case study examines the policies and programs implemented to incentivize the private sector to enter the Reproductive Health/Family Planning marketplace.

(PSP 2006)

The lack of state resources for public provision of health care in many developing countries flows from the three-way impasse created by global capitalism in which:

- A very high proportion of the population is poor and/or outside the formal economy, therefore paying little or no tax

- The government is in any event constrained by global creditors such as the IMF and World Bank to keep taxes low and reduce or eliminate tariffs which might otherwise yield resources for health

- And what revenues do come through to the government are largely channelled back to the wealthier countries in the form of debt service.

(WHO 2000, Labonté et al. 2004)

The 'inefficiency' of publicly provided services in these and other countries is a stock assumption made by neoliberals, with seldom any attempt at justification. By contrast, the inherent 'efficiency' of private health providers is also assumed, despite abundant evidence that the overhead costs of the private sector are much higher than publicly funded systems, that the costs of private treatment are higher and that only publicly funded systems have shown themselves able to deliver universal and equal access to services (Hart 2003, PNHP 2003b, Laurell and Arellano 1996).

However, if there are problems managing a publicly funded service, logic suggests the same weak and poorly resourced government would have just as many – if not more – problems in seeking to 'regulate' the activities of a relatively powerful and autonomous private health-care sector – a task which has so far eluded the administration of the world's largest and wealthiest capitalist nation. In the case of developing countries, the resources to train and sustain a skilled management structure as well as front-line service providers are constantly squeezed by the economic pressures outlined above.

The Bank has insisted that publicly funded services are 'inequitable' because the wealthy find ways to seize more than their share could be seen as an argument for progressive systems of taxes (though the Bank never raises any such suggestion): but there is more than ample evidence to demonstrate that *privatised* systems, especially those involving user fees, are even more skewed to favour preferential access for the rich while actively excluding the poor – for example, the majority of Chileans are too poor to afford to use the country's private health care (Taylor M 2003: 40).

Reforming provider payments

The tighter squeeze on public finances and the quest for cost reduction and economies in the aftermath of the 2007–8 financial crash have dovetailed neatly with the quest by private insurers to minimise their outgoings and maximise the profits they retain for distribution to shareholders. In addition, the switch from centralised and publicly provided services to a competitive market system involving a variety of private sector for-profit and non-profit providers has required some method for splitting the former public-health budget and paying out in proportion to the work done.

While Beveridge-style tax-funded systems have traditionally offered their governments the opportunity to restrict individual hospital budgets through a single centralised policy decision, in Bismarck-style systems decentralised payment mechanisms have always involved a form of 'contract' between the insurance funds and the providers of care. Theoretically, this separation of functions offers more scope to constrain the increase in costs: but in practice it has been hard to control the various purchasers of health services and even harder to control the prices charged by what is often a mix of private- and public-sector providers.

Despite this less than convincing experience, one argument for introducing a market-style system to Britain – and to countries which had centrally controlled health-care systems – was that a combination of competition and contracts would offer new mechanisms to restrain provider-led demand and inflation, thus ensuring that, in the famous words of the Thatcher NHS reforms, the 'cash follows the patient' (DoH 1989b). Following this approach, what may begin as a *market-driven* exercise to control costs can lead towards *market-style* policies and reforms – which may, in turn, deliver very different results.

Where provider-payment reforms are introduced purely in the context of cost-cutting, the alternatives include:

- Replacing fee-for-service payments by capitation-based funding for covering a designated population (prospective payment)
- Replacing flexible fee-for-service payments by fixed-price payments for particular treatments, on the basis of diagnostic related groups or the equivalent
- Payment per diem for inpatient treatment
- Payment for designated specialist services, with fixed targets.

Market-style methods might suggest the need for systems which pay hospitals only for the episodes of treatment they deliver (case-based) or the catchment population they agree to cover (capitation-based). Case-based payment can be seen as giving an incentive to respond positively to local demand – or even to compete with other hospitals for patients – while capitation-based contracts encourage hospitals to hold down costs. While it offers a way to contain costs and gives an incentive to integrate and organise services efficiently, the down-side to a capitation-based system is that it can create an incentive to cut costs at the expense of quality, to supply as little treatment as possible and even to ration care for the catchment population. Case-based contracts on the other hand can generate a perverse incentive to treat larger numbers of less-serious cases and to increase the numbers of cases treated – again possibly at the expense of quality – and possibly also increase activity beyond affordable levels (Mannion et al. 2008).

Similar pluses and minuses can be identified for systems which fund hospitals to deliver specific designated care (i.e. setting targets for cardiac or cancer treatment, accompanied by ring-fenced allocations of revenue): while it may be possible to achieve improvements in the designated service, this may well be at the expense of diverting management and staff resources from other areas of care – and reducing any local management flexibility in achieving a balanced service.

A 1998 survey of European health-care systems found that the governments seeking to pay by results were in the minority. Ten of the 16 countries examined used prospective funding systems to set budgets for hospital inpatient services – mostly global budgets, although Germany allocated prospective flexible budgets and Sweden combined prospective payments with a further payment linked to numbers treated (Maceira 1998).[8]

Since that time, there has been a substantial shift towards payment systems geared to tariffs based on the US system of 'diagnosis related groups', which are used in Denmark, Germany, Italy and Hungary. The Netherlands has a system of 'diagnose behandeling combinaties' (Nys and Goffin 2011). In England, Tony Blair's New Labour government used similar 'health care resource groups' as the basis for its controversial reform of financial flows within the English NHS which culminated in the so-called 'payment by results' system – although in practice the payments have no relationship to 'results', being pure fixed-cost-per-case tariffs (Boyle 2011). The intention of this change was clearly linked to the move towards a competitive market in health care and the establishment of 'Independent Sector Treatment Centres', use of a growing range of private-sector providers and the establishment of autonomous hospital 'foundation trusts' standing outside the management structures of the NHS (Lister 2008a).

A new and more sophisticated variation of payment by results to replace DRGs, involving a new 'bundled payment system' that pays a flat package price to cover a whole procedure from start to finish, with a 3 per cent bonus for meeting certain quality standards, is claimed to have cut the cost of hip and knee operations in Sweden by 17 per cent. However, it has resulted in public-sector hospitals carrying a more complex and costly caseload while private-sector hospitals have been able to scoop a growing share of the work (Healthcare Europa 2012).

Some have gone further and experimented with payment for performance (P4P) schemes, such as that implemented in Turkey (Performance Based Supplementary Payments) under their neoliberal Health Transformation Program from 2001, implemented together with the World Bank. This separated out purchasers and providers and gave hospitals financial autonomy, creating a competitive system (Küçükel 2009). Under Turkey's PBSP, hospital medical staff receive bonuses for increased work. One clear result of the program was a massive increase in numbers of patients treated, with 78 per cent more outpatient appointments, 30 per cent more inpatients and a huge 122 per cent increase in operations over the period 2001–6 (Sulku 2011). However, as Sulku points out, the sheer scale of these increases raises some questions over the possibility of supplier-induced demand (unnecessary treatment) and

---

8   The seven countries allocating budgets on a service-based system were Austria, Latvia, Slovakia and Slovenia (each of which paid to some extent on the basis of length of stay in hospital); England (in which payments related to service-level agreements between local purchaser and provider); Finland (with local-level service-based reimbursement); and Hungary (with a performance-related payment system) (Maceira 1998:19).

the quality of care – and concerns that patients were not being kept long enough in hospital. There would also be issues of sustainability if the very rapid increase were to continue. By contrast, linked reforms mean that primary care doctors working in the new 'family doctor' system face financial disincentives to refer people for hospital treatment (OECD 2008).

The issue of provider payment in the USA, closely linked to efforts to control rocketing health spending whilst maximising the margins of the health insurance industry, has created a voluminous and often complex literature focused simultaneously on quality of care (reducing unnecessary treatment) and value for money (see, for example: Tynan and Draper 2008, Mechanic and Altman 2009).

In many developing countries, public-sector health centres and hospitals are still funded according to historic budgets or even on the basis of numbers of staff in post, a system described by Bitran and Yip (1998) as 'the most common method of financing public hospitals in developing countries'. Not only does this replicate each year the chronic underlying lack of resources but, as the authors point out, from a management point of view the system almost inevitably promotes inefficiency, containing no incentive to alter staffing levels, reduce costs or respond to local demand for services.

Provider-payment reform is therefore a key part of the agenda in many emerging economies and developing countries including China (Coughlin 2012).

PFI/PPP and its extension internationally

The British government has pretty much pioneered the concept of the private financing of new hospital and health-care projects through the Private Finance Initiative (PFI) in the last 20 years, which has become a major contentious issue in the 'modernisation' of the British National Health Service. Meanwhile, British-based consultancy firms such as PricewaterhouseCoopers (PWC) and British-led consortia have been at the forefront of efforts to promote this approach – in many countries referred to as 'Public Private Partnerships' (PPP or 3Ps) – on an international level.

A 2010 survey by PWC's 'Health Research Institute' delighted in reports that $4 billion in hospital PPPs had been signed during the first half of 2010, including the €1.5 billion, 700-bed Karolinska in Stockholm and a €375 million, 1,465-bed new hospital in Vigo, in Galicia, northern Spain. Deals for $10 billion of health-care PPP projects in North America had been signed in the previous five years, mainly consisting of almost 50 projects in Canada, in British Columbia, Ontario (27 projects) and Quebec, including the $1.3 billion McGill University Hospital in Montreal. Brazil had opened its first PPP hospital, in Salvador, with another planned in Belo Horizonte alongside PPP-funded primary care facilities. Chile and Peru had embarked on projects. Mexico was planning eight new hospitals on greenfield sites, the first to be in Leon. And South Africa was planning to use PPP to refurbish the giant 2,964-bed Chris Hani Baragwanath Hospital (PWC 2010).

Yet these figures appear somewhat at variance with a PWC presentation of the previous year, which suggested that Canadian health-care PPPs had totalled just

$2.2 billion since 1997: of $38-billion-worth of projects identified, schemes outside Europe were estimated at £5.8 billion in total, £5 billion of which was in Canada and Australia. Among the $31.8 billion of European projects listed, the vast majority (167, worth $23.6 billion) were in the UK (almost all of these in England), 14 ($3.3 billion) were in Spain, 11 ($1.9 billion) in France, 9 ($1.9 billion) in Italy, 4 ($444 million) in Portugal and 2 ($572 million) in Germany, with two small projects, one in the Czech Republic and the other in Iceland (Wootton 2009).

However, since then a major new player has come onto the scene: the Turkish government has begun to select bids for the first of a 'large number' of major hospital projects, worth an estimated at $5 billion between 2010 and 2015. The first was the Kayseri Health Campus, in central Turkey, to include a 1,300-bed general hospital, with 200 mental health beds and 100 high-security forensic mental health beds, in a facility serving a city of almost a million people and a surrounding area with another 1.8 million. The three-year construction is expected to cost about $278 million (€215 million), to be financed over 25 years through a 'Public–Private Partnership' which will allow a private consortium to deliver a complete range of non-clinical support services such as car parking, a hotel, restaurants, a conference centre and pharmacy, taxi and transport services. More hospitals were planned for four other cities, at an estimated €250 million each (Lister 2011b).

PWC look forward to the continuation of this expanding market taking a share of what they project to be steadily rising health spending to 2020 and beyond, talking of a 'trillion dollar market for PPPs in healthcare' (PWC 2010). And more recently, building outwards from a number of projects in Australia, PWC has homed in on potential markets for PPP in south-east Asia, noting the first PPP-financed hospital in the city of Kuantan in Malaysia, the rapid economic growth rates in the region (which offer excellent potential to service hefty PPP loans) and the start of consideration of potential health-care PPP projects (PWC 2012, PWC Australia 2012).

Early in 2004, the EU changed the rules of the Stability Pact underpinning the euro, in order to encourage the use of PFI for public works, by excluding such investment from the total of public debts (as long as the private sector can be shown to be carrying the investment risk) (Murray Brown et al. 2004).

The Turkish government announced that the financing of the Kayseri project was explicitly based on 'successful examples of similar programs in some European countries, in particular the UK' although the rosy picture of the British PPP/PFI scheme is hopelessly unrealistic.

So after 20 years, the country with the highest number of PFI-financed health projects is England, where hospitals worth a total of £11 billion have been built or are under construction, according to official Treasury figures (HM Treasury 2012). However, the lifetime costs, commonly for a period of 30 years or more, are much higher – a staggering £64 billion by the time the final 'unitary charge' payments are made in 2039. The unitary charge is the combined rent and services fee paid to the private consortium that builds and provides non-clinical support services in the hospital. Other than signing off the initial contract, the government is not directly involved: financial problems arising from the constantly increasing unitary charge (generally rising by 2.5 per cent per year or by inflation, irrespective of the income of the hospital) have to be handled by the hospital trust concerned.

PFI first emerged in Britain in 1992 in the aftermath of the Conservative government's market-style reforms, which established the principle of NHS hospital trusts paying 'capital charges' on the value of their property and land assets and on any new capital borrowed from the Treasury. This policy was initially seen as a device to encourage trust managers to sell off any unused or partially used land or buildings at the first opportunity, rather than incur capital charges: but more fundamental was the notion of the NHS as *tenant* rather than landlord, occupying buildings for which it had to pay rather than simply regard as a 'free good' (Lister 2008a).

Conservative Chancellors began a two-pronged approach, which combined a steep reduction in the annual allocation of capital to the NHS with the requirement that any substantial development (initially £5 million or more) had to be advertised and 'tested' in the market under PFI, to investigate whether any private consortium might be prepared to put up the capital, build and operate the hospital, and lease it back to the NHS for a long-term (25–30 year) contract. It was described by the Treasury as changing:

> public sector organisations from being owners of assets and direct providers of services into purchasers of services from the private sector.
>
> (HM Treasury 1997, cited in Pollock et al. 1997)

For various reasons, the private sector could not be convinced to sign such contracts in the NHS until after the change of government in 1997, when New Labour, having first denounced PFI as 'the thin end of the wedge of privatisation', came to office pledged to 'rescue PFI', portraying it as 'a key part of the government's 10-year programme for modernisation'. A short Bill to open up the prospect of PFI deals was rushed through parliament in 1997 and the first hospital contracts were signed almost immediately afterwards (Lister 2008a).

The commitment to PFI became even more obsessive. In its 2000 NHS Plan, the Labour government declared its intention to establish £7 billion worth of PFI hospitals by 2010: that target was exceeded and 85 per cent of all new capital investment in the NHS (and 94 per cent of new hospitals) has since come via PFI, with public funding largely restricted to a few smaller-scale hospitals and refurbishment schemes (Sussex 2001).

As a result, an increasing share of NHS property assets have been privatised: PFI also means that an ever-growing share of NHS funding is flowing straight out of the public sector into the private sector and its shareholders, for whom (despite the rhetoric claiming a 'transfer of risk') completed PFI hospitals are seen as a virtually risk-free income stream. Once they have become PFI lease holders, NHS trusts commonly retain financial control only over those services excluded from PFI – clinical services and the payroll for nurses, doctors and other professionals. Any further financial constraints are therefore more likely to impact directly upon patient care (Lister 2008a).

PFI maintains the appearance of a publicly funded, publicly provided service while in practice diverting very substantial capital and revenue resources into the private sector. The notion that PFI hospitals represent 'value for money' despite their inflated costs has been questioned. The experience of poor quality, poorly designed and inadequately sized buildings with poor quality, privately provided support services has been highlighted in many brand-new PFI hospitals: a number have been obliged to begin extensions to add extra beds and facilities not properly planned into the original building. Management in some (such as the Edinburgh Royal Infirmary) has struggled to solve problems of ventilation and temperature control (Lister 2003a, Lister 2003b, publicprivatefinance.com 2003).

The publicly argued rationale for PFI is that it facilitates swift access to capital investment while deals that remain 'off balance sheet' appear to avoid any increase in government borrowing. When the idea was first formulated by the Conservative government in 1992, this was an especially sensitive issue, being contemporary with debate on the EU's Maastricht Treaty which sought to limit the extent of government borrowing. Advocates of PFI also argue that it transfers risk from the public sector to the private sector (although in practice all the more costly risks and all of the costs remain firmly in the public sector) and that this risk transfer has a monetary value that can mean that even schemes apparently more expensive under PFI than through conventional public procurement can be justified as representing better 'value for money' (Pollock 2004). Along with other skewed calculations that appeared to inflate the cost of theoretical 'public sector comparators' purporting to show PFI as a good deal for the NHS and the taxpayer, some of these were dismissed in 2002 by the auditor general of the National Audit Office, Jeremy Colman, who saw them as ranging from 'spurious' through 'scientific mumbo-jumbo' to 'utter rubbish':

> If the answer comes out wrong, you don't get your project. So the answer doesn't come out wrong very often.
>
> (Timmins 2002)

Most of the detailed negotiations and calculations take place in secret and remain shrouded in commercial confidentiality. This can mean that there is little if any objective scrutiny, with all the information in the hands of people with a vested interest and predisposition to press ahead with the contract. When the calculations go wrong, they can go very wrong indeed; and even some of the relatively low-cost, first-wave PFI schemes are now facing big problems.

In England, where PFI has been shown to represent very poor value for money and an extremely high-cost method of financing hospitals, the prime concern has for some time focused on the issue of affordability: although disastrous contracts now threaten to bankrupt busy hospital trusts and create chaos across a wide area, some especially disastrous schemes were reluctantly weeded out as too expensive to consider. One was a scheme to merge two specialist hospitals and a teaching hospital onto a single 'Paddington Health Campus'. This escalated in cost from £370 million to more than £1 billion and was abandoned as unaffordable; so was an £800-million scheme in Leicestershire (Lister 2008a). However, this level of common sense has not always prevailed and in East London, despite being scaled back to make it more affordable, the PFI contract signed off for the rebuild of the Royal London and Bart's Hospitals was for a building costing £1 billion for 1,000 beds − £1 million per bed − with the eventual repayments over 35 years adding up to an astonishing

£5 billion (HM Treasury 2012). Since then, local cutbacks aimed at generating 'efficiency savings' have announced that at least 200 of the 1,000 expensive beds will not be opened when the hospital is commissioned in 2013 (Health for NE London 2009).

As far back as 2005, an audit – by none other than PWC – warned that one PFI-funded hospital, the £93-million Queen Elizabeth Hospital in Woolwich, SE London, was 'technically bankrupt', having run up a deficit that was set to climb to £100 million by 2008 as a result of unaffordable unitary charge payments. The PFI deal itself was found by PWC to have added £9 million a year to the costs that would have been faced if an equivalent hospital had been funded by the government (Carvel 2005). The unitary charge amounted to 14.6 per cent of the trust's income – so that the payments for the building alone, with index-linked increases each year, came over 35 years to more than five times the initial cost of the project (Lister 2008a: 240).

In an effort to stabilise the finances, the Queen Elizabeth was merged with another costly and unaffordable PFI hospital, belonging to a neighbouring trust (the Princess Royal University Hospital in Bromley), and a nearby non-PFI hospital trust to form one giant, indebted trust covering much of south-east London: the South London Healthcare Trust. That trust, always convulsed by financial problems, is teetering on the edge of bankruptcy as this study is completed and has been placed in the hands of a government administrator (Triggle 2012).

Upwards of 20 more PFI schemes in England, many of them much more expensive than the first wave projects, are now causing significant financial instability. Repeated government interventions have been required since 2011 to keep a number of them afloat and, after a £1.5 billion bail-out proved ineffective, 'hit squads' of management consultants have been sent in during August 2012 to seven of the most wobbly to seek urgent cuts (Campbell 2012).

The situation has got visibly worse since a number of British PFI Hospitals were included among a 'Horrid Hundred' 'Flawed, Failed and Abandoned' P3 schemes reported by Ontario health campaigners in 2005, alongside nine Canadian health PPPs and Australia's disastrous La Trobe Hospital –which lost $10 million in 2000 and threatened to sue the government before being bought out of the contract (Mehra 2005). Even PWC feels obliged to admit to a number of failures in Japan:

> In Japan, there have been several instances where inflexibility in the PPP contracts led to problems later with fixed payments to the private partners for 30 to 40 years. Service provision became so expensive that the government could not continue to make the payments.
>
> (PWC 2010)

The problems work out differently in an alternative to British-style PFI, strongly promoted by PWC and by former World Bank health boss Richard Feachem from his 'Global Health Group' in the University of California. The Alzira Hospital in Valencia, Spain, which has since been the basis of further PPPs in Valencia, was built in 1999 at a cost of €61 million as a Public Private Investment Partnership (PPIP). Its contract required it to provide a full range of hospital services to the local population for a fixed capitation fee and initially promising to deliver services at up to 44 per cent below equivalent costs in Spanish and Valencia hospitals (Acerete et al. 2011). This contract proved literally too good to be true for the purchasers and was abruptly ended, to be replaced by another on more generous terms to the hospital after a lump sum of capital had changed hands.

The new contract included primary care services as well – but was still well below Spanish benchmark costs. How was this to be achieved? The key is 20–25 per cent lower running costs than public-sector hospitals. These were achieved partly by the use of new technology but, more significantly, by the reduction of health-care quality (staffing levels significantly – up to 25 per cent – lower than public-sector hospitals), reduced wage costs (73 per cent of the staff are on the hospital's lower scale of pay and benefits, working longer hours, while the remainder are still covered by their previous public-sector contracts) and by effectively selecting a less complex and costly caseload through the restriction of the range of services the hospital offers, leaving patients needing more sophisticated treatment to use public hospitals instead (Acerete et al. 2011, Bes 2009).

Similar contracts, in which the private sector constructs, maintains and delivers health services, appear to be the basis of a PPP programme for the refurbishment and management of ten hospitals in Portugal (Nikolic and Maikisch 2006).

A third variant model has been the privatised 240-bed St Goran's Hospital in Sweden, run by Capio on a six-year contract with Stockholm County Council that requires the hospital to treat only publicly funded patients and to divert private paying patients to another Capio clinic. The hospital, which had been a pilot project in local autonomy, was controversially sold to Capio in 1999 and transformed into Sweden's first private for-profit hospital: it now functions as a privately owned, publicly funded enterprise and a curious, unique hybrid version of a PPP (Nikolic and Maikisch 2006).

Capital-hungry PFI and occasionally PPP (Public Private Partnership) deals for new hospitals in the wealthy countries are a far cry from the similarly titled 'Global Public Private Partnerships' which are increasingly seen by the WHO and the UN as ways of enlisting private-sector help to carry through immunisation and other health programmes in developing countries (Buse and Walt 2000a). Around 70 such partnerships have been identified, many involving drug companies and research projects (Buse and Waxman 2001). Critics argue that the WHO is potentially vulnerable to political and economic pressure from much wealthier drug companies and private corporations, making any 'partnership' profoundly unequal (Hardon 2000), and warn of the negative impact of 'vertical programs' on basic health-care provision. Such programs have:

> weakened the infrastructure and drained the human resources required for preventing and treating common diseases (such as diarrhoea and upper respiratory tract infections) that may kill many people.
>
> (Hsiao and Heller 2007)

More detail on these 'partnerships' can be found in Chapter 5, above.

Few developing countries will find themselves in a position for PFI to become an option; and it is unlikely that those who closely scrutinise the economics and implications of the first PPIP hospital in Africa – the showpiece $120-million Queen Mamohato Memorial Hospital in Lesotho – would wish to follow the costly road of the Lesotho government or replicate its generosity to the shareholders of the South African multinational Netcare, which stands to profit for 20 year from the deal (more details of this are given above on pages 105–10).

Private-sector lenders and developers know in the high-income countries that they can count on top-sliced funding from substantial public-sector budgets, underwritten by government guarantees. There is seldom anywhere near enough uncommitted funding available in most developing countries to offer the margins that would interest PFI consortia.

Decentralisation – one size does not fit all

The call for 'decentralisation' can be found in almost all studies and reports advocating health-system reform in wealthy and poor countries alike. It is 'generally recognised as a major strategy for health reform' (Rannan-Eliya et al. 1996: 5, Valentine 1998). In abstract, the notion of 'transferring power from unconcerned and inefficient central bureaucrats to the people' is hard to oppose (Homedes and Ugalde 2005b).

Indeed, even neoliberal reformers, such as those of the British Conservative-led coalition government, make use of this populist aspect in dressing up their otherwise unpopular and far from empowering policy proposals (DoH 2012). This is not the first time a verbal change of policy emphasising local control appears to run counter to an accumulation of new central powers and a loss of local accountability in the English NHS (Goddard and Mannion 2006). Of course, from the neoliberal point of view the decentralisation of decision-making and commissioning opens up many more potential avenues for contracts and deals with the private sector – and this is the way the latest English NHS 'reforms' have gone. They remove the responsibility of the Secretary of State for provision of health services, thus giving even greater local decision-making and deniability at ministerial level when controversial policies are pushed through at local level.

An analysis of the effects of decentralising health services in Spain – where regional governments have been facing serious financial problems and found themselves driving through heavy cuts in response to the post 2007–8 banking crash – shows that in general citizens are less satisfied as a result of decentralisation. Concerns focused on primary-care services, waiting times and pressure on hospital wards (Antón et al. 2012).

At a European level, Saltman noted contradictory developments, with Central and Eastern Europe, Spain and Italy focused strongly on decentralisation, while the movement in the Nordic countries has been towards reducing the powers of local and regional government. Many European systems, he notes, 'will continue to see a tightening of state controls, especially over fiscal and quality-related matters' (Saltman 2008: 106).

Yet decentralisation needs to be geared to the specific needs and political–social realities in each country, as much as any element of the generic health-reform prescription: in some instances decentralisation may put power in the hands of social conservatives or religious fundamentalists who may restrict access to sexual and reproductive health services – with serious consequences for women, especially young women (Ostlin 2005).

While its impact depends on circumstances, it is hard to be opposed on principle to the notion of decentralisation: support for some form of decentralisation spans the political spectrum. It has been accepted both by socialists and by the New Right, by the left-leaning governments of Tanzania and Nicaragua, and by Chile's Pinochet dictatorship, as well as the World Bank and USAID.

The general assumption made by advocates of progressive decentralisation is that by breaking down centralised systems and bringing decision making closer to local people, both as providers and consumers of health care, the reform process will improve equity of access for the poor (who can be more influential at local than at national level), improve efficiency and improve quality, since more local service providers will feel more answerable to local consumers. This is not necessarily the case, as Regmi and colleagues show in their study of decentralisation in Nepal:

> The more that consumer services users make their voice heard, the better effective services should become. In Nepal however, disadvantaged and poor communities are not very effective at making their voices heard. Most decisions are still taken by a few 'elites' based in their personal and political influence.
>
> (Regmi et al. 2010: 375)

Decentralisation of a previously centralised service also assumes an availability of resources – including a developed planning and management infrastructure and human resources, in the form of skilled health managers at local level – which may well not be available in many countries (Berman and Bossert 2000, Homedes and Ugalde 2005a).

Indeed, the results of decentralisation can also prove very different from those intended, as Rannan-Eliya and colleagues found in their extensive literature review for the USAID-funded Partnerships for Health Reform:

- Control over service provision may be captured at local level by elites who are even less responsive than central government to the needs of the poor
- Urban populations are often more politically influential than rural populations and therefore better placed to keep a larger share of resources
- Decentralisation may also offer new openings for local-level corruption
- The new system may find itself struggling in the face of a lack of local managerial skills and expertise
- Decentralisation may also mean smaller scale and less well-resourced providers, which wind up delivering less training and skills for staff and a lower quality care
- Smaller organisations also lose potential bargaining power and economies of scale in negotiation with major suppliers

- And smaller scale, more local structures almost inevitably offer less scope to tackle inequalities in the terms and conditions of health workers.

(Rannan-Eliya et al. 1996: 5–6)

In countries with marked social inequalities between town and country and between rich and poor, decentralisation of services can even increase problems of equity, unless it is firmly underpinned by guarantees of adequate needs-related funding. If not, granting local hospitals and health services powers to raise local funds may liberate local entrepreneurial talent in a wealthy area but condemn poorer inner-city and rural health services to permanent under-funding and second-class status (Mackintosh 2001, Homedes and Ugalde 2005b).

According to Partnerships for Health Reform, the primary intended goal of decentralisation is to promote 'cost effectiveness', with a secondary objective of securing financial sustainability (Knowles et al. 1997). It is doubtful whether those who support the progressive aspirations of locally controlled services would also embrace decentralisation as a cost-cutting measure. In Mexico, an IDB report found that decentralisation led to a serious decline in the quality and quantity of primary and hospital services for the poor (Homedes and Ugalde 2005b: 87). Enthusiasm for decentralisation appears to have developed and survived despite the lack of evidence to show that it delivers the promised improvements to efficiency, equity, quality or accountability (Valentine 1998).

Market-style reforms, which emphasise the development of autonomous and competing local hospital units, can result in duplication of effort, wasted resources and higher transaction costs. Strengthened local control can also obstruct national-level planning and any possible rationalisation of services, as well as restricting the ability of a health system to offer a wider range of career options as a means to retain qualified staff (Bach 2000).

Bossert's comparison of three countries – Chile, Colombia and Bolivia – for Data for Decision Makers and the Harvard School of Public Health argues that, although decentralisation and health finance reform have been 'touted' by the World Bank through much of the 1990s:

> the preliminary data from the field indicate that the results have been mixed, at best, and that in some cases the backlash has included moves to recentralise services.

(Bossert 2000: 3)

Provider autonomy/corporatisation

The notion of going beyond decentralisation to establish local health-care providers as autonomous, free-standing corporate bodies in their own right achieved a certain momentum among the advocates of market-style reforms early in the 2000s (Preker and Harding 2003). This was not new: the British Conservative government's marketising measures back in 1989 separated provider units from purchasers and encouraged the creation of 'self-governing trusts', the first of which were launched in 1991. New Zealand's government also experimented along the same lines in the early 1990s, with profoundly mixed results (Lovelace 2003).

Any efficiencies that may have been secured through improved management in trusts and equivalent organisational structures were obscured by the substantial increases in transaction costs, administration and management created by the introduction of the 'purchaser–provider split' into the NHS. This appears to be the rule rather than the exception of such policies: Manning argues that:

> The successes of autonomisation in the health sector seem to be more predicted than found.
>
> (Manning 2000)

Some countries have pioneered a level of local autonomy much further than NHS trusts. Indeed, 'foundation hospitals' in Spain and in Sweden and a variant in Portugal have gone further in floating the hospital as a free-standing enterprise, 'corporatised', with their own discretion to borrow funds and conduct deals with the private sector. Britain's New Labour government copied this model in England, despite vociferous opposition from Labour backbenchers, health unions, academics and campaigners (Pollock 2003, Pollock and Price 2003b, Klein 2004).

Just over half of England's hospital trusts are now foundations, accountable only to the independent regulator Monitor and not to strategic health authorities or the Secretary of State. They have the freedom to retain any surpluses they may generate and no obligation to share this with any other NHS provider (and up to now, with a few exceptions, these have been the financially strongest NHS trusts) – although they also have no call on any public funds in the event of financial problems, which is beginning to be an issue for some foundations with large, unaffordable PFI commitments.

Although their staff (at present) remain NHS employees (and are therefore covered by the NHS pension scheme and other important, hard-won terms and conditions), Labour legislation also gave them freedom to set their own local pay, varying from the national pay scales agreed for other NHS staff. As this study is completed, a cartel of foundation trusts in the south west of England is preparing to force through local pay scales considerably worse than the existing national agreement as a way to generate apparent 'efficiency savings' and, allegedly, to protect jobs (Mountjoy 2012). In theory, foundations are also free to borrow from the private sector – banks and money markets – although up to now this has been restricted by various regulations and by a reluctance of the more canny foundation chief executives to run up substantial debts that could prove a long-term liability.

In addition, Labour's 2003 legislation, which only just passed through parliament with a wafer-thin majority, included late concessions to those who were concerned that foundation status would be used as a pretext to expand private treatment and commercial activity, while also being urged by Monitor to pull out of delivering services which do not yield a surplus – effectively, to run as private hospitals on a business basis. While foundations were free to make 'partnership' agreements with private-sector organisations, they faced a strict limit on the proportion of their income that could be derived from private sources, which was restricted to no greater percentage than was the case before foundation status (Lister 2008a). This limit has been effectively removed by the right-wing coalition government, whose Health and Social Care Act 2012 now specifically permits foundations to generate as much as 49 per cent of their total income from private sources (Collis 2012).

As with St Goran's hospital in Stockholm, this type of autonomy may yet prove to be simply a transition point on the way to full-scale privatisation (Busse et al. 2002).[9] In the aftermath of the sale of St Goran's to Capio, the Swedish government enacted legislation to forbid any further privatisation of health services: the company's current contract forbids the sale of the hospital (Nikolic and Maikisch 2006). As discussed above, Spain's four foundation hospitals have been accused of making staff work longer hours and of 'cream skimming' the more lucrative treatments, leaving other hospitals to pick up the remainder (Nash 2003, Bes 2009).

The enthusiasm for this type of reform from the World Bank's Preker and Harding cannot hide the very mixed results of the relatively limited experiments that have taken place with hospital autonomy in the poorest countries: their book collects a handful of examples from low- and middle-income countries, including Argentina, Chile, Uruguay, Ecuador and Tunisia, not all of which have succeeded – and Indonesia, where the autonomous hospitals failed to improve financing, access for the poor, personnel management, service quality or patient satisfaction, but did succeed in raising fees and increasing revenues at the expense of patients (Preker and Harding 2003: 525–6).

In other developing countries the corporatisation of hospitals has taken the form of the establishment of major teaching hospitals as 'parastatal' organisations (Kenya's Kenyatta National Hospital) or autonomous 'self-governing' bodies (Ghana's Korle Bu and Komfo Anokye hospitals). One immediate difficulty in these circumstances is the disproportionate share of resources already allocated to these hospitals, which also tend to embody some of the country's most powerful medical professionals, and which governments cannot readily scale down. On four evaluative criteria of efficiency, equity, public accountability and quality of care, research by Govindaraj and colleagues (1996) concluded that the experiment in Ghana had not delivered many of the hoped for benefits, 'although there have been some isolated successes'.

The market-style reform agenda increasingly recognises the need to 'manage' competition and restrain the 'entrepreneurialism' of decentralised, ever-more-autonomous, public- and private-sector health-care providers (Saltman et al. 2002). Indeed, it might appear that in an increasingly decentralised system there is only a marginal distinction between, on the one hand, the local powers granted to what the World Bank calls 'semi-autonomous health facilities' providing contracted services to a publicly funded health-care system and, on the other, the same public system buying similar services from a private provider.

---

9   Saltman (2002) disagrees, claiming that the majority shareholder control of this hospital is still in the hands of public-sector organisations and arguing that no substantial privatisation of providers has yet taken place in Western Europe.

Patient choice and 'consumerism'

'Choice', like decentralisation, is one of those loaded concepts that it is impossible to disagree with in principle. In many varying contexts, the freedom to choose, to select from options, can be seen as fundamental, even crucial to the delivery of acceptable services. In the context of the rampant, institutionalised individualism of the US health-care system, the notion of choice as promoted by the opponents of any collective ('socialised') health care is one that keeps the government out at all costs (neatly ignoring the central role of government funding and the Medicare system which provides for senior citizens). The insistence upon individual choices and solutions helps to maintain a system which inflicts ruinous costs on so many.

In driving through a new, decisive stage in the marketising reforms in Britain (where the continued availability of socialised medicine is the notion that is politically damaging to challenge), Tony Blair famously insisted that choice should be a central principle for reform. Beginning with the argument that choice should be a weapon of last resort when established public services failed (Blair 2001a), later he neatly argued that this was an egalitarian measure, designed to give people on low incomes some of the choices of the wealthy:

> We know what makes good healthcare. Quick access; committed care; clean, comfortable surroundings. But what happens if you can't get them? If you've the money, you buy better. That is an affront to every progressive value we believe in.
>
> There's a great myth here: which is that we don't have a market in services now. We do. It's called private schools and private healthcare. But it's only open to the well-off.
>
> There is another myth: choice is a New Labour invention. Wrong. Choice is what wealthy people have exercised for centuries. The Tories have always been comfortable with that. But for Labour choice is too important to be the monopoly of the wealthy.
>
> (Blair 2005)

This approach is reminiscent of President Obama's Affordable Care Act, which offer subsidies and new structures to ensure that Americans on the lowest incomes also have the right to be ripped off by avaricious health-insurance corporations with low-premium policies that offer little real protection against inflated health-care costs. It reinforces the market and has the potential to deepen the inequalities it claims to address.

Blair's argument echoes the neoliberal logic of Julian Le Grand, who elevates the notion of choice into an all-encompassing principle:

> It fulfils the principle of autonomy, and promotes responsiveness to users' needs and wants; it provides incentives for providers to provide both higher quality and greater efficiency; and it is likely to be more equitable than the alternatives.
>
> (Le Grand 2007, cited in Hunter 2008: 92)

But this final assertion is challenged by critics, including Fotaki and colleagues, who argue strongly that:

> Providing more choice increases inequity. This is partly because the better off are more able to exercise choice when it is offered. ... At the very least, choice policies have the potential to increase inequity.
>
> (Fotaki and Boyd 2005, cited in Hunter 2008: 94)

The main focus of Blair's 'patient choice' agenda was on the issue of waiting times and choice of provider for elective surgery: the opening move was to give patients more choice over the dates and times for appointments, and a choice of provider if they were kept waiting longer than the target time (6, Perri 2003). By 2006, this had developed into a policy insisting that all patients should be able to choose where to go for their elective surgery – whether or not they wanted or felt equipped to exercise that right, and regardless of the fact that, in most cases, patients' choice was to ensure their local hospital was raised to the highest quality, rather than merged with another, and that local services wouldn't be closed if they failed to attract sufficient patients in this new market for health care (Adams 2012b).

The market-style, New Public Management approach, emphasising the role of the individual patient as 'consumer' in a commodified health service, coupled with the separation of purchaser and provider that prevails in many European healthcare systems, can seriously undermine planning. A shortfall in resourcing for one public-sector provider which results in a delay in treatment becomes in this situation a pretext for the transfer of resources to a rival provider – whether public or private sector.

Enthoven showed a number of ways in which consumerism could easily be utilised by a largely deregulated private sector to drive up costs (and thus profits). The key factor in his list of potential problems is: 'Free choice of provider: "destroys the bargaining power of insurers"' (Enthoven 1997: 196). It was to forestall this, and similar destabilising factors, that health maintenance organisations (HMOs) and 'managed care' were introduced in the USA in the 1990s: they aimed both to contain costs and improve quality – by *restricting* the level of patient choice to a limited range of providers, contracted by the HMO. This came top of the list when Enthoven (1997: 199) summed up the four principles of managed care as:

- Selective provider contracting
- Utilisation management
- Negotiated payment
- Quality management.

Any return to an untrammelled right of the individual patient to seek treatment wherever he or she chooses could generate a new round of medical cost inflation and the danger of reduced levels of monitoring and poorer quality care. As Enthoven points out, this was the process that eventually undermined the 'managed care' system, as insurers tried to compete against each other by offering progressively greater levels of patient choice.

In publicly funded services, already struggling to supply sufficient care for a rising level of demand, the apparently innocuous suggestion of 'patient choice' can prove an impossible target or, more accurately, a potentially open-ended commitment to fund private-sector treatment at the expense of closing failing public-sector providers. In England and in other health services, such as those of Denmark and Norway, where reduced waiting times have been linked with extending patient choice, the policy has been linked with the expansion or establishment of (more costly) private-sector providers, to be funded from the collective, public purse (Lister 2011b).

To offer all patients a choice of where to seek treatment requires an expensive expansion of capacity to ensure that a surplus is always available within any provider to accommodate those who 'choose' to transfer from a competitor – and a potentially substantial and open-ended increase in budget. This also reduces the efficiency of operators with spare, costly capacity.

Yet the public sector – increasingly as a result of market-style reforms – tends to receive revenue funding only on the basis of the workload it treats, leaving little if any room for prospective investment. Because any patient exercising the choice to seek their treatment from a private provider will also necessarily take with them the funding to pay for their treatment, patient choice therefore also implies breaking down the boundaries between public and private sectors. The primacy of 'patient choice' also implies that even scarce publicly trained professional and other staff should be made available to private-sector providers if needed to grant the patient his or her choice – regardless of the consequences for the public sector (Lister 2003a).

There are also questions over the capacity of the individual to make informed choices, particularly when confronted by the confusing proliferation of apparently similar policies from a variety of health insurers under President Obama's Afford- able Care Act – or in any other context where choice is commonly viewed as a burden rather than an empowerment by the patient who requires treatment but lacks the knowledge required to choose.

Taken to its logical conclusion, patient choice, as the epitome of consum- erism and the opposite of planning, sets the choices of the individual against the stability of a system that should have an obligation to care for the whole population. And of course, all these 'choices' incur substantial overhead costs in terms of the management, advertising, promotion and partially used capacity that result from a competitive system.

Another consequence as the policy is rolled out for an wider range of specialties is that the public sector will increasingly wind up dealing with the more expensive or complex cases, the most elderly and frail patients – and generally those cases less financially attractive for the private sector. In the US, this problem of 'cream- skimming' by the private sector – and in particular by the 265 highly profitable 'physician-owned hospitals', most of which have minimal if any emergency facilities, little or no out-of-hours medical staffing and often only skeleton crews of nurses available to cope with urgent problems – emerged as a bone of contention with the most powerful bosses of the largest US hospitals (Pearlstein 2005, Kahn 2006).

This resulted in 2010 in the Obama reforms incorporating clauses to prevent groups of doctors investing in any new physician-owned hospitals. In other words, where their market share and profits are at stake, the big players opt for government intervention and less competition, rather than more: or to put it more accurately, the big hospitals objected bitterly to the new 'niche' hospitals, 80 per cent of them specialist hospitals and many taking few if any Medicare patients, maximising their profits by dumping the less-profitable caseload onto them (Lee 2008, Whelan 2010). This situation gave US hospital bosses, the most powerful of whom run enterprises each of which has a turnover of billions of dollars, a taste of the frustration felt in other OECD countries by public-sector hospital bosses faced with one-sided competition from small, specialist private hospitals with no emergency departments, no full-time medical staff and the freedom to pick which specialist services to offer.

Together with the sky high and still rising costs of health care in the most expensive and inefficient health-care system in the world, the emphasis on individual choices and options seems to have been a driving force in the development of medical tourism, as increasing numbers of dissatisfied or excluded Americans begin to search the world for affordable treatment rather than face bankruptcy from health bills from US hospitals (Pafford 2009).

Medical tourism seems to have become a subject of debate and to have grown in popularity early in the twenty-first century. It has mushroomed into a multi-billion dollar industry, with thousands of what the *Economist* has dubbed 'medical refugees' flying from the US to international facilities in India, Thailand, Singapore, the Philippines and elsewhere for treatment at a small fraction of US tariff costs. Health insurers have recognised the potential cost savings to be made and begun to support, fund and organise these visits: ironically, with such large potential savings even after the costs of transporting patients long distances to exotic locations,[10] there are concerns that more insurance companies could start to coerce patients into travelling for cheaper treatment, especially for heart surgery and other treatments costing $20,000 or more in the US. By 2009, Aetna was offering financial incentives to those who got high-cost operations in cheaper facilities abroad and Blue Cross/Blue Shield in South Carolina was actively encouraging patients to do the same (Pafford 2009: 811). Employers, too, have begun to offer employees the option of medical travel to save thousands of dollars in co-payments (*Economist* 2008).

One US hospital group has also followed the growing trend and bought up a chain of hospitals in Mexico. It offers these as alternatives for patients who would otherwise be treated in Lousiana and Texas. Concerns over the quality of care have been answered by the rapid development of high-quality skills and brand new, purpose built and state-of-the-art systems that mean the best hospitals in Asia and Latin America are at least as good as most in the US: with reports suggesting errors and adverse events in US hospitals contribute to the deaths of up to 180,000 patients a year, while medication errors alone harm 400,000, there is no basis for a huge level of public confidence that US standards are better than the alternatives (Wilson 2010, National Academies 2006).

The result of the outflow of medical business could be a loss of $162 billion in potential income for US health-care providers in 2012, while representing around $21 billion of income for the providers in developing countries.

---

10 Costs of comparable treatment in India are on average one-eighth to one-fifth of those in the West (Hazarika 2010). Gupta (2008) argues that the differential is even greater, with open heart surgery in India's best hospitals coming in between one-twentieth the cost in the UK and one-fiftieth the US cost.

The US has led the way but increasing numbers of patients from 55 countries are seeking treatment abroad, with numbers estimated to reach 10 million by 2012 (*Economist* 2008).

One concern highlighted by US critics is the fact that patients who travel abroad for treatment are waiving the legal rights and protections they enjoy at home, and may not be able to share any comparable rights where they receive their treatment (Cortez 2008). Others, like Richard Smith, argue that most of the literature on medical tourism is 'data free', with no real details on outcomes or assessment of the extent of unnecessary treatment or other issues. Smith urges the academic sector, international organisations and governments to commission research (Smith 2004). Cortez (2008: 74) argues that the development of truly 'portable' health insurance would require new 'market mechanisms' to 'mitigate moral hazard, monitor fraud and abuse and encourage quality care'.

This underlines the fact that medical tourism represents a major boost for private medicine and potentially a further drain on collective health budgets in countries which finance patients to travel for treatment. It is correctly summed up by Pocock and Phua (2011) as 'an individual solution to what is traditionally considered a public (government) concern'. They stress that this represents 'increasing acceptance of health services as a market commodity' – and is therefore clearly a step away from the development of health systems that share risk and offer collective cover to populations.

This in turn makes it less likely that ways can be found to use medical tourism as a means to improve the capacity of poor people in developing countries to access health services, as suggested by Blouin (2010). The private hospitals that are at the centre of the medical tourist business are pursuing commercial, not health, objectives: that's why they are located in urban areas and deliver high cost, often specialist services to a global elite which are unaffordable to most citizens. Many of the private owners are also overseas companies, so any profits are not used for cross-subsidy to poor patients in each country but remitted offshore or reinvested in further extension of for-profit private medicine. Government subsidies (in the form of land, reduced import duties and other tax breaks), which have helped to kick start the rapid growth of the hospitals, reduce the resources available to develop broader public health goals for their own citizens. This creates a 'two-tiered' system with a corporate segment concentrated on high-tech services and a public-sector segment attempting to address broader social needs (Hazarika 2010).

Public hospitals in Malaysia and Thailand are responding to the expansion of health tourism by allowing their surgeons to operate a private wing for paying patients, which incentivises them to treat high-paying foreigners rather than local people. And shortages of appropriately skilled and qualified professional staff also mean that services are provided to the global rich at the expense of the local poor (Pocock and Phua 2011): according to a government Planning Commission report in 2008, India alone is estimated to be short of 600,000 doctors, 200,000 dental surgeons and 1 million nurses. Meanwhile, a growing proportion of the staff with these qualifications cater for wealthy clients in elite private hospitals, with the private sector consuming 75 per cent of the human resources and advanced medical technology, 68 per cent of the hospitals and 37 per cent of the hospital beds (Hazarika 2010).

Another issue is the impact on health services in the countries which export patients as health tourists: the removal of these middle class and wealthy consumers means there is less pressure on public health systems to improve to meet the needs of the poor (Chee 2010).

European health tourism

Of course, the long-distance travel of medical tourists from the US to Asian high-tech hospitals is not the only development of health tourism: the neoliberals shaping European Union policy have worked to create a cross-border health-care market that has great attractions for private insurers and patients in the wealthier European countries weighing up the benefits of accessing much-lower-cost treatment in Central and Eastern Europe, and elsewhere. The EU market for cross-border treatment was estimated in 2008 to be about €10 billion per year, much of it concentrated in border regions, small member states with limited health facilities, people with rare diseases seeking highly specialised care, and of course the treatment of actual tourists taken ill abroad (Europa 2008).

After years of debate on the issue, beginning in the 1990s, an initial proposal for an EU Directive on cross-border healthcare was rejected at the last minute in 2008; it took another three years for a precise formula to be agreed upon. The proposals, adopted in March 2011 and set to come into force in October 2013, remain controversial and fly in the face of warnings from a simulation exercise at the end of 2011 which underlined the extent to which patients seeking treatment in other EU countries would be treated 'as if they are not part of the social system':

> The most striking set of conclusions from the simulation relates to the potential burden for patients travelling under the Directive. Patients will bear the responsibility for many of the elements involved in accessing planned treatment across borders. The responsibility to find potential treatments, the burden of proof in demonstrating to insurers that the treatment has been carried out and the responsibility to submit the correct documentation clearly was seen to lie with patients...

> Given the size of the burden for patients it is therefore likely that the Directive will only be used when there is really no alternative better managed option to receive the treatment, or by patients who do not understand the responsibility on their shoulders and the risks they take.
>
> (Jeffs and Baeten 2011: 6–7)

This point is reinforced by the fact that patients seeking treatment overseas would be entitled only to the equivalent cost of the procedure in a hospital in their own country and would have to make up any shortfall between this and the actual cost of treatment. Moreover, there is no requirement for them to be recompensed for additional travel, accommodation or other expenses. They will have to pay up front themselves, then reclaim the money; and in order to obtain payment, they have to jump through the bureaucratic hoops referred to by Jeffs and Baetan whilst ensuring that they have received prior authorisation for the treatment, although this should only be refused in limited circumstances. The standards of treatment will be those applied in the provider hospital, not those of their own health service. In the UK, the prediction is that no great exodus of patients is likely and that the numbers seeking treatment abroad will not increase far beyond the estimated 1,000 per year (Zanon 2011).

There is, however, still a real possibility that in some countries the new arrangements will provide a fresh impetus for private fee-for-service treatment and serve to destabilise health-care systems. This is likely to be the case where large numbers of patients are encouraged to seek treatment abroad and take the money with them or where foreign patients and their purchasers are prepared to pay higher tariffs than those prevailing in a health-care system, giving providers an incentive to prioritise their treatment rather than local patients. This brings the threat of an Indian-style two-tier system with different tariffs and care standards, in which local patients are the second-class citizens (Baeten 2011: 275). In Belgium, there have been concerns that the attraction of treating foreign patients could result in commercial behaviour from the country's non-profit private providers, who otherwise do not have 'private' paying patients (ibid.: 276).

The European-level market would build on the market-style systems already in place:

> Activity-based hospital financing and competition among providers are likely to stimulate cross-border collaboration. If hospital financing is mainly activity based and related to the number of patients, hospitals have a clear incentive to attract as many patients as possible, both national and foreign, at least up to their optimal 'justified' activity level. Reaching optimal capacity brings financial gain for hospitals and it is attractive for hospitals to 'fill up' available facilities, use resources and get paid for the services provided, instead of having unused capacity.
>
> (Glinos 2011: 237)

But from the standpoint of the patient-exporting countries, the prospect is that patients responding to weaknesses in health-care systems by travelling abroad will take the money with them. Moreover, as this happens, staff would be attracted to more successful and possibly better-paying hospitals in other countries, thus pushing the system goes into a further decline (Baeten 2011). Similar problems have already been seen in Greece and Italy in the 1990s and there must be concern for the future prospects of countries like Romania and Bulgaria. In these countries, health systems are visibly struggling to cope and even low prices for treatment are unlikely to attract many paying customers; but there are many well-heeled patients, able to pay the extra costs involved, who will be tempted to access treatment in other EU countries. There is also the danger that in less-populated areas the exodus of significant numbers of patients can lead to the closure of existing health services.

Ironically, analysts point out that to take advantage of the EU Directive 'patients need to be fit to travel'. 'In Estonia people who expressed a preference to seek treatment abroad were "relatively young, still healthy and educated"' (Baeten 2011: 267). This implies inequity in access and the exclusion of many most in need of health care.

Another dimension of systems in which 'patient choice' is used to break down barriers between public and private sectors is the pressure from regulators concerned with promoting competition at various levels, culminating globally with the World Trade Organization and the General Agreement on Trade in Services (GATS). Once it is clear that private-sector providers are not running parallel but competing with the public sector, this is likely to bring increased pressure from potential private-sector providers for markets to be further liberalised and opened up to global competition (Pollock and Price 2000).

The problem is especially serious in Europe, which is confronted not only by the blatantly undemocratic one-way squeeze of GATS and the WTO towards the marketisation of all aspects of the economy and welfare provision, but also by the emergence, unwished for by any EU member state, of increasing amounts of EU health policy. This is made on the hoof by the European Court of Justice and by the Commission without any basis in the EU treaties and intersects with what Greer describes as 'the EU's enormous body of law on the internal market' (Greer 2009: 4). The GATS definition of services to be opened up as competitive markets could be applied in principle to health systems in almost any of the European countries, since all have evolved in recent years to employ a mix of public- and private-sector providers. Only those supplied exclusively by the government are excluded.

In 2004–6, a full-scale fight was needed in the European Parliament to remove health from the fundamentalist marketising proposals of the Bolkenstein Directive. Since then, the European Court has ruled that health care can be considered a service under EU law and can therefore be subject to EU law on public procurement, state aid and competition law.

As Greer argues, the 'ratchet effect' (which effectively blocks any moves to reverse liberalisation policies) creates the danger that these regulations will cumulatively open up the $1-trillion EU health-care market to full-scale competition. This is especially serious because:

> Many EU health systems only achieved universal coverage by using legal mechanisms (such as nationalisation of hospitals or imposed structures for setting medical pay rates) that would not be permitted under EU law today.
>
> (Greer 2009: 6)

Once health-care systems are fragmented and opened up to the full rigours of competition, there is no legal way back to planned systems based on the health needs of the population.

Policies to expand private insurance

Although much of the international debate on user fees for health care has focused on their impact on low-income families in the low- and middle-income developing countries, the issue of user fees (co-payments, deductibles or other 'out of pocket' expenditure by the patient to access care) continues to re-emerge time and again in the OECD countries. As Bob Evans and colleagues famously summed up:

Like zombies in the night, these ideas may be intellectually dead but are never buried. They may lie dormant for a time – in the late sixties, for example, or the late eighties – but when stresses build up either in the health care system or the wider public economy, they rise up and stalk the land.

(Evans et al. 1993: 3)

In the current highly stressed context of post-2008 recession, with unresolved questions over national solvency in Portugal, Ireland, Greece, Spain and Italy, plus major economic crises in other parts of Europe, the zombies are again on the move, with user fees being introduced or increased as part of the prescription for financial balance in Greece, Spain and Portugal. However, these moves quite clearly flow not from marketising reforms but primarily from cash-cutting and austerity. This section will specifically address the issue of user fees as a means to drive more people towards voluntary health insurance (VHI) and through this to private, commodified health care.

In the context of European health-care systems, which generally offer universal coverage, it can be hard to build a substantial private health-insurance market. Ireland, with almost half its population covered by health insurance in 2008, is unusual in having cultivated a widespread fear of hefty costs for those who have the money to insure themselves[11] and yet do not do so: fear of large medical bills was cited as the most frequent response to a survey on reasons for paying private premiums (Turner 2009).

In Eastern and Central Europe and in many developing countries, the World Bank and other agencies have pressed for the introduction of user fees not as a means to raise serious resources but as a way of reducing demand – by simultaneously deterring the poorest and persuading the middle classes to seek out insurance schemes – and as a device to open up a private sector (Klugman and Schieber 1996). The Bank's International Finance Corporation has focused on developing private insurance schemes targeted at the 'lower middle and middle classes in countries without risk pooling', which is seen as contributing 'to the strengthening of the middle class' (IFC 2002: 4, 5).

Private health insurance has remained a marginal factor in the financing of health care in the European Union, amounting to less than 10% of total health expenditure in every country except France and Slovenia (with 12.8% and 13.1% respectively) and less than 5% of spending in two-thirds of EU member states. Indeed, the only sector where market coverage is significant is for insurance policies covering statutory user charges: in France and Luxembourg, over 90% of the population has this coverage, while in Slovenia and Belgium it is over 70%. In this context, the imposition of user fees in publicly provided health-care services (co-payments for drugs, consultations or hospital admission) can prove a useful spur to encourage the middle

---

11 The statistics in Ireland, like many elsewhere, show a sharp gradation of levels of take-up of private health insurance according to income: while 89 per cent of the top two social class categories (A and B) subscribe to PHI, this falls to just 65 per cent for C1, 42 per cent for C2 and 18 per cent of the lowest income and unemployed classes (D and E) (Turner 2009: 217).

classes to take out private insurance (Thomson and Mossialos 2009: 7).

Germany expects the highest earners, civil servants and the self-employed to 'opt out' of the statutory health system and take out private health insurance (PHI); and indeed, the largest amount of premium income is collected in Germany, which accounts for almost half the private health insurance premiums in the EU. There are 'opt-out' provisions for the wealthy in the Netherlands and Spain but, in general, private insurance has been squeezed out by publicly funded schemes.

One problem for insurers is the lack of substantial waiting lists and the high quality of public health-care services in many European countries. Shortage of capacity in Ireland's public hospital system, generating long waiting times, created the second most popular reason for paying for private insurance, which was that people expect (and the statistics show) that those with private insurance get treated most quickly (Turner 2009). It seems that only the real and present danger of facing catastrophic bills for hospital treatment will induce large sections of the EU population to opt for private medical insurance: in Greece, despite the high level of charges faced by those who fall ill, voluntary schemes cover only 12 per cent of the population (Thomson and Mossialos 2009).

By contrast, in Britain, where waiting times were once notorious, expansion and improved performance by the NHS since 2000 has meant that, despite extensive marketing efforts by private health insurers offering swifter and more luxurious treatment, numbers of individuals covered have been static or falling: the latest figures show the lowest ever rate of penetration of the UK population by private medical cover, down to 10.9 per cent. Analysts Laing and Buisson report a further 4.2 per cent reduction in numbers of individual-paid policies and only minuscule growth (1.2 per cent) in company-paid medical cover, while the numbers covered by these schemes actually fell in 2011 (Laing and Buisson 2012b). Average premium payments were squeezed down slightly, after years of inflation, while insurers paid out fewer claims, leaving their margins actually improved at 22 per cent. The message is clear: 'record low take-up of private medical cover by individuals, despite a wide choice of low-cost policies and downgrade options, highlights continued vulnerability in this area.' On the brighter side for the insurers, 'expected cracks in NHS performance under constrained funding may provide some medicine to halt and possibly reverse this trend...' (Laing and Buisson 2012b).

The health insurance market is becoming increasingly dominated by monopoly, with numbers of insurers varying from five or fewer in some states to 100 – or in the unique case of France, over 1,000. In 2006, in most member states the three largest insurers between them controlled more than 50 per cent of the insurance market (Thomson and Mossialos 2009: 7).

Some EU governments have attempted to pump-prime private health insurance through generous tax concessions, notably in Ireland which, since the late 1990s, has been spending millions each year on what was effectively a subsidy that reduced the cost of premiums by 32 per cent – even though most subscribers to voluntary health insurance are high earners. The cost of these subsidies, overt and covert, continued to increase over ten years from €79 million a year to an estimated €300 million in 2007 (Turner 2009). In 2010, research from Dr Anthony Staines, Professor of Health Systems at Dublin City University, estimated that the total of overt and covert subsidies for private care in Ireland could be as high as €700 million a year. This included €260 million on tax relief for health-insurance premiums; €90 million paid out for publicly funded treatment in private hospitals of people who had waited too long for treatment; and €100 million in subsidies for private patients in public hospitals. At the same time, the Health Service Executive budget was expected to lose around €600 million in 2010 (Hunter 2010).

The extent of these final hidden subsidies was underlined when ministers, as part of an austerity budget at the end of 2011, announced plans to scrap the system of designating public hospital beds as for public or private use and impose charges of €889–€1,000 per day for private patients occupying either category of bed. Such large numbers of private patients have customarily been treated without charge in non-designated beds that insurers immediately protested that the change could lead to premium increases of at least 50 per cent almost immediately. It could put the cost of a family premium for a couple with two children up by €1,000 per year (Pope 2011).

But even while this subsidy is cut, the more expensive subsidy for private health insurance remained intact and appears to be untouchable, even though PHI accounts for just 8.4 per cent of total health spending and just over a third of private-sector spending (WHO 2008d, cited in Turner 2009: 221). The Irish government calculated in 2007 that just 17 per cent of beds in public hospitals are designated as private, amounting to a larger total of beds than in the country's private hospitals, and that the public sector does not receive the full economic cost of the private beds.

Despite these costs and problems with the private sector and health insurers ripping off public-sector hospitals, the Irish government has been eager to move towards the Dutch model of 'universal health insurance', introduced in 2006 which involves mandatory health insurance chosen by the subscriber from a choice of providers. The Dutch system also centres on extensive subsidies to the private health insurers, paid as a 'health insurance allowance' to people on low incomes. These are paid to 60 per cent of households, rising to 70 per cent in 2010, and calculated to cost around €4 billion in 2009, up from €2.5 billion in 2006. One year after the reforms, one health insurer made a bid to get round the formal ban on selecting subscribers by 'cream skimming' younger subscribers in good health, offering them a lower-cost premium in exchange for a restricted range of 11 hospitals. The competition between insurers became ferocious, with some offering discounts of up to 10 per cent for employer-based group insurance – in many cases cutting the price below cost to generate a net loss (Maarse 2009a).

The Dutch system requires all citizens to take out UHI but also allows Voluntary Supplementary Health Insurance, which covers services not covered by the basic policy, such as eye and dental care, various therapies, cross-border care and some preventive care (Thomson and Mossialos 2009). But 231,000 were uninsured at the end of 2007, with another 240,000 in default on payments and not covered – almost 3 per cent of the population. Premium increases (41 per cent since the new system was introduced and predicted to double by 2014) have pushed costs per household to between €4,500 and €5,600, while the 'excess' not covered by insurance has risen from €150 to €210, with more increases expected: top-up fees for drugs also apply as a result of a government cap on reimbursement, increased as part of the Netherlands austerity budget. Bureaucratic and other costs, which had been falling prior to 2006, have risen sharply – as has doctors' pay – with little compensating advantage for patients (Haugh 2011).

The Dutch reform also involves lifting the ban on for-profit hospital care and price competition between hospitals, and has triggered major financial problems in more than 50 per cent of hospitals. Meanwhile, the projected benefits of competition between health insurers have not materialised: subscribers, after a flurry of switching in 2006–7, have proved increasingly reluctant to change insurer, while the larger companies have increasingly been able to carve up the market between them and use the price cuts secured from the hospitals to push up profits rather than to cut premiums (Haugh 2011).

Other governments around the world also offer overt or hidden subsidies to private insurers,[12] as in Australia, where the government paid out $3 billion in 2004–5. What value do the governments get back for their generosity? Cheng (2012) calculates that the cost of increased public health services that might flow from cutting these subsidies is just $1.38 million, shooting down the endless claims that those who pay private premiums are saving the state money. So an annual net subsidy of upwards of $1.5 billion is the obvious cost in Australia, plus the distortion of the health-care system and the loss of highly skilled staff trained with public resources:

> these results suggest that eliminating subsidies could potentially yield substantial public sector savings. This conclusion is in line with the growing evidence internationally that subsidising PHI in countries with universal public health systems is likely not to result in fiscal benefits to the public sector.
>
> (Cheng 2012: 24)

Cheng's conclusions, based on detailed calculations, correspond with warnings by Davoren (2001) that Australian subsidies to private insurance would not benefit public hospitals: he also pointed out that those who rely most on public hospitals are the least likely to be able to afford private insurance, most of whose subscribers are young and healthy and don't use hospitals anyway. Davoren also cites another study which shows the higher cost of the same treatment 'with the same equipment and the same technical and nursing staff' in a private hospital room compared with a public hospital next door. The impact of Medicare payments and drug costs mean that the private patient costs the government $500 more. The money allocated to subsidies was not well spent:

> Two and a half billion dollars a year could open and operate an extra sixteen 500-bed public hospitals. It absolutely dwarfs any monies the Coalition are putting into improving healthcare in rural and regional Australia.
>
> (Davoren 2001).

---

12 According to Nicolás and Vera-Hernández (2004), tax incentives are offered by Australia, Austria, Belgium, Canada, France, Germany, Greece, Ireland, Italy, Luxembourg, Mexico, the Netherlands, Portugal, Spain and the USA.

Other research shows that costs are increased by the fact that in Australia (as in other countries) patients with PHI tend to need fewer health-care services but make more use of them. Public hospitals are more efficient than private, so between 3 and 12 times more health care could have been provided if the money subsiding private insurance had been spent in expanding the public sector. Colombo also notes that in OECD countries private health insurance encourages greater use of physician services by wealthier groups, who are more likely than poorer groups to visit a specialist in Ireland, Italy, Portugal, Spain and the UK (Colombo 2007: 223). In other words, private insurance encourages access to health care to be expanded without any correlation to medical need.

A review of PHI in Australia, Canada, Chile, France, Germany, the Netherlands, the UK and the USA concluded that it's more expensive, not least because of the additional costs of marketing, increased risk and underwriting (Hindle and McAuley 2004); while Colombo also points out that the private sector pays providers more than they could earn in the public system (2007: 224).

Nicolás and Vera-Hernández carried out calculations for Spain and again drew a similar conclusion: subsidies for private health insurance, whether through income tax or tax relief to employers, are not self-financing: it costs more than it can be seen to save and there is no evidence of PHI coverage helping to reduce waiting times for publicly funded patients (Nicolás and Vera-Hernández 2004).

Thomson and Mossialos also sum up the experience in the EU countries:

> Most countries use tax incentives to encourage the take up of PHI, although these have been abolished or lowered in several countries in the last five to ten years, without much negative effect on demand for PHI. While generous tax subsidies have succeeded in fuelling demand for PHI in a few countries (notably Hungary and Ireland) they are unlikely to be self-financing and lower equity in financing health care.
>
> (Thomson and Mossialos 2009: 9)

Hsiao and Heller go further, arguing that although many countries have tried regulatory remedies to correct market failures in the private health insurance market 'no country has succeeded'.

> Often macro economists assume erroneously that the private sector production of health insurance and health services is more efficient than public sector production. This is not so. Studies have consistently found that the cost of private insurance is higher than public insurance...
>
> (Hsiao and Heller 2007: 23)

Worse, the existence of PHI 'undermines other health policy objectives, even where the market is carefully regulated'. Allowing public-sector providers to charge higher fees to privately financed patients 'creates strong incentives to prioritise these patients at the expense of publicly funded patients.' (Thomson and Mossialos 2009: 10)

Even this accumulated weight of evidence has not been enough to trigger any enlightenment among IMF researchers. Kanzler and Ng suggest naively that:

All governments should consider whether private insurance can play a greater role in alleviating fiscal burdens and resolving other issues, such as the widespread lack of health care coverage in developing countries...

(2012: 56)

Or even, without a shred of explanation or evidence:

In all locations private insurance could potentially play a role in solving many problems. For example it could help reduce OOP expenses in emerging and developing countries, thereby making healthcare more affordable and accessible.

(Ibid.: 58)

This is just not what private health insurance does. Nor, because of its unequal access and general exclusion of the poor, is it a handy tool for health promotion, public health or preventive programmes. Yet the same authors apparently believe private health insurance could also help prevent the spread of communicable diseases and high infant mortality rates (ibid.: 61), even though on the next page they admit that private payers' ability to manage cost is 'severely limited' and their administrative costs are higher: in the USA, the largest private health insurers selling primarily to employers spend 15–25 per cent of premiums on marketing, administration and profits; smaller companies selling to individuals can soak up between 35–45 per cent. By contrast, they regard every cent spent on delivering health care to their subscribers as 'medical loss' (Cheng and Reinhardt 2012).

In fact, private insurance can only work at all if there is a 'strong regulatory system' in place to override the primal forces of market competition (Kanzler and Ng 2012: 62).

In similar fashion, Colombo has also stressed the costs of PHI and the patchy coverage it can offer, warning developing countries that:

Even in some middle income OECD countries with partial health coverage or high out of pocket spending, a PHI market is struggling to emerge. In other OECD countries PHI markets have difficulty expanding in rural and other areas with less prosperous economic conditions. ... Government interventions to stimulate or expand PHI markets have significant implications for administrative costs.

(Colombo 2007: 233)

Bringing a welcome note of realism into the IMF volume, Cheng and Reinhardt implicitly counter Kanzler and Ng, pointing out that competition between insurers can lead to increased health-care prices because each separate competing insurer has a smaller share of the market and smaller leverage over hospitals and other providers (Cheng and Reinhardt 2012: 82). Colombo (2007) has also noted that a proliferation of varied insurance products, segregating the market according to risk level, can make it harder for patients to obtain coverage.

Tyson and colleagues, again in the same volume, want it both ways, claiming against most of the evidence that private insurance helps to hold down 'excess cost growth' – but then admitting that there are considerable market failures flowing from private insurance markets (Tyson et al. 2012: 117).

But even the most extreme eagerness of the IMF researchers to come up with positive arguments for health insurance in developing countries is completely eclipsed by the zeal of the World Bank's Alex Preker, who has been churning out massive tomes of material arguing this case for several years, even though he has to admit from the start that private voluntary health insurance plays only a small role in the developing world, with coverage rates generally below 10 per cent of the population, and that this share is only growing in a few middle-income countries (South Africa, Uruguay, and Lebanon) (Preker et al. 2010).

Preker makes no secret of his determination to keep social reality and principles out of his analysis at all costs and promises sensitive neoliberals early on that they will hear nothing scary or annoying. All the principles are to be those of basic neoliberalism:

> Notions of solidarity, social health insurance, social protection, universality, and other values laden terms will be avoided in this volume.
>
> (Preker et al. 2010: 4)

He moves swiftly on to suggest that some developing countries might like to consider introducing the costly and wasteful subsidies for private health insurance that have consistently failed to deliver as required in the OECD countries:

> Under another approach, health insurance is introduced for a broader segment of the population by applying a demand-driven approach, involving paying for or subsidizing the premium of the poor and low income informal sector workers [patient-based subsidisation]. This allows a more rapid expansion of coverage, by using resources that are freed up from the contributing part of the population to subsidize the premium of the poor and low income informal sector workers rather than their service providers.
>
> (Preker et al. 2010: 14)

Drechsler and Jütting, in a paper boasting some antique statistics, appear more grounded, pointing out the marginal role of private commercial health insurance in low- and middle-income countries, meaning that PHI 'depends heavily on the government's involvement in this line of business'. They cite 2002 figures (apparently the latest they have) to show insurance penetration amounted to only 0.11% in Africa, 0.14% in the Middle East, 0.29% in Eastern Europe, 0.34% in Asia and 0.4% in Latin America. These developing and emerging countries have 85% of the world's population and generate 23% of GDP, but all six regions covered in their analysis account for a mere 10% of global insurance premium income (Drechsler and Jütting 2007: 39).

Not only is the distribution of private health insurance resources unequal but so too are the societies in which PHI is best able to flourish, for the simple reason that the rich are more likely (and more able) to buy coverage. So it is no coincidence that countries where PHI is more than 10 per cent of health spending are those with the greatest inequality in income. And even where the insurers have come along, the result has not 'yet' been more lower premiums: the market remains 'uncompetitive'. Even in Latin America where 'managed care' organisations have emerged, they have focused on cherry picking the healthier patients, leaving the sickest to gravitate to whatever public-sector provision there may be.

> It is very doubtful if the private commercial insurance industry will cover marginalised individuals without accompanying public regulation.
>
> (Drechsler and Jütting 2007: 40–4)

In East Europe and Central Asia, it's a familiar story of a nascent and largely irrelevant and unaffordable private insurance sector reaching only a wealthy elite in low-wage economies; only Russia and Turkey draw more than 1 per cent of health spending from private insurance. In Azerbaijan, voluntary health insurance covers less than 0.1 per cent of the population, with insurance premiums ranging upwards in price from $600 a year while the average annual per capita income is just $700. Estonia, after a false start, has 'renounced all attempts to increase the share of PHI' (Drechsler and Jütting 2007: 69).

The inequalities deepened by private insurance are stark: in South Africa, 50 per cent of health spending is channelled to health insurance but just 18 per cent of the population is covered by it; and 80 per cent of these are in the top two income quintiles, while the lowest income groups make up only 2 per cent of the insured (Drechsler and Jütting 2007: 61).

Elsewhere in Sub-Saharan Africa, an even smaller fraction of the population is covered by commercial insurance: most schemes extend no further than relatively small groups of formally employed workers in urban areas. Instead, the focus is on non- or low-profit schemes, although many of these are too small to provide a proper risk pool (only a few have more than 10,000 members) and extremely low contributions mean that they hardly amount to insurance at all.

Learning nothing from the problems and failures of small-scale experiments in the 1990s (Musau 1999), even smaller schemes have been taking shape as 'mutual health insurance' or 'mutuelles', of which it is claimed that there are 366 registered programmes in West and Central Africa. 80 per cent of them have fewer than 1,000 people covered and half have fewer than 650 – putting the microscopic into what has become known by academic and World Bank proponents as 'micro-insurance'. Their tiny size and resources make them barely sustainable and of little or no use in covering catastrophic costs of illness. Only rarely do they cover expenses for specialist treatment or hospital care and they rely on co-payments for anything other than the smallest risk (Drechsler and Jütting 2007: 62–5).

In other developing countries and emerging economies the picture is also of a marginal, largely insignificant private health-insurance sector that caters to a rich elite and excludes the majority, making occasional token efforts at catering for the poor through community schemes and other token or pointless forms of micro-insurance. Bangladesh and Sri Lanka spend 'negligible' amounts on PHI and Sri Lanka also has a widely praised system that delivers health care to the majority without recourse to the Preker and World Bank proposals.

India had less than 10 per cent of its population covered by private health insurance in 2007, though fortunately even the Indian government after years of inaction has begun thinking rather more ambitiously and progressively than the World Bank's academics, who seem blinkered and rooted to the notion of insurance as the answer. Announcing bold plans for a new system of universal health coverage, the High Level Expert Group commissioned by the Planning Commission argues that:

> for such a vision of the UHC to be realized, a tax based system of health financing is essential. This is also the global experience, wherein countries which have introduced UHC have mostly depended on general revenues rather than on unsteady streams of contributory health insurance which offer incomplete coverage and restricted services.
>
> (Planning Commission of India 2011: 2)

Selvaraj and Karan also underline the inappropriateness of even publicly financed health insurance schemes in the Indian context, despite an extremely rapid expansion of this cover from 75 million in 2007 to 322 million in 2010. They warn that the insurance offered covers only limited hospitalisation, with no cover for primary care and care outside hospitals. It is framed around the private-insurance approach:

> Private providers find it lucrative to turn simple ailments into hospitalisation episodes, which otherwise would have been treated at the outpatient care level. … Healthcare is not viewed as a continuum of care, rather seen as compartmentalised care. …
>
> Market forces appear to have come alive in recent times, sensing immense opportunity to 'commodify' and 'medicalise' the 'health market'. It is the same market forces which were bent on preventing and denying every opportunity for the government to intervene in healthcare financing and provision.
>
> (Selvaraj and Karan 2012: 67)

They go on to insist that any policy for developing universal health coverage must also break from this model and give primacy to promotive and preventive care.

> Primary care must take precedence over secondary and tertiary care. … Significant and sustained investment in the public health system is the need of the hour.
>
> (Ibid.: 68)

This lesson needs to be learned also in many East Asian countries, where the Preker volume explains that health insurance is both marginal and irrelevant:

> PHI has not yet entered the health care market. This may be partly due to the role of the state in Asian health financing systems, which offers and generally requires public health insurance.
>
> (Drechsler and Jütting 2007: 49)

China, too, is following its own distinctive path to a more accessible health-care system for its vast population, largely ignoring the Preker and World Bank advice to extend private insurance – as are Indonesia (where community schemes and micro-insurance experiments collapsed in the 1990s, leaving US-style, for-profit, managed-care HMOs covering a mere 500,000 people from a population of 238 million) and the Philippines.

The Indonesian government has been committed to rolling out universal health coverage by 2014 – through a social security scheme covering up to half the population who are not eligible for government-funded health plans covering civil servants and formal sector workers. In 2012, with over 36 per cent of the population still not covered, the Indonesian government earmarked funding of $3.2 billion towards the costs (Hitipieuw 2012), with $708 million to fund health insurance for the poor in 2012. However, it has now been announced that the scheme will only begin in 2014, making upwards of 96 million people (40 per cent of the country's poor population) eligible for cover. Those on higher pay will still have to pay for their own insurance. The completion date for universal care has been pushed back to 2019 (*Jakarta Post* 2012a).

The Indonesian plan, Jamkesta, is effectively a vast single-payer health insurance scheme that will leave private-sector providers and public hospitals as they are: inequalities remain too, and a pilot scheme in West Java in 2011 issued Jamkesta cards to informal and low-wage workers, making them eligible for medical care in 'third class hospitals' (*Jakarta Post* 2011). There have also been complaints that the Jamkesta scheme is paying out less in claims, and doing so more slowly, than the other two schemes – Askes, which covers 18 million civil servants, and Jamsotek, which covers 27 million formal-sector workers (*Jakarta Post* 2012b). The per capita government subsidy has been as low as $6 per year, leaving those with substantial health needs, even in third-class hospitals, with substantial out-of-pocket bills if they access treatment (Tangcharoensathien et al. 2011). There have been warnings that despite the government's efforts to improve the health of the poor, up to half of the spending so far has 'leaked' to higher-income groups, and that 10 per cent of the insurance aimed at the poorest went to the 30 per cent richest, leaving a rich–poor gap (Utomo et al. 2011).

In the Philippines, too, the government-subsidised PhilHealth insurance scheme for poor households covers an estimated 85 per cent of the population of 94 million, charging them a yearly fixed premium of $26. But it does not cover outpatient services and it caps the level of reimbursement for inpatient care, leaving many patients to face hefty bills: in fact, the share of health spending covered by social health insurance actually fell from 11 per cent in 2005 to just 8.5 per cent in 2007, as the scheme reached more people. The free choice of provider comes with a substantial price tag. By contrast, Thailand's three tax-funded insurance schemes, respectively covering the formal sector, civil servants and the remainder of the population, have succeeded in almost halving out-of-pocket payments between 2001 and 2008 (Tangcharoensathien et al. 2011).

The Thai system is one of those highlighted in the conclusions of the ambitious Equitap project ('Equity in Asia-Pacific Health Systems'), a collaborative research project of 17 institutional partners from the UK, Europe and Asia, which spent three years assessing equity in the health systems of 16 Asian nations. Principally funded by a EU INCO-DEV research grant, it received additional funding support from DFID, the World Bank, the WHO, the UNDP, the Rockefeller and Ford Foundations, and the governments of Hong Kong SAR and Taiwan. It found that publicly funded health care sufficient to mitigate the worst inequalities could be provided in Sri Lanka, Thailand and the Philippines for less than 2 per cent of GDP, funded through taxation (Rannan-Eliya and Somanthan 2005b: 11). The authors identify the systems that appear to have delivered positive results for the poor as those of Sri Lanka, Thailand since 2000 and Malaysia. What do they have in common? In each case, their national policies reject targeting, two-tier systems and all forms of health insurance in favour of universalism and systems which levy no, or very low, user fees.

> It is a legitimate question, given this experience, whether any pro-poor health strategy can be considered realistic as long as official policy continues to maintain user charges for health spending.
>
> (Rannan-Eliya and Somanthan 2005b: 11)[13]

The most equitable Asian services also rejected the World Bank, neoliberal approach of providing only an 'essential package' of health services centred on primary care, and allocated a much larger share of spending to hospital and inpatient services to provide substantial risk protection (ibid.: 12).

It is conspicuous that Preker's plethora of arguments for health insurance and insistence upon various unproven systems that run counter to these findings appear completely oblivious to the Equitap project and the evidence it has presented. Time and again it is clear that the very existence of private health insurance helps to divert scarce government resources in the form of subsidies and regulatory activity away from the priority of providing for the poorest and the whole population into a system that benefits a small wealthy elite.

This can also be seen where governments accept responsibility for wide but thin coverage – leaving room for the continuation of some private insurance, at public expense. Even in Thailand, for instance, which has offered universal health care since 2001, half of the insurance premiums for a voluntary risk-sharing scheme promoted by the government are paid from public subsidies (Drechsler and Jütting 2007: 52).

Francesca Colombo, summing up lessons from the OECD experience of private

---

13 The authors point out that many of the approaches used in this Equitap report 'were originally developed by UK researchers (Adam Wagstaff, Julian Le Grand) in the ECuity project, a fifteen-year ongoing collaboration of European researchers examining equity in European health systems' (van Doorslaer 1993). The Equitap project involved 'the application of standardised methods and tools for assessment of equity in all participating countries, to enable reliable comparison of health system performance.' The dimensions of equity that have been examined 'include equity in payments, delivery of health services, protection against catastrophic impacts and health status.' The authors state that the 'work of the Equitap study represents the most comprehensive and systematic assessment to date of the available empirical evidence of health system equity performance in Asia' (Rannan-Eliya and Somanthan 2005b: 2).

health insurance for developing countries, manages to find some plus points in a 'strikingly heterogeneous' experience, but concludes that it insurance is 'unlikely to address the financial and protection needs of the poor' (Colombo 2007: 211).

A Joint statement by NGOs five years ago argues that PHI is of little value in extending coverage to the poor in developing countries:

> In countries where PHI has shown strong growth, its contribution to universal access to health care has been insignificant, or has even had an adverse effect by increasing inequalities. … The costs of regulating PHI and the fragmentation of risk pools make this an inefficient and expensive way of improving health access.
>
> (Berkhout and Oostingh 2008: 2)

For-profit micro-insurance schemes 'have low premiums but offer limited benefits packages', with most schemes in India excluding childbirth, pregnancy-related illnesses and HIV. Community-based health insurance schemes have reached just 0.2 per cent of the African population and tend to leave poor people dependent upon out-of-pocket payments.

Bond (2007) also argues strongly against the use of micro-insurance, warning that in the health and social care sector, 'microcredit evangelism' is especially dangerous.

The global view offered by Drechsler and Jütting further underlines one key point: because PHI largely succeeds best where it can offer cover to the middle class and wealthy for services that are 'excluded or not fully covered by the state' (2007: 81), it is fundamentally incompatible with genuinely universal and accessible health-care services.

Whereas some aspects of public health care can always survive because of the exclusion of the poor from PHI, PHI itself can only really flourish where public services are poor or non-existent – and even then, it requires costly government subsidies to generate any substantial level of coverage. In other words, all of the arguments that attempt to link the idea of private health insurance in any form with equity and social inclusion are baseless: private insurance companies are not a partner but a parasitic detriment to public provision and public funding.

Medical savings accounts

This particular, exceptionally regressive, version of health insurance was keenly debated in the 1990s, but only implemented in Singapore (where the idea originated), the USA and, in limited experiments, China and South Africa (Mossialos et al. 2002, Thiede and Mutyambizi 2010). It is an ideal vehicle for neoliberal reform, allowing the wealthiest to insure themselves against catastrophic health costs without making any contribution to the health care of anybody else and while pocketing the bulk of the money at the end of the process.

MSAs first evolved in Singapore in the 1980s, based on the principle of self-reliance and individual accountability. They require subscribers to save a proportion (6–8 per cent) of their income every month in a designated account to meet health-care costs – hospital admissions and costly outpatient procedures. From these accounts a premium is deducted to cover catastrophic illness insurance, with high deductibles and co-payments to keep premium costs down. By 1992, these accounts covered 92 per cent of Singaporeans. However, they did nothing to constrain supplier-induced demand in a high-tech and increasingly costly health-care system, and eventually the government was obliged to intervene to structure and regulate the health-care system (Mossialos et al. 2002: 121–2).

MSAs were first proposed in the US in 1996, offering the most benefits to high-rate taxpayers and operating alongside traditional high-deductible policies. As such, they have been of most appeal to younger and healthier subscribers. The Medicare Modernisation Act of 2003 made it a permanent option and the Bush administration attempted to widen the use of MSAs, passing the Health Savings and Affordability Act, which was estimated to cost the federal government $174 billion in tax concessions over the next ten years (Families USA 2003). Savings deposited in MSAs would be tax-deductible and any earnings from stocks and bonds held by an MSA would also be tax-free. While tax would have to be paid on any withdrawals for non-medical purposes, this only applies up to the age of 65, from which point withdrawals carry no tax penalty. The scheme has all the makings of a convenient tax shelter for the well-to-do.

In 1999, an upbeat briefing summed up the merits for Ohio consumers, their state having been one of those that exempted MSAs from state income taxes:

> Imagine a health plan that allows employees to purchase the health care services they want, and then gives them money back at the end of the year. The plan also reduces employer health insurance expenses and gives workers more, not fewer choices over doctors, hospitals and treatments.
>
> (Buckeye Institute no date)

But online customers with Wells Fargo Bank are still being urged in 2012 to subscribe to a version of MSA – a Health Savings Account:

> Now is the time to consider a Wells Fargo Health Savings Account (HSA). Learn how to save and pay for your medical expenses tax-free.
>
> (Wells Fargo 2012)

As such, MSAs have been branded by opposing campaigners in the USA as:

> a tax cut targeted toward healthy, affluent people that increases health insurance [costs] for the sick.
>
> (Park and Lav 2003)

The theory behind MSAs asserts that in case of lesser illness (incurring costs up to $1,500 or even $3,000), the funds in a patient's MSA could be used, if required, to cover costs not covered by insurance. Any money that is not used in this way could be invested in stocks and bonds, eventually to be withdrawn by the individual as an additional income in retirement (Maynard and Dixon 2002).

However, as Hsu (2010b) points out, high costs of medical care in the US mean that most medical procedures cost in excess of $2,000 and are thus likely to be covered through the catastrophic costs policy rather than drawing on the MSA – suggesting that the main savings account is seldom if ever going to be used and the tax subsidies that sweetened the deal for the subscriber might have been more wisely spent.

Claims that MSAs give consumers a strong financial incentive to control their own health-care costs find little evidence to support this theory from the US, China, South Africa or Singapore (Hsu 2010b, Hanvoravongchai 2002).

Advocates of the scheme also argue that MSAs can help offer coverage for the uninsured: but many uninsured workers earn too little to pay federal taxes and cannot afford to put aside savings of $2,000–$4,000. Families USA (2003) argue that MSAs could also increase costs for workers who currently have workplace health insurance, since they encourage employers to sign up for low-premium policies covering only catastrophic costs, leaving workers to pay out increased co-payments should they fall ill.

From the neoliberal point of view such a policy has many advantages, effectively breaking down any wider commitment to social solidarity or risk-sharing, and reducing health-care provision for the well-to-do to an individual matter between them, their bankers and insurers. MSAs 'take the notion of cost-sharing to the extreme, where the majority, if not all, routine health-care costs are borne by individuals' (Hsu 2010b: 4). As such, they act on demand but not need for health care and can only be an option for the healthier and wealthier elements who are confident of making minimum use of health-care services.

In Canada, the Romanow and Senate reviews of health-care financing generated a round of debate on MSAs (Gratzer 2002, Deber et al. 2002a, 2002b, 2002c, Forget et al. 2002, Solomon 2002, Shortt 2002) in which the argument was polarised: supporters of the policy argued that it reduced costs and could be an equitable system; while its opponents insisted that the opposite was the case and that the increase in costs would fall heavily on those with greatest health needs.

The strongest supporting evidence was produced by opponents of MSAs, who took a detailed look at the profile of health spending in the Canadian province of Manitoba and from this demonstrated that, while 80 per cent of the population incur health spending well below the 'average', the sickest 1 per cent accounted for 26 per cent of health spending. A logical consequence of this is that the apparent financial disciplines which might result in reduced costs and health spending would be ineffective among the vast majority of the Manitoba population, who already make less than 'average' use of services – and little more effective with those in greatest need of health treatment. Instead of reducing costs, MSAs would increase health spending on the healthiest members of the population (Forget et al. 2002, Deber et al. 2002c).

Park and Lav (2003: 4) note that another consequence could be to push up the cost of traditional health insurance schemes. This would be exacerbated by the encouragement of healthy and wealthy subscribers to pull out of traditional schemes and opt for MSA-style coverage instead, leaving a smaller pool of older and less-fit subscribers at increased risk, creating what Park and Lav describe as 'a death spiral for the employer's comprehensive coverage option'.

Chapter eight

The missing MDGs

We have discussed the focus of health policy and resources in the developing world on the eight Millennium Development Goals and the narrow approach this brings, with its concentration on HIV/AIDS and a few specific diseases, on young women of childbearing age as mothers, and on children – and its lack of attention to the billions of people outside of these categories. This chapter will look specifically at some of the billions who have not been the subject of any such push for improvement and extension of health care but whose health needs are a major issue on a global scale.

Elderly people: 'customers' nobody wants

In 2002, the Second World Assembly on Ageing declared that the dramatic growth in numbers of older people around the world was 'a triumph and a challenge'. The triumph was that life expectancy had increased on a world scale from just 45 years for men and 48 years for women in 1945 to 63 and 68 years respectively by 2000 (WHO 2002: 6).

The challenge is that the economic and political framework of a neoliberal global economy is not welcoming to this expanded population. In country after country and across whole continents, the growing numbers of older people are seen as a burden on resources, a 'demographic pressure' – in the context of growing austerity and the abandonment of welfarism.

In 2012, the IMF issued a report claiming that the global debt crisis is driven by rising spending on health care and pensions, the 'longevity risk': it warned that if individuals were to live three years longer on average than expected, 'the already large costs of aging could increase by another 50 percent'. This would amount to 'tens of trillions of US dollars'. The IMF focus is primarily on pensions but they note gloomily that additional health and long-term care costs 'will further increase the burden of aging' (IMF 2012: 2, 8). The credit rating agency Standard & Poor's underlines a point implicit in the IMF analysis: the advanced economies are less well placed to grow to absorb these extra costs than the emerging economies with their generally younger populations (S&P 2012).

The ageing of the population is not just an issue in the wealthier countries: the UN projection is that the global population of people aged over 60 in developing countries is set to rise by more than 3 per cent each year, from 510 million in 2011 to 1.6 billion in 2050 – 80 per cent of the global 60-plus population (UN 2011c). Even

Sub-Saharan Africa, despite HIV and AIDS, is expected to have 160 million people aged over 60 by 2050.But while many of the health issues affecting older people are similar in developing and developed countries, the level of resources and availability of systems and services to address them are very different.

A snapshot survey by Help Age International showed that two-thirds of older people in developing countries find it hard to access health care (with the biggest problems in rural areas) and that poverty means almost three-quarters of older people also lacked income for water, electricity, food and decent housing – the lack of which threatens to undermine their health (HAI 2011). Most international aid to low-income countries is targeted around specific programmes mainly focused on adults and the young (HIV/AIDS), or on the Millennium Development Goals, none of which relate to older people.

In the 'club' of richest countries, the OECD, the percentage aged 65+ more than doubled to 13.85% (164 million people) between 1960 and 2005 and is expected almost to double again to 25% by 2050. A rapidly growing proportion of these are more dependent people aged over 85, up from 0.5% in 1960 to 1.5% in 2005 (18 million people), and expected to hit 5% by 2050 (Rechel et al. 2009).

In the EU, life expectancy has gone on rising, from an average of 74.2 in 1980 to 80.3 in 2006. The expanded 27-country EU has fallen back a little from this, with an overall average of 79.4 in 2009 – and a substantial seven-year gap between the highest and lowest country levels (European Community 2012). Numbers of people aged 80+ are rising faster than any other segment of the EU population. Two-thirds of people of pensionable age have at least *two* chronic conditions requiring treatment. This has serious resource implications, since in England, health resource allocations assume that the average costs of the 65+ are more than double (and for the 75+, four times; for the 85+, almost nine times) the health costs of those of working age, 16–44 (DoH 2005, Rechel et al. 2009: 11).

A study of eight OECD countries found that between a third and a half of all health spending was on older people (Coyte et al. 2008). In England, the over-65s account for two-thirds of hospital bed-days. However, sick older people *not* close to death are no more costly to care for than younger patients with similar conditions (Thomson et al. 2009: 6 fn). A 2007 survey of 20,000 Europeans aged 50+ found that hospital use peaks between the ages of 75 and 79: age discrimination may help explain what appears to be a decline in use of health services for the apparently more vulnerable 80+ age group (Rechel et al. 2009: 11). Much of the increased cost of providing health care for older patients is not the costs of medical care but a continual and substantial increase in pharmaceutical costs and new technologies (CBC News 2011).

A harsher attitude

Clearly a longer lifespan can mean a much greater chance of contracting a new and costly disease such as cancer, or degenerative conditions such as arthritis (requiring joint replacements), dementia or Alzheimer's. Medical costs will obviously be higher for those who are also obese and at increased risk. The costs of caring for the health needs of this growing population of older people have long been seen as a threat by bankers. In 1995, when the OECD launched a debate on the implications of an 'ageing society', its own researchers pointed out that this was a changed attitude from that of the early 1980s – a change that reflects the rise of neoliberal approaches in the last 30 years and continues to shape policy (Hennessy 1995).

The OECD indeed did begin to argue for a new, harsher attitude to the elderly. In place of the notion that the reward for increased productivity, an expanding economy and a lifetime of hard work would be a future of increased leisure and earlier retirement has come the proposal that – to keep the system solvent – working lives should be prolonged, at least to 70 years of age (OECD 1998a: 11).

The OECD began an earnest debate to formulate a plan to persuade older people to stay at work:

> Existing financial incentives for early retirement should be withdrawn or scaled back significantly.
>
> (OECD 1998b)

Though life expectancy has risen in the last century, such a proposal echoes the first state pension plans in Europe, introduced in Germany by Bismarck, which also fixed the retirement age at 70, on the relatively safe assumption that few workers who paid into the scheme would survive long enough to claim much – if any – of their entitlement after they finished work. The OECD debate on health and social care policies for older people began with 'a high level of agreement' across the OECD countries that ideally they should be 'enabled' to continue living in their own homes or, if that should prove impossible, they should be supported in a 'sheltered and supportive environment' as close to their community as possible (Hennessy 1995: 8).

In 2000, the European Union actively opted to remove a mandatory right to social services and social assistance that had been incorporated in the 1996 Turin Social Charter of the Council of Europe, instead adopting a formula in the European Constitution (Eurotreaties 2003) that simply recognises an 'entitlement' – which is no guarantee at all of access. Since then, the main EU focus has been on opening up the services that are available to older people to more intensive competition and privatisation (Lethbridge 2011). Older people, it seems, are every banker's problem and (despite occasional platitudes from governments) nobody's priority.

Indeed, as Kerrison and Pollock (2001) noted in England, a global model appears to be emerging in which there are two health-care sectors – the mainstream sector, focused on the young and adults of working age, dominated by collective or public funding; and another, largely private sector for older people, in which services are means-tested or paid for out of pocket, and in which huge gaps can open up between needs and available services.

In 2003, the European Central Bank Economic Policy Committee again warned of the costs of pensions and health care, and urged member states to take steps to 'limit the public sector's exposure' to rising health bills though a cap on health spending, greater use of private finance, the use of 'market forces' to boost efficiency and a restriction of public-sector health care to 'core services' (ECB Bulletin 2003). The report went on to suggest that individuals could provide 'non-essential health expenditure':

Individuals could then decide to what degree they wish to seek insurance cover for such costs. Greater private involvement in health care funding can be achieved, in particular, through patient co-payments, as already implemented in a number of countries.

(ECB Bulletin 2003: 45)

The falling birth rate in much of Europe means that the proportion of working-age to retired people is falling. Moreover, a declining working age population will generate less income for health and pension systems. In response to this, the EU 'Lisbon Treaty' opted to widen the workforce and laid plans for the whole EU to 'increase labour force participation' by older workers – make them work more years before retirement pensions.

Customers the insurers don't want

The OECD, too, has emphasised private-sector solutions and curbing the growth of spending on state pensions, health and long-term care. But while the ECB and OECD urge older people to seek private insurance, the insurance companies tend to steer clear of the elderly or to charge prohibitively high premiums to deter all but the wealthiest: the elderly are seen as a high-cost (longer-stay) demographic and a risk. In Chile, for example, the private health insurance which covers 12 per cent of the population covers just 3 per cent of over-60s (Lloyd Sherlock 2002). Private health insurance premiums for older people everywhere are much higher than for adults of working age: many elderly are also excluded from insurance through clauses on pre-existing conditions (Thomson et al. 2009).

The neoliberal, market-oriented approach to health care sees this in terms of maintaining a healthy workforce. Because the elderly are no longer part of the main workforce, most are seen as economically inactive (their pensions are effectively deferred earnings). So a year of life for an older person is valued less highly than a year in the life of someone in the 'working age' population (aged 9–55) by health economists calculating 'disability-adjusted life years' (DALYs) (Anand and Hanson 1998, Lloyd Sherlock 2002: 198, Labonté et al. 2004: 75fn).

The removal of elderly care from the mainstream, publicly provided health-care system in Britain and other countries has represented a significant step towards 'recommodifying' services which had previously been excluded from the market. Hiving off older people into long-term care in privately owned, for-profit nursing and residential homes, or consigning them to the attentions of private, for-profit domiciliary services results – even where the state continues to foot the full cost of treatment – in care being measured in cash terms in which each patient is seen as a potential source of surplus value to a provider (Leys 2001).

Hennessy shows that the package of policies which many OECD countries have imposed on services for older patients, which allow the potential for 'catastrophic' costs, have been deemed acceptable even though they fail to uphold the principles of adequacy, equity and income protection that apply to other welfare provision (Hennessy 1995: 9). Containing costs to the public purse has always been a focus of health-care strategies for older people, whose health needs are seen as less of a priority than acute services for younger adults or children. In much of Europe and the US, long-term care of the frail elderly has remained at least semi-detached from mainstream health care, often run by private or charitable organisations.

The active contribution made by many older people (for example, in the areas of childcare, informal/unpaid health care and social care, voluntary sector work and part-time employment) is underestimated and older people are seen simply as a cost, an expense. As Lethbridge (2011: 9) points out, the main impact of this falls upon women, whose higher life expectancy means they are more likely to need care services later in life; who traditionally fill many of the jobs involved in delivering care; and who, in many cases, also wind up responsible for unpaid 'informal care' of dependent relatives. While they are in work, many women receive wages and salaries that tend to be lower than those of men, often as a result of career breaks and child-rearing responsibilities; as a result, they end their working lives with lower pension entitlements and fewer assets to pay for the costs of their own care.

Passing the buck to older people

In recent years there has been discussion of the possible savings that might be achieved by delivering long-term care through 'community care' (or in the words of the OECD, 'ageing in place') (Hennessy 1995: 6). In Britain, the state has never supported the majority of disabled and older people, and long-term health care was formally separated from the NHS in 1993 as part of the 'Griffiths' proposals for 'Community Care' (i.e. care in nursing homes). Thousands of NHS 'geriatric' beds closed and the responsibility for procuring long-term care (from a range of private for-profit and non-profit providers) was handed over to local government – since when, unlike the preceding NHS arrangements, it has always been subject to means-tested charges. This often means that older people have to pay the whole cost of their care from savings and the sale of their homes (Lister 2008a).

High charges mean that institutional long-term care rapidly becomes unafford-able for individuals, even for those who are relatively well off: and no long-term care is entirely free to access. The cost can be as much as 60 per cent of average income for all but the wealthiest 20 per cent – and few older people, especially those requiring care, have access to this level of income (Colombo and Mercier 2011). In the US, a survey of the out-of-pocket expenses of people covered by Medicare found that 25 per cent of subjects' expenditures exceeded baseline total household assets, while 43 per cent spent more than their non-housing assets. The highest costs were faced by those suffering from dementia or Alzheimer's – and 56 per cent of spending related to nursing home costs (Kelley et al. 2012).

In the early 1990s, EU countries offered a variety of provision which ranged from caring for more than 10 per cent of over-65s in hospital, nursing homes or residential homes in the early 1990s, to fewer than 3 per cent (in Greece, Italy, Portugal and Spain). By the early 2000s, the highest level of institutional care was 8.5 per cent in Sweden, while only Denmark still had a majority of long-term care and home-care services provided by the public sector (Kroger 2001). Now studies in Europe show a generalised move away from institutional (residential and nursing home) care towards care in the home (Tarricone and Tsouros 2008). Denmark is the biggest provider of institutional care for older people, covering 56 per cent of beneficiaries: but five European countries[1] care for 5 per cent or fewer of their dependent older people in institutional settings (Lethbridge 2011: 4).

A 2011 OECD survey showed that the same trend away from care in nursing homes is common in many countries, as are attempts to deter patients from using them. Waiting times for admission range from 7–8 weeks in the Netherlands up to an astonishing 2–3 years in Japan, which appears especially poorly organised to deal with the exceptional longevity of its population. However, a 2006 Japanese reform did break new ground by using professional staff from residential homes to provide support for older people living in their own homes. Similar policies have been tried in Belgium. In Mexico, New Zealand, Finland and the Slovak Republic, governments have launched programmes to train informal carers. President Obama's Affordable Care Act in the US includes new incentives for community and home-based long-term care. In other countries, cash benefits are on offer to help people organise their own support at home. But perhaps the most bizarre measure was the Japanese government' policy to pay nursing homes less than their costs for caring for patients with the lowest level of need (OECD 2011: 296–300).

Neither cheaper nor better

There is evidence that a combination of good nutrition, hygiene, support with mobility, help with medication and reduced environmental hazards can help keep people out of hospital. But in the drive to cut costs by keeping older people out of expensive hospitals and institutional care, there has been a proliferation of less well-grounded schemes for 'healthy ageing'. A 2009 OECD survey pointed out that few of these schemes had been properly evaluated on cost-effectiveness and warned that some may even increase costs and worsen health! (Oxley 2009: 20) A WHO briefing also argues that systems which appear more 'efficient' may not enhance the quality of life and that the costs and risks of care at home tend to 'fall on the care recipients and their carers' (Coyte et al. 2008: 6).

A common feature of many of the more serious proposals for the better management of patients with long-term conditions is the integration of services. A WHO Policy Brief argues that 'consensus is emerging on the need for radically redesigning services in health and social care towards integrated community-based care' (Coyte et al. 2008: 6).

However, these proposals for integration run counter to competitive market models (such as those emerging in England) which aim to open up greater private-sector involvement.

It is generally accepted that better rehabilitation services can enable hospitals to discharge patients safely to their homes, especially if followed up by supportive services at home. But this requires the development of community-based services

---

1   Austria, Estonia, Latvia, Poland and Slovakia

which may not offer profit margins to attract private providers. The WHO focus is on 'more enabling interventions' such as physiotherapy and podiatry – which may also be best provided by a public sector geared to need, not profit.

If patients are to live at home, good-quality housing and well-designed living environments are obviously desirable: but where older people have retired, they may well be living in deprived areas and houses which are far from ideal. There will be limits to how far governments and health services could or should intervene to address such problems, even if the result would be improved health status: however, in a market-based health and social care system, no intervention would be possible.

Across Europe, the availability of services and the entitlement of older people to care services vary, and there are also variations within countries: in England, as local government has cut spending, some councils have imposed tighter eligibility criteria for social care than others, creating a 'postcode lottery' for older people. Early in 2012, the older people's charity Age UK warned of 'Care in Crisis', with spending having stagnated and then decreased since 2005–6 while the number of people aged over 85, the age group which is most likely to need care, had increased by over 250,000 since 2004–5.

Because of funding cuts, councils have cut back on their service provision and increasingly restricted any care to those with the most severe needs: in 2005, 50 per cent of councils provided support to people assessed as having 'moderate' needs, but by 2011 only 18 per cent could expect any support. Just to maintain the status quo, a steady increase in funding is needed; but instead, cutbacks year by year are creating an ever-widening gap between social needs and social services. Spending in 2011–12 should have risen by £200 million: instead it had fallen by £300 million – creating a £500 million gap. As a result, 40 per cent of the 2 million older people in England with care-related needs were receiving no support from public- or private-sector agencies (Age UK 2012).

Retreat from universalism

Especially at times of austerity and constraints on government spending, there are debates on whether support for long-term care should be universal or offered only to the poorest pensioners. One way to lay the basis for 'top-up' payments by service users is to change from providing services to the payment of cash benefits, to be spent by the client or on their behalf.

In various countries there have been experiments or discussions on 'consumer directed payments' that allow a service user to purchase care themselves. However, this withdrawal of the public sector does not guarantee the availability or dependable quality of services from private for-profit or non-profit providers. In a market system, private providers cannot be compelled to deliver services which do not yield profit: and the quest for competition makes it impossible to plan or to match services to needs.

A major problem with paying benefits directly to patients is that the risk, responsibility and potential extra cost is transferred to the service user, who may not have the knowledge, expertise or opportunity to spend wisely. The WHO also points out that 'The quality of personal care purchased is uncertain': patients may even 'have a financial incentive to 'underuse potentially needed formal professional care that is more expensive' (Coyte et al. 2008: 13). And consumer-directed payments themselves may also prove expensive and inefficient to run. The Netherlands has pioneered this, as part of a system of long-term care covering 3.6 per cent of the population. One thing the payments have not been good at is holding down spending: the amount paid out rose from €413 million in 2003 to €2.3 billion in 2010 (Maarse 2012). In response, the government will in 2013 give stronger powers to local government, allowing them to decide how much to allocate in support payments for domiciliary services, while imposing significant spending cuts (dressed up, as so often, as 'efficiency'). Eligibility criteria have been tightened, user charges have been increased. The new coalition from April 2012 is even now looking to scrap much of the personal budget system altogether (Maarse 2012).

The onward march of market-style reforms, which fragment services and seek to open up chosen sectors to private providers, flies in the face of evidence not only on the care of older people but also on the development and improvement of health-care systems. Fotaki and Boyd (2005) analyse 'quasi market reforms' in Sweden and the UK, and conclude that they produced no improvement in quality, efficiency or effectiveness: nor did they increase choice, which had been reduced for both service users and staff. Moreover, the market approach means that 'inequalities are likely to increase' (ibid.: 241). Experience shows that the most effective way to improve the quality of services is through peer review and pressure, collaboration, and the sharing of best practice. All of these are outlawed by the rules of a competitive market.

Older people in developing countries

If dramatic words like 'shock' are appropriate at all in discussing the issues of the growing elderly population, it is in the context of the developing countries, where the rapid expansion of the over-60 age groups has been remarkable. It took France more than 100 years for the population of over-65s to double from 7 per cent to 14 per cent: but in Brazil, China and Thailand the same transformation will take just 20 years. And while, as we have seen, the wealthier countries have failed over a much longer timescale to ensure adequate and equitable provision for older people's health needs, the question will be posed much more quickly in the developing world (Tran 2012).

Of the world's 400 million people aged over 80, 80 per cent will live in these countries by 2050 – 100 million of them in China. Yet few studies have looked at the health issues facing older people in Sub-Saharan Africa, where the continuing fight against communicable diseases now increasingly runs alongside a growing toll of noncommunicable disease (NCDs) with heart disease and stroke, visual impair-ment, hearing loss and dementia among the major issues (WHO 2012b). NCDs are now the biggest causes of death among the over-60s in developing countries as well as the OECD.

The rising numbers of older people are significant because, as might be expected, international comparisons show sharp increases in the average cost of health care for older age groups, with average expenditure levels from three to five times higher than for people aged under 65 (Anderson and Hussey 2001). The expansion of the most potentially vulnerable age group, with the highest levels of morbidity and use of health services, places huge new demands on available health-care resources. Yet despite 'an era of unprecedented, rapid and inexorable global ageing', the older population has remained a largely 'invisible' factor on the policy agenda (HAI 2002). Until recently, the issue of health policy for older people rated relatively low on the scale of political priorities for health-system reformers: even now, the leading NGO raising the demands of older people on an international level feels obliged to argue that adjustments are needed to ensure that ageing is no longer the 'missing dimension' or 'blind spot' in data collection, and that action on ageing forms part of the future development agenda (UNPFA and Help Age International 2011: 162).

Misconceptions of needs and costs

Lloyd Sherlock (2002) shows that the World Bank's limited interest in the care of the elderly only developed during the mid-1990s. Indeed, the Bank's new-found interest in the issues of ageing came too late to influence its input to the 1994 Cairo International Conference on Population and Development, where its submission, in line with much of the discussion, was largely focused on issues of reproductive health (World Bank 2001b). The Bank now admits that it was slow to recognise the scale of poverty amongst the older population; but even when it did begin to take up issues of ageing, the Bank's initial focus centred on the establishment of pension schemes for workers employed in the formal economy. In 1999, five years after the Cairo conference, when the Bank prepared a follow-up paper on the changing demographics of the world, issues of ageing and the implications 'were mentioned' – though once again ageing 'was not the central focus' (ibid.).

In part, the Bank's reluctance to discuss expanded and improved services for older people in developing counties is due to the false impression that very large numbers of older people are likely to require expensive and complex treatment. Many of the treatments most needed are relatively cheap and effective. Visual impairment takes the greatest toll in years lost to disability among the over 60s in low- and middle-income countries: cataracts are one of the most common problems and an expansion of treatment for cataracts could prevent blindness in up to 150 million people, two-thirds of them aged over 60: the operation is cheap, safe and cost-effective (WHO 2012b). Studies show that between 32 per cent and 80 per cent of older people have high blood pressure, while only 4–14 per cent are receiving treatment. Yet the drugs for this are an 'evidence-led' 'best buy' at a cost of less than US$1 a year per person in low-income countries (WHO 2012b: 19).

In fact, quality data on the health problems and needs of older people in developing countries is largely absent, again underlining the lack of priority that has been accorded this area of health policy (Lloyd Sherlock 2002: 200). Basic skills and resources are lacking. Even a relatively prosperous middle-income country like

Chile turns out to have just six geriatricians for the whole country (Shetty 2012). Nursing-home facilities, even in the Argentine capital, are of questionable quality and likely to exclude some of the most vulnerable older patients (Lloyd Sherlock and Redondo 2009).

Governments and international agencies are increasingly looking to reforms based on market models, or promoting insurance-based systems and user charges, or seeking ways of maximising 'efficiency', containing costs and restricting public spending.

With media headlines focused on the MDGs, high levels of child mortality and the grim toll of HIV/AIDS, the agenda of issues relevant to the care of older people has been seen as tangential even to the campaign for Health for All 2000 (HFA) promoted by the WHO in the world's poorest countries. The focus of HFA and other WHO programmes, and much of the rationale of World Bank 'targeted' measures, has generally centred on mothers, reducing child mortality, promoting health through vaccination of the young, and buttressing the health of the working population.

While these are perfectly legitimate goals, they appear to leave little in the way of resources for the care of older people. As Lloyd Sherlock argues, the primary-health-care (PHC) focus of the WHO reform campaign effectively sidelines the needs of the elderly:

> Whilst age discrimination was never an explicit goal of PHC, it inevitably entailed a reduced prioritisation of services which principally benefited older age groups.
>
> (2002: 197)

This generalised, tacit downgrading of the priority of care for the elderly can be compounded at local level by ageist, discriminatory policies, including age limits, and sometimes by the prejudices and negative stereotypes which may shape the attitudes of health-service workers to older people seeking treatment (UN 2002: §70).

Overview: the economics of elderly care

Many World Bank policies for establishing an infrastructure of basic health care in developing countries start from a calculation of the economic costs of ill health in terms of lost production. For those who seek an economic justification for investment in health care, there is thus the argument that securing a healthier workforce will reduce poverty through enabling economic growth or, as Cohen argues, that:

> A healthy population is an engine for economic growth. ... Healthier workers are physically and mentally more energetic and robust, more productive and earn higher wages. A healthy workforce is important when attracting foreign direct investment. ... Ill health may leave persons able to work, but reduce their productivity, shorten their working lives, and increase the numbers of days lost to illness.
>
> (Alleyne and Cohen 2002:5, 8)

From this standpoint, health promotion among younger adults is a sound business investment. By contrast, providing health care and decent living standards to the older population is not only an irrelevance but potentially a drag on the expansion of the economy. Even before the MDGs narrowed the focus of donors to specific issues relating to women, children and the young,[2] four of the five main 'agency goals' set out in the USAID Strategic Plan 1998–2003 related to issues of unwanted pregnancy, childbirth, child nutrition and HIV transmission – and none of them take account of older people (USAID 1999).

The evident lack of concern for reforming the care of older people demonstrates that the pattern of health-care reform is not driven by the progress in medical and pharmaceutical technology; nor does it flow organically from attempts to tackle problems and pressures within health care. Instead, the menu of health-care reforms is derived from a separate political and ideological agenda. This approach, as the previous chapters have sought to show, starts from the wrong questions and almost inevitably winds up advocating the wrong answers.

Markets and mental health

Prominent among the key noncommunicable diseases taking a toll on older people in the high-, middle- and low-income countries alike is dementia, the mental deterioration often linked with old age. It is second only to visual impairment in the toll it takes in years lost to disability (WHO 2012b). Data suggests that in 2010 there were almost 36 million people living with dementia and 7.7 million new cases each year: 58 per cent of dementia sufferers live in developing countries. This is set to rise to 71 per cent of a much larger total of 115 million by 2050 (WHO 2012b: 16).

The 'treatment gap' between the probable incidence of dementia and the numbers diagnosed is very wide. It is estimated that as few as 20 per cent of cases, up to a maximum of only 50 per cent, are recognised and documented in high-income countries, while one study in India showed 90 per cent of cases had not been identified. Mental health services in 17 low- and middle-income countries leave large numbers of people with anxiety and mood disorders and substance misuse without treatment (Wang et al. 2007). Campaigners project from this type of performance that 28 million of the 36 million with dementia have not been diagnosed, even though various forms of treatment, if delivered early, can delay the onset of the disease and improve cognitive function, as well as encouraging caregivers (Alzheimer's Disease International 2011).

One factor in low levels of diagnosis and treatment is the issue of funding. Like other aspects of health care, mental health care is subject in many countries to user fees, with high costs for prescription drugs. Moreover, it is likely to be excluded from most insurance policies that might be affordable to those on low incomes. Since mental illness sufferers the world over tend to be on lower rates of pay, if they are

---

2   While largely ignoring the high mortality and disease burden resulting from under-nutrition of nursing mothers and children, which is estimated to result in 2.2 million deaths a year and 21 per cent of disability-adjusted life years for children under five (Black et al. 2008).

in employment at all, they are not attractive customers for private insurers – which are primarily focused on young, fit, affluent people of working age who are likely to make minimal claims and generate maximum profits. Publicly funded health-care systems and social health insurance in the wealthier countries tend to give low priority to mental health provision, and under the impact of austerity there are growing gaps in cover that leave those requiring drugs and treatment with the unacceptable choice: pay up or go without (Funk et al. 2007).

Even in this context, there seems to be a deep-seated blind spot on the issue of dementia, where patients are even less likely to be able to pay an economic market fee for their care or be covered by private insurance. Even though the WHO in 2008 made dementia one of its seven priorities for its Mental Health Gap Action Plan, a major WHO document on 'Mental Health systems in selected low- and middle-income countries' failed even to mention its existence (WHO 2009).

However, constraints on resources and lack of political will to put appropriate services in place are problems that apply not just to the mental health problems of old age but across the board. The combined disability burden of mental illness, neurological disorders such as epilepsy, and substance abuse (collectively known as MNS) represents 14 per cent of the global burden of disease measured in DALYs: the treatment gap between incidence and treatment is as wide as 75 per cent in many low- and middle-income countries, which have most of the burden but few resources to deal with it. A WHO study found that even in high-income countries, 35–50 per cent of serious MNS cases had received no treatment in the previous 12 months, while 76–85 per cent in less-developed countries had received no treatment at all.

On a world scale, it is estimated that a third of schizophrenia cases, more than half of the cases of depression and three-quarters of alcohol abuse went untreated. In many low-income countries, 95 per cent of people with epilepsy receive inadequate treatment if they get any at all. The gap is a very big one: around the world it is estimated that between 12 and 49 per cent of people will suffer some form of MNS issue during their lifetime, and between 8 and 29 per cent in any given year; and that MNS represents a massive 30 per cent of the burden of noncommunicable disease (mhGAP 2008). More recently, the WHO and Alzheimer's Disease International have teamed up to declare dementia a "public health priority" (WHO and ADI 2012).

If discussed at all in the context of developing countries, mental health care has until the last few years been largely dealt with as an adjunct to the more central issue of establishing a minimum package of primary-health-care services and setting up new structures of user fees as a device to establish various forms of health insurance. Perhaps because it doesn't easily fit into any market-style reform package – and does not feature in the MDGs or attract funding from the big donor organisations which have concentrated exclusively on medical interventions for specific physical diseases – mental health has also remained largely neglected as a subject for policy research by the otherwise-active global agencies and consultancies. A search of the World Bank's 14,000 online publications for the term 'mental health' early in 2003 drew just 19 references, none dealing in any depth with policy issues.

Even now, as the WHO and other specialists try to kick-start a serious initiative to plug glaring gaps in mental-health services, the list of funding organisations playing a leading role conspicuously lacks any mention of the World Bank (although the African Development Bank is involved), USAID or the Bill & Melinda Gates Foundation. Indeed, even the WHO has reservations about the extent to which mental health can be promoted and prioritised alongside other noncommunicable diseases (NCDs). A 2011 meeting in Moscow, which happily heard from a pharmaceutical-company boss arguing that the private sector wants to be seen as a key partner in initiatives to combat NCDs, also heard the WHO's 'Assistant Director-General for Noncommunicable Diseases and Mental Health' set out reasons why mental health should not be added to the four main diseases to be targeted in a high-profile campaign (WHO 2011).[3] One reason was that mental health had already been omitted for the past ten years or more since the Global Strategy on NCDs had been launched in 2000; another was that the four priority areas all take a high death toll – accounting for 80 per cent of deaths from NCDs – while mental illness brings relatively few deaths; the third reason was that the four diseases 'share the same main risk factors, so prevention approaches are similar' (WHO 2011: 14).

It's hard not to conclude from this response that there are more deeply seated reasons why mental health, and MNS in general, are not given higher priority by governments. Perhaps the collective indifference of the Gates Foundation, the World Bank and the other big money organisations, together with the limited opportunity for profitable private-sector involvement[4] and the grudging and reluctant involvement of governments[5] that have dragged their feet and made minimal allocations of resources, are more decisive in watering down the enthusiasm for mental health services.

Whatever the explanation, whether it lies in politics, economics or ideology, the mismatch between the resources allocated to MNS and the burden of disability it brings is considerable: WHO figures show that on a world scale mental health disorders alone account for 11.5 per cent of DALYs, but spending by governments averaged just 3.8 per cent of health budgets. Average mental health spending per capita in low- and middle-income countries is just US$0.3 per capita, compared with the US$3–4 suggested by the WHO. There is even a significant inequality between low-income countries and upper-middle-income countries, with the latter spending an astonishing 70 times more per capita, providing 24 times more beds per 100,000 population and offering 8 times more mental health staff (WHO 2009: 8). Despite the best efforts of mental health activists, absence of funding 'remains the dominant reported impediment' to implementing plans to 'scale up' services for mental health in low- and middle-income countries (Eaton et al. 2011: 1,598). A third of countries

---

3   The four targets are cardiovascular disease, diabetes, cancers and chronic respiratory diseases.

4   Significantly, the WHO's Mental Health Gap Action Programme specifies that schizophrenia and other psychotic disorders should be treated with 'older antipsychotics'. These are available very cheaply as generics and offer little towards the dividends of big pharma's grasping shareholders (WHO 2008: 11).

5   Reports from more than ten countries out of 44 surveyed identified poor awareness and low priority or poor commitment by political leaders as major barriers to the development of mental health services. Half of survey respondents said securing funds for mental health was no easier than in 2007, while some said it was harder (Eaton et al. 2011: 1,594, 1,599)

don't even have a specific budget for mental health and 21 per cent of those that do allocate it less than 1 per cent of health spending (mhGAP 2008: 8). Lower funds were given by government donors in 2008 than in 1995 and WHO spending on NCDs (including mental health) was cut by a third between 2002 and 2008 (Eaton et al. 2011: 1,599).

Mental health is another clear example of the inverse care law: the countries with the greatest burden of disease are the least well equipped to deal with it, lacking the money, the professional staff and any infrastructure of training to fill the gaps. In many middle-income countries, where some investment has been made in mental health it has followed archaic models of care from the nineteenth century in Europe, building large, costly mental hospitals located primarily to serve urban populations and showing reluctance to move towards a modern system of community-based and decentralised delivery of mental health services that could reach deprived rural populations.

The WHO's Mental Health Gap Action Programme prioritises eight MNS conditions for specific intervention: depression, schizophrenia, suicide, epilepsy, dementia, drug abuse, alcohol abuse and child mental health problems (mhGAP 2008: 4). A few of the evidence-based interventions turn out not to be health care at all, but public health, preventative measures, improved care in pregnancy and childbirth, and education of carers (for dementia sufferers). It's clear that mental health services can only function effectively in a public-health framework and that the factors generating mental illness are generally social and external, and are exacerbated by poverty, discrimination and other aspects of deprivation. While mental illness itself clearly has an economic cost to those affected, the economic and political contexts also affect mental health – and potentially limit the resources available to deliver mental health services.

The problems in achieving an effective mental health service in the low- and middle-income countries, other than lack of financial resources and government commitment, include: overcentralisation – not least in the continued reliance on large psychiatric hospitals which also consumed an average 80 per cent of mental health budgets (WHO 2009: 8); the challenge of integrating mental health care into primary care (a core recommendation of the WHO's special *World Health Report* on mental health, 2001); a shortage of public-health expertise; and shortages of trained mental health personnel (Eaton et al. 2011: 1,599).

Staff shortages are a major limitation: low- and lower-middle-income countries have hardly any psychiatrists, even fewer psychologists or social workers, and a tiny handful of psychiatric nurses (mhGAP 2008, WHO 2009). In Chile, gearing up to widen access to evidence-based care for depression required a hefty 344 per cent increase in the number of full-time psychologists employed in primary care centres (Eaton et al. 2011: 1,598). Without a minimum of mental health facilities and staff it is impossible to deliver community health care. In the absence of qualified staff or any mechanism to train them, the urgency of delivering some support to those suffering mental illness means that there has been discussion of using volunteers as well as families and carers to fill the gap, although policy experts warn that it could have unintended consequences. Seeing unpaid volunteers as a substitute for the proper provision of professional services could prevent the development of a working system for mental health care and reduce choices for service users (Eaton et al. 2011: 1,597).

Mental health in the wealthier countries

That mental health does not fit neatly or obviously into the framework of market reforms is underlined by the general lack of focused and convincing research and policy discussion from the OECD. A three-year OECD health project, begun in 2001 and intended to confront the growing challenges facing health policy and health-care systems, designated long-term care for frail elderly persons as a specific area of study but made no reference at all to mental health (OECD 2001b, 2001c). The European Commission published an 86-page report on the state of mental health in the EU which was also largely restricted to general comments for the lack of appropriate comparative data: even such a basic measure as the level of use of psychotropic drugs in treatment seemed to be lacking (Europa 2004: 20).

In 2005, the WHO in Europe published a wordy and worthy declaration and an action plan for Europe, largely lacking in concreteness and commitment to any specifics (WHO 2005a, 2005b) – although a declaration at Helsinki in January 2005 did take the positive step of affirming the responsibility of European governments to ensure that there are:

> sufficient resources for mental health, considering the burden of disease, and to make investment in mental health an identifiable part of overall health expenditure, in order to achieve parity with investments in other areas of health.
>
> (WHO 2005b: 5)

There is little indication that the commitment to this policy has driven much change in European countries: mental health consistently emerges as the poor relation of health care when it comes to budget allocations and policy priorities, receiving a widely varying percentage of total health spending. Before the 2008 financial meltdown, this ranged in Western Europe from 3.5 per cent in the Czech Republic and 4 per cent in Portugal to 13 per cent in England and Luxembourg, with lower levels in Eastern Europe (Knapp et al. 2007).

A more serious subsequent analysis of mental health policy and practice in Europe found a worryingly high proportion of costs of care in Central and Eastern Europe coming from out of pocket payments and health insurance. Furthermore, it found that insurance companies were either excluding mental health from cover or charging excessively high premiums, which clearly has serious implications for equity in access for service users who are likely to be poor (Knapp et al. 2007: 69). The authors also note the impact of market-style reforms, which have resulted in increasing numbers of publicly funded mental health services being delivered by private for-profit or non-profit providers, opening up new avenues for private-sector involvement. Experience from the US showed the danger of the cream-skimming of relatively prosperous clients with less severe levels of mental illness by the private insurers, while limited private-sector provision, sometimes further restricted by public-sector spending cuts, also leaves state provision struggling to cope with the most severe and chronic problems.

User payments for mental health care are widely applied, with the Mental Health Economic European Network reporting out-of-pocket charges for some specialist mental health provision within publicly funded health-care systems in 8 of the 17 West European countries. These can be applied without reference to the ability of the service user to pay: care free of charge in Ireland was restricted to the bottom third of the income scale and insurance cover is limited. Charges are also a factor in East and Central Europe (Knapp et al. 2007).

The inverse relationship between level of illness and ability to pay is as wide, if not wider, in mental health than any other area of care. Between 10 and 30 per cent of psychiatric service users with severe needs utilise as much as 80 per cent of the services available (Torrey 1997, Lien 2003). These are also the people least likely to be covered by insurance or able to pay fees to cover the sometimes extremely high costs of their care, which may be required for many years. This means that the greater their level of health need, the less attractive a mental illness sufferer is as a client to a for-profit private-sector provider; and the less easily such needs can be met within a market-style health-care system or 'managed care' (Chisholm and Stewart 1998). There are also indications that poverty and unemployment can serve to prolong the duration of a mental illness, resulting in even higher costs of care (Weich and Lewis 1998).

The focus for policy makers and service providers therefore tends to switch away from those with the greatest to those with the least need, those with the most manageable problems and those already within the system. As one senior executive of a for-profit mental health service provider in the US summed up: 'You don't go looking for people who are going to be the highest risk unless you want to go bankrupt' (Torrey 1997: 125).

Across Europe, one challenge that has been facing mental health-care systems has been to organise a transition from exclusive reliance on costly, low quality and oppressive treatment in large institutions, consuming up to 70 per cent of mental health budgets, to more accessible, local and empowering community-based services, with sufficient resources to deal with the minority of more severe cases that require some form of hospital care. Progress has been uneven, hindered in some case by funding formulae which privilege the large hospitals; and Russia in particular has given more generous funding to the very large psychiatric hospitals with over 1,000 beds. Even where the larger hospitals are closed down, the transition to a system based on community health services can be complex. Funds generated by the savings made within, and eventual closure and sale of, psychiatric hospitals can 'leak' from mental health into acute care and other sectors (Knapp and McDaid 2007: 80–1).

Even much of the literature on mental health provision is lop-sided in the current market context, with a heavy bias towards papers focused on pharmaceutical treatments rather than psychotherapy, 'little on service reorganisation and almost nothing on mental health promotion.' The new atypical antipsychotics and other recent developments in (more costly and profitable) drugs to treat schizophrenia has ensured that these have become the central element in drug trials, many of them sponsored by big pharma, while there are comparatively few studies of treatments for child and adolescent mental health problems, anxiety disorders or personality disorders (Knapp and McDaid 2007: 83).

The impact of market-style reforms and the emphasis on the role of the private sector has also had the effect of fragmenting provision, allowing private providers to cherry pick aspects of mental health care they see as profitable. Meanwhile, the major focus of health-care systems has also been swivelled even more obsessively towards acute medical and surgical services, leaving inadequate resources for mental health.

This latter aspect is clearly argued in an important new study in the UK, 'How Mental Illness Loses Out in the NHS' (CEPMHPG 2012), which sets out the stark disparity between the scale and impact of mental illness (causing almost half of all ill health among under-65s; generally more debilitating than most chronic physical conditions) and the level of access to treatment (just a quarter of all those with mental illness are receiving treatment 'compared with the vast majority of those with physical conditions') – and the fact that it receives just 13 per cent of the NHS budget. The report explains why increasing the spending on mental health care would more or less pay for itself by reducing costs for the provision of physical care for patients whose condition is worsened or even triggered by mental health problems, and getting millions of people with depression or crippling anxiety conditions into productive, paid work (CEPMHPG 2012).

By contrast, UK mental health charities have been warning for some time that spending cuts in the NHS, local government, housing and social services are having a combined and detrimental impact on mental health services and their service users, undermining the effectiveness of systems and resulting in care that is unfit for purpose (Lakhani 2011, MIND 2011). An investigation by mental health charities has helped to underline the fact that, while demand for mental health support is increasing, some services are shrinking. Even though the government's mental health strategy for England ('No Health without Mental Health') is 'well regarded':

> There is little evidence, as yet that the strategy is being used systematically to guide local decision making; this is currently dominated by cost reduction, leading to reorganisation and cuts in service.
>
> (Centre for Mental Health et al. 2012)

The report found 'considerable evidence' of cuts in the support available for people with mental health problems in both statutory (health and local government) and voluntary-sector organisations, with the loss of specialist services and those tailored to the needs of especially marginalised groups. Services for older people and for children, which have always been under-funded and left out of earlier strategic plans for mental health, are now sharing in the cuts: older people's services are also hit hard by cuts in social service spending by local authorities. A survey of members of the NHS Confederation, which represents NHS providers, found that 23 per cent of organisations responding thought the quality of care would decrease (twice as many as thought acute care quality would suffer), while even more community and mental health providers thought cuts would be 'extremely problematic'. More than half the child-and-adolescent mental health providers and commissioners who responded said they planned to cut spending on services; and local authorities were planning to cut up to 25 per cent. To make matters worse, the Conservative coalition's massive market-style 'reforms' of the NHS were widely expected to bring increased fragmentation of services and disruptive organisational and structural changes (Centre for Mental Health et al. 2012).

The worrying findings of the charities' survey were further reinforced by a Department of Health report which revealed the first actual real-terms fall in mental health spending in England for ten years, dropping by 1 per cent to £6.63 billion, with the cuts falling hardest on crisis resolution, early intervention and outreach – three of the key services for minimising the hardship and suffering of those with severe mental illness (Ramesh 2012b).

The picture in England seems consistent with the general situation in Europe. In the Netherlands, 40 per cent of people with bi-polar disorder are estimated to have no contact with mental health care; and a study of the Netherlands and five other countries[6] found that there was inadequate use of mental health services for the prevalence of mental illness, with the lowest rates of treatment in Italy and Belgium (Knapp and McDaid 2007: 85). Sweden spends just 8 per cent of its health budget on mental health but is opening up a share of this for private operators: psychiatric and addiction services in Stockholm have been contracted out to two companies, Carema and Cooperative Praktikertjänst (Healthcare Europa 2011). In the UK, patients publicly funded by the NHS account for the lion's share of the £1.1 billion private for-profit psychiatric hospital sector, mainly through use of medium secure beds and other inpatient places, at an annual cost of £975 million (Lintern 2012).

The problem of inadequate access to treatment is also a large and growing one in the USA, where mental health services are being sharply cut back. A 2010 survey by the Substance Abuse and Mental Health Services Administration found that 40 per cent of adults with serious mental illness were not receiving any treatment and that mental health spending, although rising in cash terms, had fallen back as a share of all health spending from 7.2 per cent in 1986 to just 6.1 per cent in 2005. And the market was not meeting the levels of need: by 2005, public sources of coverage, notably Medicaid, the safety-net service for those on the lowest incomes, accounted for more than 50 per cent of mental health expenditure (SAMHSA 2011). A 2008 survey found that private health insurance paid for less than a quarter (23.8 per cent) of mental health inpatient treatment measured by discharges, significantly lower than its share of just over a third (34.1 per cent) of all discharges (Saba et al. 2008). A considerable proportion of potential US mental health 'patients' are being 'cared for' in the hostile surroundings of state prisons and jails: 24 per cent of state prisoners and 16.9 per cent of jail inmates, along with an estimated 70 per cent of youth in juvenile centres, live with serious mental illness (Finkel 2012).

However, in the US, as in Europe, a squeeze on mental health spending is creating what the National Alliance on Mental Illness calls a 'continuing crisis':

> Increasingly emergency rooms, homeless shelters and jails are struggling with the effects of people falling through the cracks due to the lack of needed mental

---

6   Belgium, France, Germany, Italy and Spain

health services and supports. States such as California, Illinois, Nevada and South Carolina, which made devastating cuts to mental health services previously, have made further cuts for fiscal year 2012, putting tens of thousands of citizens at great risk. States have cut more than $1.6 billion in general funds from their state mental health agency budgets for mental health services since FY2009, a period in which demand for services increased significantly.

(NAMI 2011: 1)

The five largest cuts recorded in this NAMI report are in South Carolina (39.3 per cent since FY2009), Alabama (36 per cent), Alaska (32.6 per cent), Illinois (31.7 per cent) and Nevada (28.1 per cent). As a result of these and other cuts, in some states, 'entire hospitals have been closed: in others, community mental health programs have been eliminated. Some 4,000 psychiatric hospital beds have closed since 2010' (NAMI 2011: 2–3, 6). California has gone so far as to shift responsibility for all provision for residents with serious mental illness to county level and slashed back on state-level staff who might be expected to monitor the resulting services.

As the cuts have continued and escalated, some high-profile problems involving mentally disordered offenders have highlighted the damage that has been done to services, to society and to individuals who are denied the support they need to cope. In Arizona in January 2011, Jared Lee Loughner went on a shooting spree killing six people and leaving 13, including Congresswoman Gabrielle Giffords, severely injured. He was arrested, but only when documents were filed in court in April was it revealed that he had received treatment at Sonora Behavioral Health Hospital in Tucson (Martin 2011). New coverage in the aftermath of the shooting picked up on the fact that mental health services for children and adolescents in Arizona are few and far between, unaffordable to middle-class Americans and available on an emergency basis only to the poorest families: medication too is costly, with the bills falling on service users and their families. Therapy for teenagers can be obtained privately at $80–$120 per hour or more, meaning that for a family of modest means like the Loughners the bill for twice weekly sessions could be 20 per cent of the household income (*Wall Street Journal* 2011). Others point out that Arizona, with 6.6 million people, up to 396,000 of whom are likely to have a serious mental illness, has mental health beds for just 6,851 people and limited outpatient provision based mainly around family therapy and drug and alcohol issues: but it has 1,318 gun shops, eager to sell to punters no matter how mentally ill they may be (Pein 2011).

Arizona's mental health laws include some of the strongest in the US for involuntary treatment: but its mental health services had been cut back by 37 per cent in the run-up to the shooting, meaning that 12,000 adults and 2,000 children could no longer get the branded medication that they had been taking (Frum 2011). The cuts, to fill a $1 billion hole in the state's finances, had been forced on Governor Jan Brewer, and brought a reversal of her initial attempt to restore funding to mental health and drug treatment services that had previously been cut (Santa Cruz and Powers 2011).

As this study is completed, another, similar episode shows that the issues of mentally disordered young people, access to weaponry and desperate shortages and gaps in mental health services are by no means restricted to Arizona: another tragedy in Colorado saw 58 wounded and 12 die in a gun rampage by another young man whose mother had tried to get treatment for him (Fitzpatrick 2012).

Brutal cuts in US mental health keep coming: in May 2012, Louisiana announced cuts of $270 million from mental health services, childhood care and breast cancer treatment. Among the hardest hit will be the homeless people eking out an existence in shelters, 80 per cent of whom are thought to be living with mental illness and/or substance abuse. A large psychiatric hospital was also predicted to close (Masson 2012). By July the cuts target had been increased to $329 million, a quarter of the state's annual health budget, slashing health insurance cover for 1.2 million people, most of them children. Louisiana State Hospital, a psychiatric hospital, was to be closed (Barrow and Adelson 2012). One spin-off of the mental health cuts is of course the failure to treat many people with serious mental illness, causing concern in the already-violent city of New Orleans, where detox beds, a quarter of inpatient beds and ten emergency beds have been axed (Maldonado 2012).

Similar fears have been raised in New York State, which has been emptying out its psychiatric hospitals after the governor decided it should stop providing treatment to people with serious mental illness, claiming they can get the same services elsewhere. New York's mental health capacity has been reduced from 599 psychiatric beds per 100,000 people to fewer than 28, while 14,000 offenders with serious mental illness were imprisoned. One New York jail, Riker's Island, now houses more mentally ill people than all of the state's hospitals (Jaffe 2012).

One conspicuous area of underinvestment, the impact of wide-scale drug abuse, and its knock-on effects on law and order in the USA have frequently been discussed in the mass media. The now-defunct National Drug Intelligence Center (2011) estimated the costs to society at $193 billion in 2007, $11.4 billion of which were direct health-care costs. However, spending on drug-abuse treatment amounted to just 1 per cent of health insurance costs (Cartwright 1999).

Disability – the hidden giant

One billion of the world's seven billion people live with one or more physical, sensory, intellectual or mental impairments, and one household in four contains a disabled member: yet the issue of disability is not mentioned in any of the eight Millennium Development Goals, or the related 21 Targets or 60 Indicators. This omission is described by the UN as:

> a lost opportunity... Indeed this lack of inclusion is more than a lost opportunity
> – a growing body of opinion and data argues that unless persons with disabilities
> are included, none of the MDGs will be met.
>
> (UN 2011a: viii)

The UN analysis argues that this may be because people with disabilities have incorrectly been seen as people whose lives are defined by medical and rehabilitative needs, or as individuals appropriate for charity: but it is impossible to avoid the fact that one reason they are ignored in such brazen fashion is that the majority are poor, and therefore do not constitute an attractive or lucrative market for the private sector. The WHO *World Report on Disability* discusses at length the extent to which people with disabilities are ignored or excluded:

> Misconceptions about the health of people with disabilities have led to assumptions that people with disabilities do not require access to health promotion and disease prevention. Evidence shows that health promotion interventions such as physical activities are beneficial for people with disabilities. But health promotion activities seldom target people with disabilities, and many experience multiple barriers to participation.
>
> (WHO and World Bank 2011: 60)

The UN has attempted to revisit their status and importance by redefining disability in the 2008 UN Convention on the Rights of Persons with Disabilities to set disability in the context of the relationship between the individual and the:

> social attitudes and the physical, economic and political environment that hinders the full equal participation of persons with disability in society.
>
> (UN 2011a: viii)

Disability was explicitly included in the 2010 *MDG Progress Report* discussing education of children with disabilities and recognised by the UN in a 2011 resolution on 'Realization of MDGs for persons with disabilities for 2015 and beyond'.

However, the UN report readily concedes that although disability issues may (as with other health issues) be implicit in the MDGs, and 'all MDGs are relevant to persons with disabilities and all MDG efforts must include persons with disabilities and evaluate this inclusion' (UN 2011a: xi), the lack of any specific reference to them or commitments to deliver improvements makes it much harder to include them in the related efforts to develop health and other services. It also acknowledges that, although some progress can be made, in reality there will be no significant changes in the MDG goals and targets at such a late stage.

Interestingly, prior to this new upsurge in interest in addressing problems of disability, the most frequent reference to it in global health policy debates was not centred on the actual issue of disability itself but on the World Bank's 1993 formulation of the notion of 'disability-adjusted life years' (DALYs) as a proxy measure for the cost-effectiveness of various health treatments (Arnesen and Nord 1999, Gwatkin and Guillot 2000, Ollila and Koivusalo 2002). If anything, the focus on the dismal pseudo-science of health economics has diverted attention from the key issue of assessing the prevalence of disability and the development of appropriate programmes to support and empower people with disabilities.

The underlying roots and causes of disability include inherited impairments, accidents, cardiovascular and pulmonary illness, psychiatric illness and chronic pain, conditions such as hypertension and diabetes; and in the developing world, malnutrition, communicable disease (including HIV/AIDS, tuberculosis, malaria and measles), violence and poor perinatal care (Murray and Lopez 1996, WHO

2004b). Preventable environmental factors that can cause or worsen disability include unsafe water and poor sanitation, air pollution and road accidents. Global burden of disease estimates suggest that two-thirds of disability is attributable to age-dependent, chronic noncommunicable disease, the vast majority of this in the developing countries. Dementia is the largest single factor but the after-effects of stroke and arthritis are also important (Sousa et al. 2009).

As the WHO points out:

> Disability is a development issue, and it will be hard to improve the lives of the most disadvantaged people in the world without addressing the specific needs of persons with disabilities.
>
> (WHO 2011: 12)

People with disabilities encounter barriers when they attempt to access health-care services: studies in India (Uttar Pradesh and Tamil Nadu) and South Africa have found that cost, lack of locally accessible services and transportation were the top three barriers to using health facilities. The issue of cost is paramount, according to the 2002–2004 *World Health Survey*, which also found it was a problem that affected a far higher proportion of people with disabilities than non-disabled people needing the same treatment. People with disabilities experience lower rates of employment, are more likely to be poor and are therefore less likely to be able to afford private health insurance – even if it is offered to them. But even employed people with disabilities may be excluded from private health insurance because of pre-existing conditions or be 'underinsured', facing large potential out-of-pocket costs (WHO 2011: 67). The countries where some of these barriers to health insurance have been reduced are those where governments subsidise insurance for certain categories of disabled people, effectively neutralising some of the market's bias against the poor and disadvantaged.

In some high-income countries, special additional incentive payments are offered to doctors and primary care organisations to cover people with disabilities who would otherwise be ignored. But as the WHO report points out, even removing fees does not guarantee access to services, whether this be for mental health patients feeling the barriers of stigma or for people with mobility difficulties accessing treatment at a distance from their homes (WHO 2011: 70). For some service users there is a correlation between the distance they have to travel to a clinic and their adherence to regular treatment, which can be a particular problem in rehabilitation: there are real benefits in working to integrate services to minimise costly and difficult journeys (WHO 2011: 114).

The Convention on the Rights of Persons with Disabilities highlights the environmental factors that restrict the participation of people with disabilities, in particular:

- Inadequate policies and standards
- Negative attitudes
- Lack of provision of services
- Problems with service delivery
- Inadequate funding

- Lack of accessibility
- Lack of consultation and involvement of disabled people in planning services
- Lack of data and evidence.

(WHO 2011: 262–3)

Perhaps the key recommendation coming out of this is number six: 'provide adequate funding and improve affordability'.

While many of the health problems of people with disabilities could be addressed by the roll-out of health care based on primary health care and community-based treatment and rehabilitation, the predominant focus on disease-specific programmes and donor-funded vertical programmes (intervening from the outside and developing little or no infrastructure of health or social care) offers little benefit (Gillam 2008). But the failure to mobilise even the resources required to achieve the MDGs, and the pressures to focus what funds there are on the eight MDG goals, mean that there is unlikely to be a transformation in attitudes to disability any time soon.

Chapter nine

It doesn't have to be this way – alternative approaches

The preceding chapters have told the sorry tale of the years since the 1978 WHO Assembly in Alma Ata, a succession of missed opportunities to reshape the world's health-care systems along progressive lines and of the historic reverse inflicted by neoliberalism. Fleetingly, the realisation of a global vision seemed possible – a vision of health care no longer viewed and delivered as a commodity, a commercial service like hairdressing or manicure, but built upwards from local needs and local access to primary health care; a vision of health care encompassing, where necessary, more complex and high-tech medicine through hospitals and services; and driven by the interests of patients, populations and communities, by a determination to combat discrimination and inequalities, and by a concern to improve health rather than generate profit.

Of course, even then the apparent consensus was an illusion, hiding the profoundly different core assumptions of the US – even though the full power of the developing 'medical–industrial complex', which has since effectively hijacked government and shaped American health policy in its own short-term interests, was then only beginning to take shape (Relman 1980). In 1978, US health spending was just over 8 per cent of GDP: that share has since more than doubled, with more than one dollar in every six in the giant US economy flowing through the health-care system – and into the pockets of people who like the system as it is, and are determined to keep it that way (OECD 2012a).

Under their pressure and that of similar forces in other countries, the Alma Ata vision has been tragically and wastefully supplanted by a mean-spirited, divisive, profit-focused approach, in which patients are seen (or dismissed) only as potential customers, and public and collective funding is a target for appropriation by avaricious corporations and grasping individuals determined to turn health into their business. Equity concerns go out of the window once market forces are allowed to predominate: even the most fragile semblance of equity can only be secured within competitive markets by costly government intervention and subsidies to incentivise professionals and companies to do the right thing. Along with other managerial and administrative overheads from an inefficient system, this pushes up costs and drains the limited pools of funding available to commission care for the poorest.

The poorest bear the heaviest cost everywhere, in the form of the disease burden, unaffordable charges and a lack of access to care; but it's not just the poor who lose out from this perverted system, which at every level applies the 'inverse care law'.

While the availability of good quality health care is inversely proportional to the need for it (leaving rural populations, the elderly, the mentally ill, the urban poor and vulnerable minorities everywhere desperately under-served), the concentration of power and decision-making is almost invariably in the hands of those most remote from the services and systems they are shaping.

In this type of system, even the wealthy can find themselves at risk. A failure to invest in immunisation and in the treatment of communicable disease means that these diseases remain a potential threat to everyone: a brief glimpse of the rapid spread of a disease across the modern globalised world could be seen in the SARS outbreak of 2002–3 (Knobler et al. 2004) and in the spread of the H1N1 swine flu 'pandemic' in 2009, which appeared to originate in Mexico but rapidly became a global panic. There are concerns that incomplete immunisation, especially of the most deprived rural populations, together with the failure to eradicate diseases like polio, can leave the danger of new outbreaks (Goldberg 2012).

The wealthy may not like to recognise that they share the same planet as the poor and sick, but that is the reality. When an emergency strikes, even the wealthiest cardiac patient can find that their country's health-care system, long under-funded and run down to keep their taxes low, lacks the basic medical expertise and technical resources to meet their health needs.[1] Countries with high levels of ill health are unhealthy for all: in Uganda, child mortality rates are 192 deaths per 1,000 live births for the poorest fifth of households – but 106 per 1,000 even for the richest (WHO 2008c).

The option to plan luxurious medical tourism to India and elsewhere is not much consolation for middle-class Americans requiring emergency resuscitation, belatedly discovering that their platinum plated, so-called Cadillac health insurance does not cover all the costs of the treatment they need; nor for wealthy English people who find that the private sector they have favoured for its luxury, speed and convenience offers no real emergency services. Even relatively prosperous sections of the middle class in the USA can be wiped out by the sky-high costs of substantial hospitalisation, bringing the misery of third-world experience into juxtaposition with the world's most extravagant and wasteful health-care system. The ruinous cost of health care was also a major issue for middle-class families in the UK prior to the 1948 National Health Service.

The difficulty is that even where there are objectively good reasons why it is in the interests of the middle classes and the wealthy to support universal access to health care, the prevailing political ideology, reinforced through consensus between

---

1   Van der Gaag (1995) noted (in an educational article for the World Bank promoting 'public and private initiatives') the inequity of some public provision. While his stress is on the rich snatching publicly funded services intended for the poor, his examples show that in Côte d'Ivoire less than one-quarter of the rural poor who were sick received any form of medical care – but only half of the urban rich could access care either, meaning half potentially went without. And in Peru while only 20 per cent of the poor received care, 43 per cent of the rich also went without. He failed to explain in what way the private sector is any more equitable for the poor, although obviously it may prove more responsive to the rich, assuming that they are able to cooperate by only suffering the kind of health problems the private sector finds it profitable to treat.

the establishment political parties and much of the mass media, imposes the narrow political blinkers of neoliberalism. This encourages short termism and selfishness and cultivates conditioned responses of hysterical aversion to any form of progressive taxation, which has meant that many can be persuaded to think, act and vote against their genuine long-term interests. Many more are not so much persuaded as unable to see an alternative.

It is the lack of a substantial and organised alternative view that makes the problem so intractable. The 'Third Way' neoliberal political degeneration has rendered traditional social-democratic parties – which were already tied comprehensively to a reformist perspective of working within and upholding the capitalist system – even more impotent. Most establishment parties embrace the same world view: and with few, mainly short-lived exceptions, the more radical socialist left has lacked sufficient popular base and political ambition to mount an effective challenge. There are some welcome signs of exceptions to this rule: in Greece, the socialist Syriza coalition came very close to winning the second general election in 2012, on a platform of rejecting the austerity measures and restoring health and other key public services (Lister 2012d). In the Netherlands, the radical left Socialist Party appeared until the week of the elections to have a real chance of winning, again on a progressive platform (Coman 2012). There are substantial and influential left-wing alliances in Portugal and in Denmark (Bensaid et al. 2011). In a less organised and politically conscious movement, there have been spontaneous outbursts of radical rejection of neoliberal and regressive 'reforms' in Romania, which forced back controversial health reforms early in 2012 and continued to destabilise the government (Holt 2012). Trade unions in many countries continue – if only sporadically and without much conviction from their leaders – to resist cutbacks and privatisation in health care, although too often health workers are left to fight back alone. Union leaders can seem more preoccupied with preserving their political alliances at the top than defending their members and the services they deliver. But division on the left is sadly more common than unity; and the articulation of socialist perspectives, or even the core values of social solidarity which underpinned the great movement towards welfarism and universal access to health care in much of Europe after the Second World War, is very much relegated to the margins.

It doesn't have to be this way. The left does not have to take such a low profile or allow such a regressive agenda to predominate. But in many countries the radical left has barely, if at all, outgrown the economistic and 'workerist' approach of the 1960s and 1970s, which focused on the industrial proletariat that was largely seen to consist of male manufacturing workers; whilst the predominantly female workforce in health, education and other services was seen as less interesting, its struggles less important. It's time to grow up, to recognise that in many countries now the public-sector workforce is more organised than the private sector, more combative than much of the private sector, and taking the brunt of the cuts inflicted through the austerity drive in Europe and beyond. The left has failed to address these issues with the necessary seriousness, and its failure is part of the ongoing failure of leadership that confronts working people.

This book, focused on health policy, does not offer a detailed critique of the socialist left, which has little to say in any detail about the subject: but in addressing the issue of alternatives we need to consider who might usefully advocate these policies to make them a reality. Ideas themselves must be the start of practical action if they are to have any serious impact. The alternatives to be discussed will be dismissed by some as too radical; whereas some on the left will no doubt see them as a concession to the status quo, because they do not explicitly call for the overthrow and replacement of capitalism: I make no apology on either front.

For those who see the solution in a more modest tweaking of the system, there is nothing ahead but prolonged disappointment as the system adjusts to ensure that the profits still flow – and the poorest continue to lose out. For a classic example of this, look at the Obama reforms in the US, which have begun to extend health cover to some of the previously uninsured – but only by compelling millions on low pay to buy rip-off, apparently lower-cost, 'bronze' insurance plans that effectively leave them holding much of the risk of any serious illness in the form of 'deductibles' and 'coinsurance' of up to 40 per cent (True Cost 2012). The insurers are smiling: but they would have been smiling as broadly if Mitt Romney had won the 2012 election and carried out his pledge to reverse the ACA, because they and the medical–industrial complex are securely rooted in the US political establishment.

For those who want more explicit calls for socialist revolution, the answer is simple: how do we get to the point where this is a realistic perspective rather than a frustrated empty slogan? A revolution might well emerge as the consequence of a growing mass campaign for lesser demands, with rising levels of political consciousness, triggering a crisis in the government and opening an opportunity for a determined socialist movement. But there is no chance that a socialist revolution in an advanced capitalist country would precede the development of a substantial party of committed socialists, and much more advanced awareness and demands for a new system, including a new vision in which health care is genuinely recognised as a human right. In other words, any solution premised on socialist revolution jumps over the necessary steps to secure one: this is propagandism, not serious revolutionary politics.

Some of the alternative approaches discussed in the following sections may be seen as propaganda, as idealism or simply as wishful thinking. But it's possible to imagine alternative ways of financing, planning and organising health care, and it can be useful to have an idea of how it might look, even if we don't immediately have the levers to hand to secure the outcome we would like. Some ideas are more feasible than others: all of them at some point or other bring those fighting for them into conflict with the limitations of the existing capitalist system and its reliance upon profit, exploitation and inequality. At the end of the day, universal access to comprehensive health care and capitalism are incompatible. While we are a long way from the possibility of moving beyond the shackles of the current system and reaching the ultimate modernisation of health care, and its definitive liberation from the market, we can try to imagine what might be achieved and to look for ways in which we might advance in the right direction by the actions we take here and now.

Planning – to meet health needs

The starting point has to be the need for planning – not markets – as the means to organise health-care systems and allocate resources for the utmost efficiency, eliminating the colossal waste and unproductive bureaucracy of existing market mechanisms. This also means streamlining fragmented insurance-based systems to create single-payer systems: this one change alone could save enough in the US to cover all of the uninsured and deliver additional savings (PNHP 2012).

To make health care accessible to the poorest we also need risk sharing on the broadest possible basis – universal coverage – and the elimination of elitist opt-outs for the wealthy, which would also ensure that those with the greatest power to force changes have an interest in securing high-quality health care that will not only benefit them. To make health systems affordable, resources must be raised, not simply by cutting waste, taxing or levying subscriptions from those in the formal workforce, but also by raising a tax levy on all the main economic and financial players in each country. Sadly, there are few success stories at implementing this approach among the low- and middle-income countries: Costa Rica and Sri Lanka are normally the favourite two examples (McIntyre 2007).

To ensure that adequate resources are raised requires steeply progressive income taxes that also tax share income, company profits, rent and other forms of reward which mainly flow to the well-to-do. In some less-developed countries where multi-nationals trade, manufacture or extract raw materials whilst exploiting cheap labour and paying minimal tax – or manipulate the books to export profits to tax havens elsewhere – this means imposing turnover tax on the economic activity in the country, on pain of confiscation of assets.

Coordinated international action is also needed to stem massive tax evasion (Mathiason 2012) and shut down the tax havens which enable the tiny super-rich minority to bilk billions of people and to starve public budgets of the resources to run services (Shaxson 2011). It's estimated that by 2010, a staggering $21–$32 trillion has been invested virtually tax-free through over 80 offshore havens: 139 low-middle-income countries that have been put through IMF 'structural adjustment' programmes turn out not to be indebted at all, but net lenders, through their corrupt ruling elites, of up to $13 trillion (Henry 2012) – although they seem to have taken their cue from the anti-tax philosophy of the American right (Robin 2011). Illicit financial flows out of developing countries are enormous and have been growing at 18 per cent per year since 2000: the estimate is that in 2008 alone, illicit outflows amounted to between $1.26 and $1.44 trillion, 44 per cent of it from Asia (Kar and Curcio 2011).

While this colossal amount of tax evasion and fraud – and how to recapture the trillions that have been stolen away – is seldom discussed, World Bank researchers have been among those who have actively discussed additional radical measures to raise resources for health care. Some of their suggestions are calculated to create apoplexy among the more highly strung neoliberals and profit-hungry, tax-averse bankers and speculators: a tax on currency transactions (Tobin tax[2]). The World Bank researchers, looking to raise funds for global financing of health care in developing countries and working from conservative estimates, suggest that a Tobin tax at the level of 'one or two basis points' (0.01–0.02 per cent) on foreign exchange market transactions of $300 trillion per year would generated $15–$28 billion annually (Gottret and Schieber 2006: 129). More radical campaigners have calculated that a similar 'Robin Hood' tax on transactions in the US, levied at 0.5 per cent, could raise a staggering $350 billion each year. They also point out that the US enforced a similar tax for over 50 years from 1914 to 1966, taxing every sale or transfer of stock. Supporters of reviving this approach include the largest US nurses' trade union, Jeffrey Sachs, former Goldman Sachs executives, Nobel Laureate Joseph Stiglitz, over 1,000 leading economists, financier George Soros, entrepreneur Warren Buffet, former Democrat Vice President Al Gore and Ronald Reagan's former budget director David Stockman (robinhoodtax. org 2012). Microsoft founder Bill Gates discusses the proposal approvingly in a report to G20 leaders in November 2011 (Gates 2011).

It's clear from the mixed bag of support in the US that there is no simple divide between left and right on the issue of the financial transaction tax: in Europe, too, support comes from all sides, although the opposition to it is consistently from the neoliberal right wing. The French government of François Hollande has pressed ahead unilaterally with a doubling of the transaction tax imposed by President Sarkozy on purchases of shares from 109 French companies valued at €1 billion or more from 0.1 per cent to 0.2 per cent – with the increase estimated to raise an extra €500 million in a full year and the levy set to raise $1.6 billion in 2013, a minimum of 10 per cent of which is committed to the global fight against disease and pandemics (Fouquet and Cimino 2012, Hollande 2012). A fresh campaign to bring in a financial transactions tax in the EU has been launched, led by the French and German governments, despite Britain's David Cameron's vociferous opposition and pledge to fight it 'all the way' (AFP 2012a, 2012b).

Other ways to raise funding for global health objectives include levying a tax on airline tickets, to be collected by airlines and controlled in each participating country: the World Bank projections suggested in 2006 that this could raise about €5 per ticket; with €20 extra on business-class and first-class tickets, it could raise €10 billion a year. In fact, the airline tax has become a major part of the funding stream for UNITAID, contributing 70 per cent of the $1.3 billion it has raised since 2006 and implemented by nine of UNITAID's 29 member countries.[3] UNITAID works with other, bigger, donor organisations, using its bargaining power to negotiate down

---

2   Named after economist James Tobin, who first proposed a tax on speculative currency transactions in 1972 and has developed the idea since. There are various permutations on how the tax might be implemented, at what level and how effective it might be; while the opponents, as with any tax, have of course screamed in hysterical fear that the entire edifice of capitalism could be thrown into chaos by taxes as low as 0.005 per cent. Interestingly, the alleged sensitivity of the financial institutions to such microscopic levels of taxation stands in contrast with the austerity programmes imposed by Western governments since 2008, inflicting double-digit cutbacks in pensions, public-sector pay and public-service budgets.

3   Cameroon, Chile, Congo, France, Madagascar, Mali, Mauritius, Niger and South Korea

the cost of drugs to treat HIV/AIDS, malaria and tuberculosis. Again, France has been one of the most consistent and vigorous in imposing the tax, with no other European countries joining in: it's clear that neoliberal governments, despite the adherence of some of them to UNITAID's call for 'innovative development funding', have no appetite for Hollande's call to 'globalise solidarity' (Hollande 2012).

Of course, with their on-cost of pollution, airlines are only one of the 'global bads' that could potentially be taxed to generate funding for international health projects. Proposals have been floated for a global carbon tax (which even if imposed only on high-income countries, could raise \$60 billion a year (Gottret and Schieber 2006)) or a global tax on arms sales, raising money for social good while making it more expensive to do global harm. Tobacco taxes, especially if substantial, could serve both to deter smokers (and thus improve health) and raise revenues. It has been acknowledged by IMF researchers that price increases on cigarettes are highly effective in reducing demand (Jha et al. 1999).[4]

But while tobacco sales have been soaring in Asia, generating a huge health issue of smoking-related deaths,[5] the Chinese government has been especially unwilling to use taxation on cigarettes as a means to fund health care, despite estimates that a tax increase of 6.5 per cent could finance essential health services for the poorest 100 million in China (Saadah and Knowles 2000: 9). Far from pressing for progressive action on this, and ignoring information it has itself published previously, the IMF has instead pressed developing countries to lift restrictions on tobacco consumption and to privatise state-owned tobacco industries, including these among its conditions for loans. The resultant accelerated market promotion of tobacco products by profit-hungry multinationals has fuelled the use of tobacco, imposing a massive burden on health and health services in already poor countries (Gilmore et al. 2009).

Of course, there is a problem shared by the Tobin tax, financial transaction tax and taxes on tobacco: the economy, and health care and other services funded this way, can become 'hooked' on the global bads, needing to maintain revenue from dangerous or damaging activities, while the taxes raised are not large enough to deter the harmful industries or make a serious dent in their sales and profits. It's like reformist politicians clinging desperately to the capitalist system, opting to preserve it in defiance of mass – even revolutionary – movements, rather than side with those pressing for an alternative way forward.

---

4 Attempting to promote the tobacco companies' alternative approach to this, and to argue why more people smoking can boost government treasury coffers, a report by Arthur D. Little for tobacco giant Philip Morris made the unwise argument that the company's products are highly effective at killing their customers (CNN.com 2001). Arguing against tax increases on tobacco in the Czech Republic, the report famously argued that the increased health costs of the illnesses generated from tobacco consumption were more than compensated by the cash benefits to government of early deaths among smokers:

reduced health-care costs, savings on pensions and housing costs for the elderly – all related to the early mortality of smokers. Among the positive effects, excise tax, VAT and health care cost savings due to early mortality are the most important.

(Arthur D. Little Inc 2000)

5 From 2000, smoking became the most common cause of death in China: Bhushan (2001) estimated that one in six Chinese could expect to die in this way.

In fact, it seems that the squeals of anguish from companies and governments objecting to such progressive imposition of taxes greatly exaggerate the negative impact on demand for global 'bads'. This leaves the problem that if other, more hard-hitting policies were introduced – for example, to restrict and reduce airline traffic or tobacco use – the tax take would in turn be reduced, and the problems of funding health care and other necessary social goods would have to be resolved in other ways. Even in an ideal world in which tobacco consumption could be scaled right back or eliminated, the cost benefits in the form of reduced health-care requirements will take some time to come through.

Tax funding – and tax evasion

However, even where 'innovative' sources of funding are rejected, there are plenty of progressive options on more conventional tax gathering – because the evidence is that the most cost-efficient way to raise the funding for universal health care is through progressive taxation, even in developing countries (Rannan-Elliya and Somanathan 2005b). Tax funding incurs the lowest levels of overheads, makes use of administrative machinery that is already in use, and can make use of the powers of government to make sure people pay up.

The problems of course begin when the wealthy set out to avoid and evade tax: in the UK, the civil service union PCS has calculated that simply collecting the unpaid tax, without any additional increases, could raise £120 billion per year,[6] easily enough to wipe out all deficits and cancel further austerity measures (Murphy 2012). In addition to this, very low levels of taxation on corporate profits also point to ways in which substantial revenues could be raised by governments with a progressive agenda without dumping additional costs and charges on the poor and middle classes: in the UK, corporation tax, at 24 per cent, is 40 per cent lower than it was when Margaret Thatcher was in office: simply restoring that level would bring in more than £18 billion a year.

The consistent underlying reluctance of big business and the wealthy to pay their share of general taxation is consistent with their endless quest for ways to evade contributing to collective provision of health care. Between 2001 and 2010, the US borrowed over $1 trillion to give tax breaks to the wealthy: in fact, the accumulation of vast wealth without proportional contribution to taxes is another reason for the widening gulf between the very rich and everybody else in the US and UK. In the US, the wealthiest 400 Americans have more wealth than the poorest 150 million. In 2010, 25 of the 100 largest US companies paid their CEOs more than they paid in US taxes – largely through use of offshore tax havens (Collins 2012). In total, over $10 trillion is held by wealthy individuals in offshore accounts: tax havens are 'the most important single reason why poor people and poor countries stay poor' (Shaxson 2011). Wealth on this scale easily buys the compliance of governments, few of whose political leaders even from social-democratic parties have any clear or

---

6   Comprising £25 billion of tax avoidance a year, £70 billion of tax evasion a year and £25 billion of tax paid late at any point in time.

developed critique of capitalism or any genuine commitment to tackle privilege and inequality: the Hollande government is a recent exception to the rule of European governments imposing the heaviest austerity burdens onto the poor and working people while pampering the rich and offering them 'incentives' through continual tax cuts.[7]

Clearly, any real steps to put health care on a sustainable basis need to get to grips with this highly organised and systematic milking of the wealth of countries by an already hugely wealthy elite.

How to spend it: the right pharmaceuticals

The Alma Ata policies set out the basic requirement for an infrastructure of primary health care, which remains indispensable to ensure local access to health-care systems for the rural and urban poor as well as those on higher incomes. This remains a task to be accomplished, interrupted as it has been in the developing countries by unwise policy impositions from the World Bank and IMF, and interrupted as it is now by sporadic efforts at delivering aid through unconnected, individual vertical programmes, funded and controlled from outside the recipient country, often dislocating existing services and, as we have seen in Chapter 5, often luring away scarce health professionals and skewing the allocation of resources.

To be effective, primary care needs the support of hospital services, specialist mental health and, of course, an effective coordination of public health and preventative measures to minimise risks to health and educate on diet, lifestyle issues (smoking and alcohol), sexual and reproductive health and healthy ageing.

A dependable supply of the right mix of affordable and effective drugs is also necessary to ensure that many treatments can be delivered at an early stage at primary care level and control diabetes, hypertension, asthma and a variety of problems that can escalate into more serious illness, requiring more expensive and intensive treatment at a later stage if they are uncontrolled. This means confronting the vested interests of the drug companies, which continue to regard it as their right to secure generous subsidies to cover their R&D costs whilst pocketing any resulting profits and retaining total control over the research agenda, directing much of it to 'me too' drugs that prolong patents or cash in on lucrative markets, often for trivial issues (Angell 2005, Carrier 2008). Drug companies also have a direct interest in treating rather than preventing disease and therefore act as an obstacle to the proper development of cost-effective public health and preventive measures.

The long-term solution requires public-sector ownership and control of drug companies and their R&D, to eliminate the distorted priorities of commercial and profit-seeking behaviour and open up the possibilities of a more socially responsible agenda – although there are still issues with ensuring that public-sector bodies

---

7   'The new budget increases the top marginal income-tax rate to 45 per cent from 41 per cent and contains a special tax on incomes above €1 million ($1.3 million) a year, with about 1,500 individuals consequently subjected to an overall rate of 75 per cent. They will pay on average €140,000 more in taxes next year, the government said' (Parussini and Horobin 2012).

prioritise health need rather than financial advantage. But of course, the biggest problem is a political one: securing governments with the commitment to pursue radical policies in the teeth of the massively powerful and well-resourced lobby of the drug corporations (which in the US employ more than two lobbyists for every member of Congress, with lobbyists including almost 500 former federal officials and 40 former members of Congress)[8] (Drinkard 2005). Few political parties even formally embrace the basic principles of nationalising or in any way challenging the drug companies, and few of those that do have any real intention of doing so. Even where drug companies are caught red-handed in breach of the laws regulating their behaviour, they simply pay up even the biggest fine, make a ritual apology – and carry on the same way.

Recent examples include GlaxoSmithKline, fined $3 billion in summer 2012 by the US Justice Department for marketing drugs for unapproved uses, paying kick-backs to doctors and the Medicare system, and downplaying known risks of certain drugs. GSK sold Paxil, an antidepressant, to children for whom it was not shown to work. They sold Wellbutrin, another anti-depressant, as a pill for weight-loss and erectile dysfunction. They sold the anti-diabetic pill Avandia whilst concealing data that showed it increased cardiac risks.

But the giant corporation had already made $11.6 billion on Paxil, $5.9 billion on Wellbutrin and $10.4 billion on Avandia, a total of $27.3 billion – more than nine times the fine they paid to settle the investigations. Pfizer paid up $2.3 billion in 2009 to settle a similar investigation. The drugs involved were Bextra, Geodon, Zyvox and Lyrica (Varma 2012). But each drug had already made hefty profits, so the drug giant, with a turnover of $67 billion, was able to pay up and still come out on top. Its huge profits have allowed the drug industry to overtake even the arms industry in its level of defiance of laws and regulations (Macalister 2012). Even the regulators have proved to be toothless and biased towards big pharma, turning a blind eye to safety issues and rubber-stamping the distribution of new drugs with minimal, if any, scrutiny (Rosenberg 2012).

In this context, perhaps a slightly more feasible starting point for intervention would be to press for a comprehensive opening of the books of the drug companies so that committees of experts could vet the work they are doing and their activities in marketing and promoting their products. Even if a 'nationalisation' is complex in the context of such large and powerful multinationals, it's important to take steps to rein in their power, beginning with an end to any government subsidy for the development of 'me too' drugs that replicate the effects of existing patented or generic drugs.

There should be no subsidies or support for research into any lifestyle drugs – not least because, if these prove effective, they will have an immediate potential market amongst the prosperous classes and will not require a subsidy. They are unlikely to contribute to health objectives. Any subsidies that are paid for specific research should be tied firmly to strings stipulating the projects they are to be used for, the

---

8   'At nearly $266.8 million, the pharmaceutical and health products industry's federal lobbying expenditures not only outpaced all other business industries and special interest areas in 2009, but stand as the greatest amount ever spent on lobbying efforts by a single industry for one year' (Opensecrets 2010).

pricing of the eventual product and the bulk price to public health services. Governments seeking to force down the costs of generic drugs should consider the 'Kiwi' model, which uses competitive market forces to play generic drug manufacturers off against each other, thus securing the lowest price (Flood 2011).

A new lease of life for professionalism

Treatment and drugs must be delivered by skilled professionals – who must be trained. This requires an expansion of training efforts and a global strategy to halt the drain of doctors, nurses and other professionals towards the high-income countries, stripping lower- and middle-income countries of the personnel to deliver even basic services (Packer et al. 2009). Once properly organised – by gearing services to social and clinical need and ensuring access to health care of those in most need – health services that break from the perverse incentives and logic of commercial medicine can offer a new lease of life for the professionalism which has been so sidelined by the brutish commercialisation of health care. Staff freed from the pressures of profit-seeking companies and competition can return to early principles[9] and begin to develop new, twenty-first-century ethical values based on solidarity, equity, the generalisation of best practice, and improvement through collaboration and cooperation rather than divisive competition.

The combination of a global shortage of qualified health professionals and the global surplus of labour offers a historic opportunity for the development of a system that shares the expertise developed in health-care delivery in high-income countries. Cuba has shown the enormous benefit of attracting and training health professionals from around the world; and even if they lack the unique Cuban integration of primary care, public health and high-tech medicine, the OECD countries can benefit from a recruitment and training of student doctors and nurses who can return after a period of work to develop health care in their own countries. Such staff could then work with governments in developing countries to enable them to develop their own, modern medical and nursing schools drawing on twenty-first-century knowledge and techniques (De Vos et al. 2008). This would offer the developing countries the valuable chance to skip over the developmental stage of large-scale psychiatric hospitals and geriatric hospitals, to work directly in community-based models of care and to learn from twenty-first-century public health and preventive expertise.

Professionals in management roles must be required to act as health professionals first and foremost, and held to account for any actions that pressurise or compel staff

---

9 Eliot Freidson refers to the Sesquicentennial Code of 1847, the year in which the American Medical Association was formed, which set out the ethics of the clinical encounter, norms for behaviour between professional colleagues, norms to regulate competition and economic relations between professionals, and set minimum fees while requiring physicians 'cheerfully and freely' to provide care without charge to those who could not afford to pay. The same Code prohibited the patenting of 'any surgical instrument or medicine or dispensing any formula whose composition was secret' (Freidson 1999). A bigger contrast with the grim reality of today's reactionary AMA and its shameless, mercenary alliance with the most exploitative for-profit providers and insurers against single payer and any form of collective or socialised health insurance is hard to imagine.

under their control to breach the basic codes of professional conduct (through lack of adequate staffing levels or material resources). Only through proper resourcing, proper staffing and the right skill mix is it possible to work consistently to improve the quality of health care and tackle those problems and poor practice that have developed as a result of chronic shortages, defective management and dysfunctional systems. The proper financing of health care through tax funding and other collective means can eliminate cash payments, and the proper reward of professional and other staff can also eliminate the corrupt practices of 'informal payments'.

A first step towards reintegrating a fragmented health-care industry and rebalancing its priorities can be the imposition of tough regulation. This should raise and equalise levels of pay and terms and conditions for private contract, private-sector and public-sector health workers, and eliminate the financial benefits to private providers of 'cherry picking' the least-complex caseload, possibly by reducing payments for all publicly financed patients by a risk premium. Once the possibility of securing easy profits while dumping more serious problems onto public-sector providers is eliminated, most of the for-profit private providers are likely to withdraw from the market (as private support-service companies withdrew from hospital services in Scotland once unions secured equal pay and conditions for staff with their public-sector equivalents (UNISON Scotland 2002)).

Another area of private-sector involvement in public health services is also likely to require government-level intervention: the Private Finance Initiative (Public Private Partnerships) and equivalent arrangements have always been a thinly veiled licence for the private sector to print money at public expense. All contracts signed under these schemes need to be immediately reviewed to question value for money and the skewed financial criteria under which they were agreed in the first place. Those which reveal excessive levels of profits being accrued in excess of the interest and costs that would have been payable to finance a scheme through public-sector means must be brought into public ownership, with minimal, if any, compensation to pension funds and other possible secondary victims. This issue also has an environmental angle, since the new hospitals built by the private consortia through PFI/PPPs are also designed by them (most apparently to a fairly limited standard template of curves, coloured panels and other features which recur in almost every PFI hospital): although some of the hospitals have been proclaimed to be 'energy efficient', architect Sunand Prasad has pointed out that not one of the 100 new hospitals in England can be held up as a real exemplar of sustainable design (Taylor 2012).

Hospitals consume and generate energy, consume vast amounts of water and generate waste – some of it hazardous, some of it potentially infectious – in huge quantities. The challenge of recycling and establishing the carbon-neutral hospital is an important one. The development of a wide range of disposable, single-use medical equipment (notably syringes) replacing previous sterilisation processes has generated profits for suppliers but wastes raw materials on a massive scale. The provision of sterile supplies has in many cases been outsourced to generate private profits, leaving hospitals no longer self-sufficient in these services. Health-care systems need urgently to launch projects involving staff at every level in collaboration to streamline the work and recycle wherever possible to ensure that hospitals, clinics and other services are sustainable. Similar exercises need to be conducted in the big pharmaceutical manufacturing plants, appraising environmental impact, pollution and potentially hazardous waste.

On another level, the centralisation of hospital services, requiring more and lengthier patient journeys by car or by other forms of transport, and the re-provision of community health services in patients' homes, requiring professional staff to make many more journeys, often at times of peak traffic, also need to be revisited in terms of their environmental impact, as well as the problems posed for patients who are less than perfectly mobile. (Such policies, eagerly promoted in abstract as a pretext for hospital closures and rationalisation, also have implications for financial costs and staffing.)

On a global scale, the priorities for allocating funds and resources for key services – notably mental health and the care of older people – need to be reviewed and adjusted upwards to meet levels of need and eliminate user fees. Basic standards and human rights – in terms of minimum levels of treatment, staffing and access to therapeutic care – must be introduced and a crash programme of training additional specialist professional staff to fill gaps in care must begin in each country. A major investment is required in community-based teams delivering psychiatric services and support for the frail elderly, with appropriate bases, resources and support from hospital services where required. The elimination of wasteful bureaucracy in market-based systems to focus health-care resources on front-line delivery of care should facilitate this change without undue detriment to acute and other services.

This must be part of a programme of international action to plug the visible gaps in the Millennium Development Goals, addressing issues of disability and the burden of con-communicable disease in the low-, middle- and high-income countries.

Democracy

The emphasis of market-based systems and reforms on the concept of the consumer serves to underline the fact that these policies offer no serious element of account-ability or democratic control: all that's promised is the 'right' of the customer to complain (after the event) about a faulty product or substandard service. Customers of supermarkets, burger chains and other consumer businesses have no influence over the allocation of services, which are decided in management meetings and boardrooms, and relentlessly follow the logic of profitability and identified target markets – and have little if anything to do with social need.

On one level, health care is widely seen as a different, unique type of service; but the commercial exponents of medical practice are driven by the same logic as their other commercial counterparts. That's why substantial private hospitals are seldom located in deprived urban areas or rural locations, and why their size is constrained by the narrow range of services they wish to offer to a selected, well-funded clientele, and the limited number and mix of staff they employ to deliver this, and nothing more.

Publicly funded and provided health-care systems have the opportunity to rise above these limitations, to make themselves much more open and approachable for local communities and responsive to the health needs of deprived and sometimes neglected or forgotten groups – such as ethnic minorities separated by language issues, frail older people, mental health service users, people with learning difficulties, unpaid carers and the desperately poor struggling to scrape by. Addressing these health needs offers the possibility of tackling long-term issues of prevention, public health and continuity of care to ensure minimal use of expensive and unfriendly hospital facilities. But none of this can be done if key decisions are to be taken by politicians at national level or as the prerogative of a bureaucratic hierarchy lacking local roots and working to abstract policy blueprints rather than proven local needs.

Decentralisation of health-care systems can bring problems if it is not accompanied by the necessary resources and a genuine degree of local flexibility in responding to local problems and issues. But if they are coupled with a basic right to minimum levels of appropriate care and a basic standard of treatment, local services can benefit from a system allowing the election and recall of management boards. This is especially the case if staff are also given democratic rights to involvement in decision-making and policy formulation, allowing issues of quality and organisation that concern them to be raised and resolved in collaborative fashion. What I am proposing is a variation of the 'participatory democracy' pioneered in the Brazilian city of Porto Allegre (Bruce 2004) and the Venezuelan Barrio Adentro system (Mooney 2012). It is quite different from the Cuban model of local organisation firmly under the centralising control of the Cuban Communist Party, a model which also has many strengths in its delivery of a remarkably successful health-care system, but is not one which many would seek (or be able, in other circumstances) to emulate.

Various possible ways exist for giving more democratic control and accountability to local communities; but they are in clear contrast to the many spurious parodies of engagement and accountability that have been developed in an effort to give the impression of inclusion. One such is to be found in the ludicrous, tokenistic trappings of democracy in autonomous hospitals (foundation trusts) in England, in which patients, staff and the public are urged to become 'members' and to vote for representation on a governing council, to go through the motions of various meetings and ostensibly democratic processes – while all the real decision-making takes place at the level of the Board of Directors, with little if any concern to the views or engagement with others (Lister 2008a). Another English example is the fraudulent establishment of 'social enterprises' – non-profit private businesses set up to take over services previously delivered in the public sector. These have been foisted on staff who find themselves dragged with minimal pretence at consultation into a new employment contract by managers proclaiming – in defiance of the evidence – that staff are to be 'empowered' and set free to deliver improved quality services (Lister 2012c).

The 1970s campaigning for 'workers' control' of production, to facilitate an improvement in quality of services, is long overdue for revival in the NHS. A combination of management arrogance, financial pressures limiting staffing levels, and competitive and market pressures have worked to undermine NHS morale and to alienate staff from their own professional skills, and from their obligations and commitment to the patients.

The 2013 Francis Report in England, drawing conclusions and 290 recommendations from a lengthy investigation into scandalous failures of care at Mid Staffordshire Hospitals Foundation Trust, which led to between 400–1,200 unnecessary deaths, has again highlighted the widespread prevalence in an increasingly cash-and-targets-led health sector of bullying, the intimidation of critics and 'whistleblowers', and cavalier decisions being taken for far-reaching cost-saving measures and staffing cuts without any attempt at a risk assessment on their implications (Francis 2013).

Shockingly, the report has been followed up with disciplinary action under medical and nursing codes of conduct against dozens of individual nurses and doctors – many of whom, having found themselves working in desperately understaffed services, no doubt failed to uphold adequate standards of care. But no action has been taken against the director of nursing, the medical director or any of the senior managers whose irresponsible decisions – driven by the quest for foundation trust status to make cuts of £10m in a year – resulted in a system that virtually guaranteed poor care. Tackling individual symptoms rather than the underlying systemic failures – and doing nothing to support those who speak out and attempt to challenge unacceptable decisions and management regimes – will not secure sustainable improvements or the quality of health care that could be delivered if staff were genuinely empowered to raise their concerns, proposals and demands.

Health care, after all, has to be much more than the heroic efforts of individuals. It has to involve the development of teams, sharing and developing skills in a multidisciplinary framework. Sadly, the wider concept of the health-care team – the free collaboration and cooperation between specialists and professionals across institutions and on an international level – runs into collision with the neoliberal quest to fragment health care into a competitive 'market' of rival businesses. Competition laws and regulations increasingly disparage any form of collaboration and cooperation, even between not-for-profit organisations delivering public services, as 'collusion' and cartels – while turning a blind eye to collusion by employers that seek to undermine the terms and conditions of health workers. (One blatant example of the latter is the cartel of NHS employers in the South West of England that is conspiring to force a break-up of the national agreement fixing pay and conditions for all NHS staff (Wells Journal 2012).)

For health workers to be given any genuine level of control over the quality of the work they deliver, and the design of the systems and services within which they work, is therefore incompatible with the market disciplines of capitalism – as is any consistent adherence by staff to professional values and codes of conduct when they conflict with the demands of the financial balance sheet of the organisations employing them. But empowering health staff to develop and improve the care they give, through cooperative effort, is also the only way in which staff can help to drive a process of quality improvement in services rather than face the frustrations of management short-termism, narrow focus, cash-driven policies, and the prioritisation of cash, surpluses and profits above patient care.

Here, too, at the chalk face of the delivery of services, global health is in conflict with private profit. Most people are clear which they would prefer to prevail and prosper. The question is whether this can be translated into political and popular action that can confront the powerful multinational forces of neoliberalism and their complex and costly ideological machinery, to secure a new system based on the collective sharing of risk, social and international solidarity, pride in professional achievement, and the ambition to preserve and prolong healthy lives for the world's diverse population.

I only hope that this book can contribute to the development of appropriate policies, political movement and activity to help us all move in this direction.

Appendix

A toolkit for testing the content of a health policy in context

In the course of the reading for this study, it has become increasingly apparent that some of the language, and especially the terminology, that is used in discussing the various reform proposals and the motivation for them can be profoundly ambiguous. Some 'reform' proposals, far from embracing an agenda of equity and progressive change, seek to dress up market-driven cost-cutting reforms, or market-style experiments, in language which is designed to defuse opposition.

Documents setting out national and regional policy proposals for the reform of health-care systems are likely to contain a variety of potentially misleading and ambiguous terminology, catch-phrases and formulations – language which may in some instances lead in a progressive direction, but in others back towards neoliberalism, inequality and costly market-style systems.

A focus on 'primary care', for example, may either:

- Imply a courageous commitment to the progressive 'Health for All' ideals of primary health care set out in the WHO's 1978 Alma Ata declaration, fighting to expand and improve the infrastructure of health care for the very poorest and most isolated

- Or be little more than a fig leaf covering a policy of withdrawing government support for publicly funded hospital services and consolidating a 'World Bank-style' two-tier system, in which only the most minimal care is available to the poor and rural populations, and hospital care is available only to those with money for private treatment.

Since the terms are themselves ambiguous, being used not only by organisations and institutions happy to conceal their principal purpose but also by those who are genuinely concerned with equity and universal access to care, it is only possible to gauge the significance of a given term in the specific context in which it appears.

A number of key questions can help determine the overall framework and approach of the document or paper in which potentially misleading phrases and terms appear. These questions seek to distinguish between positive proposals which are serious attempts to remedy clearly identified problems of equity and access, accountability and affordability; and those which are simply a window dressing of empty promises to disguise a neoliberal reform or a package of spending cuts dressed up as a restructuring or rationalisation of services.

The following table is drawn from the author's experience of researching for this study and 28 years of involvement in analysing official health-service documents in the UK. It seeks to identify the hallmarks that distinguish a proposal for progressive reform from a rhetorical device intended to obscure an essentially unpopular proposal in the populist language of equity.

Characteristics of plans centred on market-driven or market-style reforms	Elements that should be (but rarely are) visible in a progressive reform agenda
Finance-driven (either by global cash constraints on health care at national level, a structural adjustment programme or in response to price competition/market pressures) – although this will at all times be strenuously denied in public pronouncements, which will claim that proposals reflect 'clinical' concerns, 'quality' issues or giving patients greater 'choice'.	Patient- or service-driven changes – often pushing the boundaries of affordability in order to meet clearly demonstrated local health needs, remedy inequalities or address genuine and demonstrable concerns over quality of services.
New policy centred on propositions drawn from neoliberal ideology (e.g. arguing in support of the 'efficiencies' of market systems, private-sector involvement or competition).	Starting point is securing the universal right to health, and need to maximise access for local communities. Recognises and, where necessary, addresses the underlying social inequalities and environmental issues that determine ill health.
Policies are presented without supporting evidence of success.	Evidence-based policy, building on best practice or on lessons drawn by health professionals from critiques of shortcomings of existing system and provision.
'Consultation' process involves only partial disclosure of the full implications of the policy.	Transparency in presenting proposals, spelling out strengths, weaknesses, costs, opportunities and threats. Full disclosure of all working documents. Main text offers a full overview of the proposal, the motives behind it and the expected consequences.
'Consultation' documents inaccessible to key groups of stakeholders (not distributed, written in inaccessible language or not translated where this is necessary to allow minority communities to engage in discussion of their health care needs and services).	Special steps are taken to ensure that all affected groups in the community are fully enabled to take part in any consultation, engaged in the process and empowered to shape decisions.
Policies are based on contentious statistics and planning assumptions or vaguely claim to be backed by 'evidence' that either does not exist or proves not to support the plan.	Policies cite evidence from comparable studies, experience elsewhere and existing services, with references and sources clearly published to invite scrutiny.
Policies purport to be focused on addressing inequalities in health, concentrations of ill health, or the development of preventive measures and public health initiatives – but all of these concerns appear only in the opening pages and are not translated meaningfully into any of the actual proposals for action.	Inequalities and improving health are at the centre of the proposals at every stage of the argument, with practical and costed plans to address the problems identified.

Characteristics of plans centred on market-driven or market-style reforms	Elements that should be (but rarely are) visible in a progressive reform agenda
Policy flows from pressures and requirements outside of health care; it is not related to local needs and is imposed upon local structures.	Clearly located in the current context of the appropriate national and local demographic trends and/or changing profile of hospital caseload (reduced need for surgical in-patient beds often running alongside increased requirement for emergency medical beds).
Policy promises to widen access (or offer 'universal' access) to a 'basic package' or 'basket' of health cover; but this falls short of covering many forms of health care, or takes the form of some 'voucher' or cash-limited entitlement to treatment in public- or private-sector hospitals – up to a certain value. The unspoken implication is that service users may be required or may opt to pay the difference themselves through 'top-up' payments – creating a two-tier system with different levels of access dependent upon ability to pay.	'Universal' means that *everyone* is covered; user fees are eliminated to ensure that there are no barriers to access by the poor. Publicly funded care is provided through publicly owned services, thus delivering no subsidies to any private-sector companies seeking to profit at the expense of public budgets and services.

If a policy is being copied from other governments, health-care systems and providers, or other organisations abroad, is this change being made...

Under pressure from external donors to create a public–private partnership? OR **Under instruction**, as a condition of World Bank or IMF support?	Voluntarily, on the government's own initiative or at the urging of health professionals wishing to model services on best practice?

Financing issues

Proposals remain unspecific, with no costings of the revenue or capital required, and no clear statement of future costs. The business plan is incomplete, unpublished or deliberately withheld as 'commercial in confidence'.	Policy and its implementation are convincingly costed, with full implications for capital investment explained; possible sources of funding are identified.
No identified source of funding: will promised developments ever be completed?	Sufficient financial resources (capital and revenue) have been identified and allocated for the implementation of the policy.
Funding has not yet been allocated or is only promised on a short-term basis.	Funding has been allocated on a long-term and affordable basis, taking account of likely future pressures.
Evasive discussion of human resource issues or unwarranted assumptions. Key issues left unresolved – with no date for resolution. Consultation may specifically centre only on abstract 'principles' and ideas rather than details.	Sufficient human resources are in place, or training needs have been identified and incorporated into the policy proposal, with timelines and milestones to check progress. Clear structures and systems for delivery of any proposed new services, and their location, are all set out in advance.

Characteristics of plans centred on market-driven or market-style reforms	Elements that should be (but rarely are) visible in a progressive reform agenda
The plan involves improbably quick decision-making (ultimatum) or gives no projection of future timetable.	The plan includes a practicable timetable for implementation, with milestones and stages at which evaluation can take place
No identified structure of accountability.	Responsible individuals, institutions or organisations are identified as accountable for implementation, with a mechanism to review and address any shortcomings
The policy is being imposed by government against the express opposition of most health-care professionals and their organisations, concerned over quality and accessibility of patient care.	The reform responds to demands or requests from front-line health staff and local communities, and addresses serious longstanding weaknesses such as: • Elitist professional power • Unequal access to care • Gaps in service provision.

Where services are being restructured and reorganised, how do the new arrangements compare with the existing arrangements?

User fees and/or co-payments are being introduced to reduce access and use of services.	Levels of service and/or numbers of patients are expanded or at least maintained.
Services are reduced, 'rationalised', 'centralised' or 'downsized'.	Service provision is linked with patterns of local need and the demographic profile, and are focused on maximising access for those with appropriate needs.

Bibliography

6 P (2003) Giving consumers of British public services more choice: what can be learned from recent history? *Journal of Social Policy* 32(2): 239–70

Abbasi K (1999) The World Bank and world health: Interview with Richard Feachem. *British Medical Journal* 318: 1,206–8 (1 May)

Abrantes A (2003) Contracting public health care services in Latin America. In Preker and Harding 2003

Abt Associates (1999a) Health insurance and access to care. *Healthwatch* IV(1): 1, 2, 6 (Fall)

Abt Associates (1999b) Regulating quality in US nursing homes. *Healthwatch* IV(2): 3–4 (Winter)

Abt Associates (2003a) *Iraqi health system strengthening*, http://www.abtassociates.com/Page.cfm?PageID=8400&OWID=2109766999&CSB=1#before [accessed 12/09/06]

Abt Associates (2003b) *Tenets for Iraqi Ministry of Health (MOH) Working Groups*, http://www.abtassociates.com/collateral/ACFCAAWBaWtG.pdf

Acerete B, Stafford A, Stapleton P (2011) Spanish healthcare public–private partnerships: the 'Alzira model'. *Critical Perspectives on Accounting* 22(6): 533–49 (August)

Adams S (2012a) Breast implant scandal 'inevitable' due to MHRA failings: *The Lancet. Telegraph*, 18 January, http://www.telegraph.co.uk/health/healthnews/9020818/Breast-implant-scandal-inevitable-due-to-MHRA-failings-Lancet.html [accessed 10/12/12]

Adams S (2012b) Giving patients choice 'will drive hospital closures'. *Telegraph*, 16 May, http://www.telegraph.co.uk/health/healthnews/9269830/Giving-patients-choice-will-drive-hospital-closures.html [accessed 10/12/12]

Adler A (ed.) (1980) *Theses resolutions and manifestos of the first four congresses of the Third International*. Ink Links, London

AfDB (2010) AfDB and Investment Fund for Health in Africa Sign Euro 10 Million Equity Investment. African Development Bank, http://goo.gl/ayGWF [accessed 25/01/13]

AFP (2012a) David Cameron promises to fight financial transactions tax 'all the way'. *Telegraph*, 24 May, http://www.telegraph.co.uk/finance/financialcrisis/9286541/David-Cameron-promises-to-fight-financial-transactions-tax-all-the-way.html [accessed 13/01/13]

AFP (2012b) France, Germany revive EU financial transaction tax plan. France24/com, 29 September, http://www.france24.com/en/120929-france-germany-revive-eu-financial-transaction-tax-plan [accessed 29/09/12]

Africa Public Health Alliance (2012) Special Joint Conference of African Ministers of Finance and Health, Tunis 4–5 July. Media/Public Statement, 10 July, http://www.pambazuka.org/en/category/advocacy/83534 [accessed 10/12/12]

African Capital Markets News (2011) Aureos Africa Health Fund invests $2.5m in Kenya healthcare. 21 November, http://www.africancapitalmarketsnews.com/1460/aureos-africa-health-fund-invests-2-5m-in-kenya-healthcare/ [accessed 22/09/12]

Age UK (2012) Care in crisis 2012. Age UK, http://www.ageuk.org.uk/Documents/EN-GB/Campaigns/care_in_crisis_2012_report.pdf?dtrk=true [accessed 10/12/12]

AHA (2012) New report finds that sequester of Medicare spending could lead to more than 750,000 jobs lost. American Hospitals Association, AHA-AMA-ANA press release, 12 September, http://www.aha.org/presscenter/pressrel/12/120912-pr-jobsreport.pdf [accessed 10/12/12]

Ahiuma-Young V, Obinna C (2012) Nigeria: Enrollees Disagree With Hygeia Over Health Care Plan. *Vanguard*, 3 January, http://allafrica.com/stories/1201032085/html [accessed 14/5/12]

Aid Watch (2010) The World Bank's 'horizontal' approach to health falls horizontal? 10 June, http://aidwatchers.com/2010/06/the-world-bank%E2%80%99s-%E2%80%9Chorizontal%E2%80%9D-approach-to-health-falls-horizontal/ [accessed 25/01/13]

Akazili J (2012) Is healthcare financing and delivery in Ghana equitable? *Global Health Check*, August, http://www.globalhealthcheck.org/?author=24 [accessed 02/03/13]

Akpofure I (2009) IFC's investment operations around the world – an overview. http://goo.gl/iGA07 [accessed 25/01/13]

Alcock P, Craig G (eds) (2001) *International Social Policy*. Palgrave, Basingstoke

Alleyne GAO, Cohen D (2002) *Health, Economic Growth, and Poverty Reduction*. The Report of Working Group 1 of the Commission on Macroeconomics and Health, WHO Geneva, http://whqlibdoc.who.int/publications/9241590092.pdf [accessed 02/03/13]

Almeida C, and 17 other international academics (2001) Methodological concerns and recommendations on policy consequences of the World Health Report 2000. *Lancet* 357: 1,692–7 (26 May)

Altsassets Private Equity News (2012) Aureos invests in West African private hospital Clinique Biasa. 4 July, http://www.altassets.net/private-equity-news/by-news-type/deal-news/aureos-invests-in-west-african-private-hospital-clinique-biasa.html [accessed 27/07/12]

Alzheimer's Disease International (2011) World Alzheimer Report 2011, The benefits of early diagnosis and intervention. ADI London, http://www.alz.co.uk/research/WorldAlzheimerReport2011.pdf [accessed 02/03/13]

Amanfo J (2006) Ridge hospital detains baby over ¢3.2m. *Public Agenda*, 20 January, http://www.ghanaweb.com/public_agenda/article.php?ID=4740

AMI (no date) Healthcare Portfolio. http://www.amiplc.com/index.php?action=healthcare [accessed 14/5/12]

Anand S (2012) Where are private equity investors putting money? *Wall Street Journal, Deal Journal India*, 21 June, http://blogs.wsj.com/dealjournalindia/12/06/21/where-are-private-equity-investors-putting-money/ [accessed 26/08/12]

Anand S, Hanson K (1998) DALYs: efficiency versus equity. *World Development* 26(2): 307–10 (February), http://www.sciencedirect.com/science/article/pii/ S0305750X97100195 [accessed 25/01/13]

Anderson GF (2009) Missing in action: international aid agencies in poor countries to fight chronic disease. *Health Affairs* 28(1): 202–5, Doi: 10.1377/hlthaff.28/1/202 [accessed 12/05/12]

Anderson GF, Hussey PS (2001) Trends in expenditures, access and outcomes among industrialised countries. In Wieners 2001

Angell M (2005) *The Truth About the Drug Companies*. Random House, New York

Antón JI, Muñoz de Bustillo R, Fernández-Macías E, Rivera J (2012) Effects of health care decentralization in Spain from a citizens' perspective. Munich Personal RePEc Archive, http://mpra.ub.uni-muenchen.de/39423/

Apax Partners (2012) Apollo Hospitals. Apax.com, http://www.apax.com/sectors/healthcare/ our-investments/apollo-hospitals.aspx [accessed 26/08/12]

Appleby R, Crawford R, Emmerson C (2009) How cold will it be? Prospects for NHS funding: 2011–2017. The King's Fund, London, UK, http://discovery.ucl. ac.uk/18311/1/18311/pdf [accessed 25/01/13]

Armey D (2001) Just gotta learn from the wrong things you done. Heartland Institute, 9 January, http://www.heartland org

Armstrong P, Glyn A, Harrison J (1984) *Capitalism since World War II, The making and breakup of the long boom*. Fontana Original, London

Armstrong P, Armstrong H, Coburn D (2001) *Unhealthy Times, Political Economy Perspectives on Health and Care in Canada*. Oxford University Press

Arnesen T, Nord E (1999) The value of DALY life: problems with ethics and validity of disability adjusted life years. *British Medical Journal* 319: 1,423–5 (27 November)

Arthur D Little Inc (2000) Public Finance Balance of Smoking in the Czech Republic. http://edition.cnn.com/2001/BUSINESS/07/16/czech.morris/study.doc [accessed 02/03/13]

Associated Press (1987) Thatcher Sets New Charges For Health Service Treatment. AP News Archive, 25 November, http://www.apnewsarchive.com/1987/Thatcher-Sets-New-Charges-For-Health-Service-Treatment/id-1a4d189c2f431332c59faf510b742f75 [accessed 28/07/12]

Athens News (2012) Medicine? Cash only say pharmacists. 31 May, http://www.athensnews. gr/portal/9/55969 [accessed 21/09/12]

Attaran A, Sachs J (2001) Defining and refining international donor support for combating the AIDS pandemic. *Lancet* 357(9,249): 57–61 (6 January)

Aubrey ME (2001) Canada's fatal error – health care as a right (part 1). *Medical Sentinel* 6(1): 26–8, Association of American Physicians and Surgeons, Macon Georgia

Audit Commission (2006) Learning the lessons from financial failure in the NHS. Audit Commission, London, http://www.audit-commission.gov.uk/SiteCollectionDocuments/ AuditCommissionReports/NationalStudies/financial_failure_nhs.pdf [accessed 25/01/13]

Aureos Capital (2012a) Abraaj Capital Announces Acquisition of Aureos Capital. 20 February, http://www.aureos.com/pressreleases/20-02-2012-abraaj-capital-acquisition [accessed 22/09/12]

Aureos Capital (2012b) Aureos managed Africa Health Fund invests US$5 million in Nigerian assisted reproductive centre. 2 April, http://www.aureos.com/pressreleases/02-04-2012-ahf-therapia-health-acquisition [accessed 22/09/12]

Aureos Capital (2012c) The Africa Health Fund managed by Aureos invests in Togolese private hospital. 2 July, http://www.aureos.com/pressreleases/02-07-2012-ahf-togolese-private-hospital [accessed 22/09/12]

Aureos Capital (2012d) Abraaj Capital announces completion of acquisition of Aureos Capital. 24 July, http://www.aureos.com/pressreleases/20-02-2012-abraaj-capital-acquisition [accessed 22/09/12]

Aureos Capital (2012e) Africa Health Fund invests US$4.5 million stake in Ghanaian hospital. 28 July, http://www.aureos.com/pressreleases/28-07-2011-ahf-investment_in_ghanaian_hospital [accessed 22/09/12]

AusAID (2006) Australia's aid program. Global Education website, http://www.globaleducation.edna.edu.au/globaled/go/pid/24

Axelsson H, Bustreo F, Harding A (2003) Private Sector Participation in Child Health: A Review of World Bank Projects, 1993–2002. Health, Nutrition and Population (HNP) Discussion Paper, World Bank, May

Bach S (2000) Decentralisation and privatisation of municipal services: the case of health services. Sectoral activities programme Working Paper ILO, Geneva, November

Baeten R (2011) Past impacts of crossborder health care. Chapter 8 in Wismar et al. 2011

Baeza C, Klingen N (2011) The growing danger of non-communicable diseases. World Bank, Washington DC, http://siteresources.worldbank.org/HEALTHNUTRITIONANDPOPULATION/Resources/Peer-Reviewed-Publications/WBDeepeningCrisis.pdf [accessed 14/01/13]

Baggott R (2000) Understanding the New Public Health: towards a policy analysis. In Hann 2000

Bain & Co. (2012) Global healthcare private equity report. Bain & Company Inc, 8 March, http://www.bain.com/publications/articles/global-healthcare-private-equity-report-2012/aspx [accessed 14/01/13]

Baker B (2012) Debating the World Bank Report on Fiscal Constraints – A return to the 90s? *Global Health Check*, 28 March, http://globalhealthcheck.org/?m=201203 [accessed 10/07/12]

Baker BK, Ombaka E (2009) The danger of in-kind drug donations to the Global Fund. *Lancet* 373: 1,218–21

Baker R, Caplan A, Emanuel L, Latham S (eds) (1999) *The American Medical Ethics Revolution*. Johns Hopkins University Press

Balabanova D, McKee M, Pomerleau J, Rose R, Haerpfer C (2004) Health Service Utilization in the Former Soviet Union: Evidence from Eight Countries. *HSR: Health Services Research* 39: 6, Part II (December)

Bale M, Dale T (1998) Public sector reform in New Zealand and its relevance to developing countries. *World Bank Research Observer* 13(1): 102–21 (February)

Ball J, Sawer P (2009) NHS chief tells trusts to make £20bn savings. *Telegraph*, 13 June, http://www.telegraph.co.uk/health/healthnews/5524693/NHS-chief-tells-trusts-to-make-20bn-savings.html [accessed 01/10/12]

Banerji D (1999) A fundamental shift in the approach to international health by WHO UNICEF and the World Bank: instances of the practice of 'intellectual fascism' and totalitarianism in some Asian countries. *International Journal of Health Services* 29(2): 227–59

Bannerjee A, Deaton A, Lustig N, Rogoff K (2006) An evaluation of World Bank research 1998–2005. World Bank, Washington DC, 24 September, http://siteresources.worldbank.org/DEC/Resources/84797-1109362238001/726454-1164121166494/RESEARCH-EVALUATION-2006-Main-Report.pdf [accessed 14/01/13]

Banrhia S (2009) Apollo Hospital served notice for charging money from poor patients, http://www.latestnewsonline.net/health/apollo-hospital-served-notice-for-charging-money-from-poor-patients/50689/html [NOT found]

Barraclough S (2005) Australia's international health relations in 2003. *Australia and New Zealand Health Policy*, 2: 3, doi:10.1186/1743-8462-2-3, http://bmc.ub.uni-potsdam.de/1743-8462-2-3/1743-8462-2-3.pdf

Barrow B, Adelson J (2012) Louisiana cuts Medicaid program to the bone. *Times-Picayune*, 13 July, http://www.nola.com/politics/index.ssf/12/07/louisiana_cuts_medicaid_progra.html [accessed 15/09/12]

Basu N (2011) Should India hand out economic aid? *Business Standard*, 13 September, http://www.business-standard.com/india/news/should-india-hand-out-economic-aid/448968 [NOT found]

Basu S, Andrews J, Kishore S, Panjabi R, Stuckler D (2012) Comparative performance of private and public healthcare systems in low- and middle-income countries: a systematic review. *PLoS Med* 9(6): e1001244/doi:10.1371/journal.pmed.1001244, http://www.plosmedicine.org/article/info%3Adoi%2F10.1371%2Fjournal.pmed.1001244 [accessed 10/12/12]

Bayliss K, Kessler T (2006) Can privatisation and commercialisation of public services help achieve the MDGs? An assessment. United Nations Development Programme International Poverty Centre, Brasilia Working Paper No. 22, July, http://www.undp.org/povertycentre [NOT found]

BBC News (2009) UK elderly fourth poorest in EU. 27 July, http://news.bbc.co.uk/1/hi/uk/8169859/stm [accessed 25/01/13]

BBC News (2012) Unions angry at health consortium's ideas for South West. BBC News Cornwall, 23 August, http://bbc.co.uk/news/uk-england-cornwall-19353569 [accessed 30/09/12]

Beattic J (2011) Organ selling firm in NHS talks. *Daily Mirror*, 9 September, http://www.mirror.co.uk/news/politics/2011/09/06/organ-selling-firm-in-nhs-talks-115875-23399313

Beavers N (2008) Pilot Polyclinics expected to get go-ahead. *Primary Care Today*, 4 June, http://www.primarycaretoday.co.uk/practicebusiness/pilot-polyclinics-expected-to-get-go-ahead [accessed 25/01/13]

Becker S, Werling KA, Carnell H (2011) Private equity investing in healthcare – 13 hot and cold areas. McGuire Woods, Chicago, http://www.mcguirewoods.com/news-resources/publications/health_care/private-equity-investing-healthcare.pdf [accessed 14/01/13]

Beckford M (2011) NHS blood bank could be partly sold off. *Telegraph*, 17 February, http://www.telegraph.co.uk/health/healthnews/8329118/NHS-blood-bank-could-be-partly-sold-off.html [accessed 20/01/13]

Beeharry G, Whiteford H, Chambers D, Baingana F (2002) Outlining the Scope for Public Sector Involvement in Mental Health. World Bank Health, Nutrition, and Population (HNP) discussion paper

Bennett S, Gilson L (2001) *Health Financing: Designing and Implementing Pro-Poor Policy.* London UK: Health Systems Resource Centre

Bensaid D, Sousa A, Thornett A (eds) (2011) *New parties of the left: experiences from Europe.* IMG Publications, London, 1 July

Berkhout E, Oostingh H (2008) Health insurance in low-income countries Where is the evidence that it works? Joint NGO Briefing Paper (bp 112), Oxfam, Oxford, 7 May

Berman P, Bossert T (2000) A Decade of Health Sector Reform in Developing Countries: What Have We Learned? *DDM Report No. 81,* Cambridge MA: Harvard School of Public Health, http://www.hsph.harvard.edu/ihsg/publications/pdf/issue-brief-decade. PDF [accessed 12/06/04]

Bes M (2009) Spanish health district tests a new public sector mix. *Bulletin of the World Health Organization* 87: 892–3, http://www.who.int/bulletin/volumes/87/12/09-031209/ en/index.html [accessed 16/01/13]

Bevan G, Skellern M (2011) Does competition between hospitals improve clinical quality? A review of evidence from two eras of competition in the English NHS. *British Medical Journal* 343: d6740, doi: 10.1136/BMJ.d6740

Bhattacharjya AS, Sapra PK (2008) Health insurance in China and India: Segmented roles for public and private financing. *Health Affairs* 27(4): 1,005–14 (July–August)

Bhushan I (2001) Health sector challenges in Asia and the Pacific: the Strategy of the Asian Development Bank. In Molina and del Arco 2001

Bhushan I, Keller S, Schwartz B (2002) Achieving the Twin Objectives of Efficiency and Equity: Contracting Health Services in Cambodia. Asian Development Bank, *ERD Policy Brief* No. 6 (March)

Bitran R, Yip WC (1998) A review of health care provider payment reform in selected countries in Asia and Latin America. *Major Applied Research No. 2, Working Paper 1,* August, PHR, Abt Associates Inc, Bethesda MD

Black D (1980) *Inequalities in Health* (the Black Report). DHSS London

Black R (1970) *Stalinism in Britain.* New Park Publications, London

Black RE, Allen LH, Bhutta ZA, Caulfield LE, de Onis M, Ezzati M, Mathers C, Rivera J (2008) Maternal and child undernutrition: global and regional exposures and health consequences. *Lancet* 371: 243–60 (17 January), DOI: 10.1-16/S0140-6736(07)61690-0

Blagys J (2012) Health of the Nation – Germany. Gesundheit! *Stockholm Network Health and Welfare Newsletter* No. 10, http://www.stockholm-network.org/downloads/publications/ Gesundheit_10.pdf [accessed 10/12/12]

Blair T (2001a) The power of community can change the world. Labour Party, 3 October

Blair T (2001b) Prime Minister's speech on public service reform. 16 October, cited in 6 2003

Blair T (2003) Where the third way goes from here. *Progressive Governance,* http://www. progressive-governance.net/php/print_preview.php?aid=35 [accessed 12/05/03]

Blair T (2005) Full text of Tony Blair's speech. http: //news.BBC.co.uk/1/hi/UK_ politics/428 7370.stm [accessed 03/09/12]

Blas E (2004) The proof of the reform is in the implementation. *International Journal of Health Planning and Management* 19, S3–S23

Bloom E, Bhushan I, Clingingsmith D et al. (2006) Contracting for health: evidence from Cambodia. Unpublished working paper, Washington DC, Brookings Institution

Blouin C (2010) Trade in health services: can it improve access to health care for poor people? *Global Social Policy* 10(3): 293–5

BMA (1997) *Leaner & Fitter.* October BMA Health Policy & Economic Research Unit, London

Böhlke N, Greer I, Schulten T (2011) World champions in hospital privatisation – the effects of neoliberal reform on German employees and patients. In Lister 2011b

Bond P (2006) The dispossession of African wealth at the cost of African health. Regional Network for Equity in Health in east and southern Africa (EQUINET) with Southern African Centre for Economic Justice, Equinet Discussion Paper No. 30, March

Bond P (2007) Microcredit evangelism, health and social policy. *International Journal of Health Services* 37(2): 229–50

Bond P, Dor G (2003) Neoliberalism and Poverty Reduction Strategies in Africa. Discussion paper for the Regional Network for Equity in Health in Southern Africa (EQUINET), March

Bonilla-Chacin ME, Murrugarra E, Temourov M (2005) Health Care during Transition and Health Systems Reform: Evidence from the Poorest CIS Countries. *Social Policy & Administration* 39(4): 381–408

Boseley S (2003a) Aids drugs scandal: toll soars. *Guardian*, 3 July

Boseley S (2003b) Diabetes creating world health catastrophe, warns leading doctor. *Guardian*, 25 August

Boseley S (2003c) Huge NHS bill for infertility rights. *Guardian*, 26 August

Boseley S (2003d) UK backs poor nations over medicine patents. *Guardian*, 8 May

Boseley S (2012a) Drug companies join forces to combat deadliest tropical diseases. *Guardian*, 30 January, http://www.guardian.co.uk/global-development/12/jan/30/drug-companies-join-tropical-diseases [accessed 10/12/12]

Boseley S (2012b) World Bank's Jim Yong Kim: 'I want to eradicate poverty'. *Guardian*, 25 July, http://www.guardian.co.uk/global-development/12/jul/25/world-bank-jim-yong-kim-eradicate-poverty [accessed 22/09/12]

Bossert TJ (2000) Decentralisation of Health Systems in Latin America: A comparative study of Chile, Colombia and Bolivia. Data for Decision Making Project, Harvard School of Public Health, June

Boulders Advisors Ltd (2011) Market Analyses of Public and Private Sector Capacities to Expand Access to Subsidized ACTs in Ghana. Project Report, Accra, Ghana, http://goo.gl/f5ZVe [accessed 25/01/13]

Bourdieu P (1998) Utopia of Endless Exploitation: The essence of neoliberalism. *Le Monde Diplomatique*, December, translated by JJ Shapiro, http:/www.forum-global.de/soc/bibliot/b/bessenceneolib.htm [accessed 24/08/03]

Bourguignon F, Bénassy-Quéré A, Dercon S, Estache A, Gunning JW, Kanbur R, Klasen S, Maxwell S, Platteau J-P, Spadaro A (2008) Millennium Development Goals at Midpoint: Where do we stand and where do we need to go? European Commission, September, http://ec.europa.eu/development/icenter/repository/mdg_paper_final_20080916_en.pdf [accessed 14/01/13]

Boyer R, Drache D (eds) (1996) *States Against Markets: the Limits of Globalisation.* London, Routledge

Boyle D, Conisbee M, Burns S (2004) Towards an asset-based NHS. The missing elements of NHS reform. February, New Economics Foundation, London

Boyle S (2011) United Kingdom (England) Health System Review. *Health Systems in Transition* 13(1), European Observatory on Health Systems and Policies, Copenhagen

Brabers AEM, van Roijen MR, de Jong JD (2012) The Dutch health insurance system: mostly competition on price rather than quality of care. *Eurohealth* 18(1): 30–3, http://nvl002/nivel.nl/postprint/PPpp4585/pdf [accessed 18/01/13]

Bradley M (2009) Egypt pledges health cover reform. *National*, 18 February, http://www.thenational.ae/article/20090218/FOREIGN/701251928/1002 [accessed 15/05/10]

Brandon RM, Podhorzer M, Pollak TH (1991) Premiums without benefits: waste and inefficiency in the commercial health insurance industry. *International Journal of Health Services* 21(2): 265–83

Braveman P, Starfield B, Geiger HJ (2001) World Health Report 2000: how it removes equity from the agenda for public health monitoring and policy. *British Medical Journal* 323: 678–81 (22 September)

Breitman G, Stanton F (eds) (1977) *The Transitional Program for Socialist Revolution.* Pathfinder Press, New York

Brekke KR, Cellini R, Siciliani L, Straume OR (2010) Competition and quality in health care markets: a differential-game approach. *Journal of Health Economics* 29: 508–23, DOI:10.1016/j.jhealeco.2010.05/004

Breman A, Shelton C (2001) Structural Adjustment and Health: A literature review of the debate, its role-players and presented empirical evidence. Paper No. WG6:6, Cambridge MA: Commission on Macroeconomics and Health, June, http://www.cmhealth.org/docs/wg6_paper6/pdf [accessed 27/05/03]

Brook PJ and Smith SM (2002) *Contracting for Public Services.* World Bank

Brouwer S (2011) Revolutionary Doctors: How Venezuela and Cuba are Changing the World's Conception of Health Care. Monthly Review Press

Brown A (2000a) Current issues in sector-wide approaches to health development: Mozambique case study. WHO Geneva

Brown A (2000b) Current issues in sector-wide approaches to health development: Uganda case study. WHO Geneva

Brown P (2002) WHO to revise its method for ranking health systems. *British Medical Journal* 324: 190 (January)

Bruce I (2004) *The Porto Alegre Alternative: Direct Democracy in Action.* Pluto Press, London and Ann Arbor

Brugha R, Walt G (2001) A global health fund: a leap of faith? *British Medical Journal* 323: 152–4

Brundtland GH (1998a) Address to the Regional Committee for Africa (48th session, Harare). WHO, 31 August

Brundtland GH (1998b) Dr Gro Harlem Brundtland: entry on duty in Geneva. WHO: office of Director General, 21 July

Brundtland GH (2001a) Globalisation as a force for better health. *Lecture at LSE*, WHO, 16 March, http://www.lse.ac.uk/collections/globalDimensions/lectures/globalisationAsAForceForBetterHealth/transcript.htm [accessed 02/03/13]

Brundtland GH (2001b) *WHO/WTO workshop on differential pricing and financing of essential drugs.* Speech, Norway, 8 April, http://www.wto.org/english/tratop_e/trips_e/tn_hosbjor_intro_e.htm [accessed 02/03/13]

Brundtland GH (2001c) Scaling up action to tackle illness associated with poverty: the global fund for AIDS and health. *World Health Assembly Technical Briefing*, Geneva, 18 February

Buckeye Institute (no date) Medical Savings Accounts. A how-to guide for Ohio businesses and employees. http://www.buckeyeinstitute./policy%20Reports/mas.htm [accessed 20/05/12]

Burrows R, Loader B (eds) (1994) *Towards a Post Fordist Welfare State*

Buse K, Walt G (2000a) Global public–private partnerships part I – a new development in health? *Bulletin of the World Health Organization* 78(4): 549–61

Buse K, Walt G (2000b) Global public–private partnerships part II – what are the health issues for global governance? *Bulletin of the World Health Organization* 78(5): 699–709

Buse K, Waxman A (2001) Public–private health partnerships: a strategy for WHO. *Bulletin of the World Health Organization* 79(8): 748–54

Business Daily Africa (2010) Private equity taps health sector growth. 26 April, http://www.businessdailyafrica.com/Corporate-News/-/539550/905644/-/14gka78z/-/index.html [accessed 15/01/13]

Busse R, van der Grinten T, Svensson PG (2002) Regulating entrepreneurial behaviour in hospitals: theory and practice. In Saltman et al. 2002

Busse R, van Ginneken E, Wörz M (2011) Access to healthcare services within and between countries of the European Union. Chapter 3 in Wismar et al. 2011

Bustreo F, Harding A, Axelsson H (2003) Can developing countries achieve adequate improvement in child health outcomes without engaging the private sector? *Bulletin of the World Health Organization* 81(12): 886–95

Cairns P (2012) The Investment Case – Liberty Holdings Ltd. Moneyweb, 26 February, http://www.moneyweb.co.za/mw/view/mw/en/page295164?oid=562943&sn=2009+Detail [accessed 14/05/12]

Caldwell K, Francome C, Lister J (1998) *The Envy of the World*. NHS Support Federation, London

Cameron A, Ewen M, Ross-Degnan D, Ball D, Laing R (2008) Medicine prices, availability, and affordability in 36 developing and middle-income countries: a secondary analysis, http://www.theLancet.com, 1 December, DOI:10.1016/S0140-6736(08)61762-6

Campbell D (2012) Hospital trusts offered £1.5bn emergency fund to pay PFI bills. *Guardian*, 3 February, http://www.guardian.co.uk/society/12/feb/03/hospital-trusts-emergency-fund-pfi [accessed 30/09/12]

Canadian Press (2011) Cost of aging population on health care 'overblown'. The Canadian Press, 29 August, http://www.cbc.ca/news/health/story/2011/08/29/grey-tsunami-aging-population.html [accessed 14/01/13]

Carlson C (2004) Mapping Global Health Partnerships. What they are, what they do and where they operate. GHP Study Paper 1: DFID Health Systems Research Centre, May, http://www.healthsystemsrc.org

Carrier R (2008) Science in the Grip of the Economy: On the Epistemic Impact of the Commercialization of Research. In Carrier and Howard 2008

Carrier R, Howard D (eds) (2008) *The Challenge of the Social and the Pressure of Practice: Science and Values Revisited*. Pittsburgh: University of Pittsburgh Press, pp. 217–34

Carson D, Clay H, Stern R (2010) Primary Care and Emergency Departments. Report from the Primary Care Foundation, March, http://www.primarycarefoundation.

co.uk/files/PrimaryCareFoundation/Downloading_Reports/Reports_and_Articles/ Primary_Care_and_Emergency_Departments/Primary_Care_and_Emergency_ Departments_RELEASE.pdf [accessed 25/01/13]

Cartwright WS (1999) Book Review: Methods for the Economic Evaluation of health care programmes, by Drummond MF et al, Oxford University Press. *Journal of Mental Health Policy and Economics* 2: 43

Carvel J (2005) Flagship PFI hospital technically bankrupt. *Guardian*, 16 December, http://www.guardian.co.uk/uk/2005/dec/16/publicservices.topstories3 [accessed 01/09/12]

Castro A, Singer M (eds) (2004) *Unhealthy Health Policy.* Altamira Press, Walnut Creek, New York and Oxford

Caufield C (1997) *Masters of Illusion, The World Bank and the Poverty of Nations.* Pan Books

CBC (2011) Cost of aging population on health care 'overblown'. Canadian Press, 29 August, http://www.cbc.ca/news/health/story/2011/08/29/grey-tsunami-aging-population. html [accessed 29/06/2012]

CBS Athens (2012) Austerity brings Greece's healthcare system to its knees. CBS news, 14 June, http://www.cbsnews.com/8301-18563_162-57453670/austerity-brings-greeces-healthcare-system-to-its-knees [accessed 19/09/12]

Centre for Economic Performance (2012) How mental illness loses out in the NHS. Mental Health Policy Group, Centre for Economic Performance, June, http://cep.lse.ac.uk/pubs/ download/special/cepsp26/pdf [accessed 14/01/13]

Centre for Market innovations (2012) Hygeia community health plan. http:// healthmarketinnovations.org/program/hygeia-community-health-plan-hchp [accessed 14/05/12]

Centre for Mental Health, Mental Health Foundation, Mind and Rethink Mental Illness (2012) The Mental Health Strategy, system reforms and spending pressures: what do we know so far? http://www.mentalhealth.org.uk/content/assets/PDF/publications/mental_ health_strategy_what_do_we_know_so_far.pdf?view=Standard [accessed 10/12/12]

CEPMHPG (The Centre for Economic Performance's Mental Health Policy Group) (2012) How Mental Illness Loses out in the NHS. London School of Economics, June, http:// cep.lse.ac.uk/pubs/download/special/cepsp26/pdf [accessed 10/12/12]

Chee HL (2010) Medical tourism and the state in Malaysia and Singapore. *Global Social Policy* 10(3): 336–57

Chen S, Ravallion M (2012) More relatively poor people in a less absolutely poor world. *World Bank Policy Research Working Paper* 6,114, July, World Bank Washington

Cheng TC (2012) Measuring the effects of removing subsidies for private insurance on public expenditure for healthcare. 11 November, Melbourne Institute Working Paper 26/11, Social Science Research Network, http://papers.ssrn.com/sol3/papers. cfm?abstract_id=1961524 [accessed 10/12/12]

Cheng TM, Reinhardt UE (2012) Perspectives on the appropriate role of the private sector in meeting health care needs. In Clements et al. 2012

Chinitz D, Preker A, Wasem J (1998) Balancing solidarity and competition in health care financing. In Saltman et al. 2000

Chisholm D, Stewart S (1998) Economics and ethics in mental health care: traditions and trade-offs. *Journal of Mental Health Policy and Economics* 1: 55–62

Christian Aid (2003) *Struggling to be heard: Democratising the World Bank and IMF.* Christian Aid, London

Clarke JH, Gewirtz S, McLaughlin E (eds) (2000) *New Managerialism, New Welfare?* Sage

Clemens MA, Pettersson G (2006) A New Database of Health Professional Emigration from Africa. Working Paper No. 95, Centre for Global Development, August

Clements B, Coady D, Gupta S (eds) (2012) *The Economics of Public Health Care Reform in Advanced and Emerging Economies*. International Monetary Fund, Washington DC

Clements B, Keen M, Perry V, Toro J (2010) From stimulus to consolidation: revenue and expenditure policies in advanced and emerging economies. IMF Fiscal Affairs Department, 30 April, http://www.imf.org/external/np/pp/eng/2010/043010a.pdf [accessed 14/01/13]

Clinton HR (2012) A World in Transition: Charting a New Path in Global Health. PEPFAR, Washington DC, June, http://www.state.gov/secretary/rm/12/06/191633/htm [accessed 10/12/12]

Clover B (2012) Exclusive: NHS or private expressions of interest sought to run 'failing' trust. *Health Service Journal*, 23 August, http://www.hsj.co.uk/news/policy/exclusive-nhs-or-private-expressions-of-interest-sought-to-run-failing-trust/5048619/article [accessed 14/01/13]

CMH (Commission on Macroeconomics, Health) (2002) Working Group 5: Improving health outcomes of the poor. WHO, Geneva, http://whqlibdoc.who.int/publications/9241590130.pdf [accessed 25/01/13]

CNN.com (2001) Morris study blasted, 16 July, http://edition.cnn.com/2001/BUSINESS/07/16/czech.morris/

Coburn D (2000) Income inequality, lowered social cohesion and the poorer health status of populations: the role of neo-liberalism. *Social Science and Medicine* 51: 135–46

Cochi SL (2012) The future of global immunization. Will the promise of vaccines be fulfilled? Center for Strategic and International Studies, Washington DC, April, http://csis.org/files/publication/111205_Cochi_FutureGlobalImmun_Web.pdf [accessed 10/12/12]

Cohen D, Carter P (2010) WHO and the pandemic flu 'conspiracies'. *British Medical Journal* 340, doi: 10.1136/BMJ.c2912 (published 3 June), http://www.BMJ.com/content/340/BMJ.c2912#alternate [accessed 22/09/12]

Cohen RA, Martinez ME (2006) Health insurance coverage: Estimates from the National Health Interview Survey, 2005, National Center for Health Statistics, http://www.cdc.gov/nchs/nhis.htm, [accessed 24/08/06]

Cohn J (2011) If Republicans are serious on health care… New Republic blog, 24 January, http://www.tnr.com/blog/jonathan-cohn/82048/if-republicans-are-serious-health-care [accessed 15/01/13]

Colgan AL (2002) Hazardous to Health: the World Bank and IMF in Africa. Africa Action Position Paper, April, http://www.africaaction.org/action/sap0204.htm [accessed 29/06/02]

Collins C (2012) *99 to 1, How wealth inequality is wrecking the world economy and what we can do about it*. Berrett Koehler Publishers, San Francisco

Collins C, Green A (1994) Decentralisation and primary health care: some negative implications in developing countries. *International Journal of Health Services* 24(3): 459–75

Collins CD, Green AT, Hunter DJ (1999) Health Sector reform and the interpretation of policy context. *Health policy* 47: 69–85

Collis G (2012) Private Patient Income Cap. UNISON Parliamentary Briefing: January, http://www.unison.org.uk/file/UNISON%20-%20Private%20Patient%20Income%20 Cap%20briefing%20-%20Jan%202012/pdf [accessed 14/01/13]

Colombo F (2007) Lessons for developing countries from the OECD. Chapter 8 in Preker et al. 2007

Colombo F, Llena-Nozal A, Mercier J, Tjadens F (2011) Help Wanted? Providing and Paying for Long-Term Care. OECD Publishing, Paris, http://www.oecd.org/els/ healthpoliciesanddata/47885662.pdf [accessed 24/01/13]

Colombo F, Mercier J (2011) Help wanted! Balancing fair protection and financial sustainability in long-term care. *Eurohealth* 17(2–3): 3–6

Coman J (2012) Dutch embrace radical left as European dream sours. *Guardian*, 2 September, http://www.guardian.co.uk/world/12/sep/02/netherlands-elections-socialist-party [accessed 14/01/13]

Cometto G, Brikci N (2009) Can private equity deliver on equity? *Bulletin of the World Health Organization* 87(10): 735 (October), doi: 10.2471/BLT.09/069492 http://www. ncbi.nlm.nih.gov/pmc/articles/PMC2755321/ [accessed 25/01/13]

Comins L (2009) First fix our state hospitals. *Daily News*, South Africa, 15 June, http:// www.iol.co.za/news/south-africa/first-fix-our-state-hospitals-1/446466 [accessed 25/01/13]

Commons Health Committee (2010) *Commissioning: Fourth Report of Session 2009–10.* Vol. I, 30 March, House of Commons, http://www.publications.parliament.uk/pa/cm200910/ cmselect/cmhealth/268/268i.pdf [accessed 25/01/13]

Connell R, Fawcett B, Meagher G (2009) Neoliberalism, New Public Management and human service professions: introduction to the special issue. *Journal of Sociology* 45: 331, DOI: 10.1177/1440783309346472

Conway T (2012) Business as usual at Earth Summit. International Viewpoint, online September, IC452 http://www.interbationalviewpoint.org/spip.php?article2734 [accessed 01/10/12]

Corporate Watch (2005) Corporate carve up: UK consultants creating a new Iraq. http:// www.corporatewatch.org/?lid=2479 [accessed 25/01/13]

Cortez N (2008) Patients without Borders: the emerging global market for patients and the evolution of modern health care. *Indiana Law Journal* 83(1), article 3: http://www. repository.law.Indiana.edu/ilj/vol83/iss1/3 [accessed 25/01/13]

Costello AM, Allen A, Ball S, Bell S, Bellamy R, Friel S, Groce N, Johnson A, Kett M, Lee M, Levy C, Maslin M, McCoy D, McGuire B, Montgomery H, Napier D, Pagel C, Patel J, de Oliveira AJP, Redclif N, Rees H, Rogger D, Scott J, Stephenson J, Twigg J, Wolff J, Patterson C (2009) Managing the health effects of climate change. *Lancet* 373: 1,693–733, 16 May

Cotlear D (2000) Peru: Reforming health care for the poor. Human Development Department LCSHD Paper, March, No. 57, World Bank, Washington

Coughlin J (2012) The eighth annual China Healthcare Forum 2012 – Universal Health Insurance: Dream and Reality. CEIBS press release, 9 June, http://www.ceibs.edu/ media/archive/103879/shtml [accessed 18/01/13]

Coulter A (1998) Managing demand at the interface between primary and secondary care. *British Medical Journal* 316: 1,974–6 (27 June)

Coulter A, Ham C (eds) (2000) *The Global Challenge of Health Care Rationing*. Open University Press, Buckingham

Coyte PC, Goodwin N, Laporte A (2008) How can the settings used to provide care to older people be balanced? WHO Policy Brief, http://www.euro.who.int/__data/assets/pdf_file/0006/73284/E93418/pdf [NOT found]

Creese A (1997) User fees: they don't reduce costs, and they increase inequity. *British Medical Journal* 315: 202–3 (26 July)

Creese A, Kutzin J (1995) Lessons from Cost-Recovery in Health, Forum on Health Sector Reform. Discussion Paper No. 2 Division of Strengthening Health Services, WHO, Geneva

Creswell J, Abelson R (2012) A giant hospital chain is blazing a profit trail. *New York Times*, 14 August, http://www.nytimes.com/12/08/15/business/hca-giant-hospital-chain-creates-a-windfall-for-private-equity.html?pagewanted=all&_r=0 [accessed 14/01/13]

Crisp N (2007) Global Health Partnerships: The UK contribution to health in developing countries. http://www.dh.gov.uk/en/Publicationsandstatistics/Publications/PublicationsPolicyAndGuidance/DH_065374 [accessed 24/01/12]

Dahlgren G (2000) Efficient equity-oriented strategies for health. *Bulletin of the World Health Organization* 78(1): 79–81

Danida (2003) A world of difference. Royal Danish Ministry of Foreign Affairs, Copenhagen, http://www.danida-publikationer.dk

Danida (2005) Africa – Development and security. Royal Danish Ministry of Foreign Affairs, Copenhagen, http://www.danida-publikationer.dk

Danziger MP (2011) Tip Sheet: Illicit Financial Flows from Developing Countries 2000–2009. Press release, 18 January, Global Financial Integrity, http://iff-update.gfintegrity.org/documents/GFI%20IFF%20Update%20Tip%20Sheet%20-%20FINAL.pdf [accessed 14/01/13]

Danzon M (2002) Foreword to Mossialos et al. 2002

Dar Al Fouad Hospital (2012) website: http://www.daralfouad.org/about.html [accessed 23/09/12]

Darzi A (2007) Healthcare for London: a framework for action. NHS London, http://www.londonhp.nhs.uk/wp-content/uploads/2011/03/A-Framework-for-Action.pdf [accessed 25/01/13]

Das J, Do Q-T, Friedman J, McKenzie D (2008) Mental health patterns and consequences: results from survey data in five developing countries. *World Bank Economic Review* 23(1): 31–55, doi.10.1093/wber/lhn010

Datzova B (2003) Health Care Reform and Inequality of Access to Health Care in Bulgaria. UNRISD, Geneva

Davie E (2011) Gateways using nurses to screen GP referrals. *Pulse*, 10 August, http://www.pulsetoday.co.uk/main-content/-/article_display_list/12511567/gateways-using-nurses-to-screen-gp-referrals [accessed 25/01/13]

Davies JB, Sandström S, Shorrocks A, Wolff EN (2008) The world distribution of household wealth. Discussion Paper No. 2008/03, United Nations University and World Institute for Development Economics Research, Helsinki, February, http://www.wider.unu.edu/publications/working-papers/discussion-papers/2008/en_GB/dp2008-03/_files/78918010772127840/default/dp2008-03/pdf [accessed 25/01/13]

Davies P (2012) *The NHS handbook 2012–13*. NHS Confederation, London

Davoren P (2001) Why private health insurance initiatives don't help public hospitals. *New Doctor* issue 75, Winter, http://www.drs.org.au/new_doctor/75/dav oren_75/html

De Ferranti D (1985) Paying for health services in developing countries: an overview. *World Bank Staff Working Papers* No. 721, Washington DC

De Ferranti D (2006) *The World Bank and the Middle Income Countries*. Brookings Institute, http://www.brookings.edu/views/papers/200603deferranti.pdf [accessed 16/11/06]

De Rivero DAT (2003) Alma-Ata revisited. *PAHO Perspectives in Health* 8(2), http://www. paho.org/english/dd/pin/number17_article1_4/htm [accessed 16/01/13]

De Vos P, De Ceukelaire W, Bonet M, Van der Stuyft P (2008) Cuba's health system: challenges ahead *Health Policy and Planning* 23(4): 288–90, first published online 2 May, doi:10.1093/heapol/czn010

Deacon B (2000) Socially responsible globalization: The challenge for social security. International Social Security Association (ISSA) Research Programme

Deacon B (2001) International Organisations, the EU and global social policy. In Sykes et al. 2001

Deacon B, Ilva M, Koivusalo M, Ollila E, Stubbs P (2005) Copenhagen Social Summit ten years on: the need for effective social policies nationally, regionally and globally. Globalisation and Social Policy Programme (GASPP) team, STAKES, Helsinki, http://bib.irb.hr/datoteka/191427/policybrief6/pdf [accessed 14/01/13]

Deber R (2000a) Thinking before rethinking: some thoughts about babies and bathwater. *Healthcare Papers* 1(3): 25–32 (Summer 2000), http://www.longwoods.com/hp/summer00/2.html [accessed 07/05/03]

Deber R (2000b) Getting what we pay for: myths and realities about financing Canada's health care system. Background papers for the Dialogue on Health Care reform, http://www.utoronto.ca/hpme/dhr/4.html [accessed 11/05/03]

Deber R, Forget E, Roos L, Shortt SED (2002a) Medical Savings Accounts: an idea that just won't die. *Globe and Mail*, 26 July, Toronto

Deber R, Forget E, Roos L (2002b) Return of the 'zombie': Are medical savings accounts a better way to meet health-care needs, or will they simply increase costs? *National Post*, 7 August, Toronto

Deber R, Forget E, Roos L (2002c) MSAs: even less than meets the eye. *Technical Report*, University of Mainitoba, http://www.umanitoba.ca/centres/mchp/hot_topic/msa.html [accessed 14/11/03]

Deeming C (2001) The decentralisation dream. *Public Finance*, 23–9 November, pp. 28–9

Defever M (1995) Health care reforms: the unfinished agenda. *Health Policy* 34(1): 1–7 (October)

Delion J, Rosen JE, Klofkorn Bloome A (2005) Lessons From World Bank-Supported Initiatives to Fight Hiv/Aids in Countries with IBRD Loans and IDA Credits in Nonaccrual. World Bank Global HIV/AIDS Program Discussion Paper, May

Democracy Now (2007) Report: Gates Foundation Causing Harm with the Same Money it Uses to Do Good, http://www.democracynow.org/2007/1/9/report_gates_foundation_causing_harm_with [accessed 25/01/13]

Denning S (2012) HCA: The Unsustainble Private Equity Bubble in US Health Care. Forbes, http://www.forbes.com/sites/stevedenning/2012/08/15/private-equity-wont-fix-health-care-either [accessed 26/08/12]

Dent E (2007) Go and tell people what it's like here. *Health Service Journal*, 7 June, pp. 24–7

Dentzer S (2009) The devilish details of delivering on global health. *Health Affairs* 28(4): 946–7 (July–August)

Department of Health (DoH) (1989a) Caring for People: Community Care in the next decade and beyond. November, HMSO, London

Department of Health (DoH) (1989b) Working for Patients. January, HMSO, London

Department of Health (DoH) (1990) National Health Service and Community Care Act 1990, http://www.legislation.gov.uk/ukpga/1990/19/contents [accessed 02/03/13]

Department of Health (DoH) (2000a) National Beds Inquiry. 10 February, London

Department of Health (DoH) (2000b) Shaping the future NHS: long-term planning for hospitals and related services. Consultation document on the findings of the National Beds Inquiry, DoH, London

Department of Health (DoH) (2003a) Chief Executive's Report to the NHS. December, DoH, London

Department of Health (DoH) (2003b) Chief Executive's Report to the NHS: Statistical supplement. December, DoH, London

Department of Health (DoH) (2003c) Departmental report 2003. July, The Stationery Office, London

Department of Health (DoH) (2003d) Agenda for Change proposed agreement. January, DoH, http://www.dh.gov.uk

Department of Health (DoH) (2004a) Hospital Episode Statistics 2002–3. http://www.dh.gov.uk/PublicationsAndStatistics/Statistics/HospitalEpisodeStatistics/HESFreeData/HESFreeDataList/fs/en?CONTENT_ID=4028328&chk=6HBoYS [accessed 23/05/04]

Department of Health (DoH) (2004b) NHS Hospital, Public Health Medicine and Community Health Service Medical and Dental Workforce Census, England, 30 September – detailed statistics. http://www.publications.doh.gov.uk/public/work_workforce.htm, 19 March [accessed 16/05/04]

Department of Health (DoH) (2005) Hospital and Community Health Services Gross Current Expenditure per Head 2002–3. http://webarchive.nationalarchives.gov.uk/+/www.dh.gov.uk/en/publicationsandstatistics/publications/annualreports/browsable/DH_5340460 [accessed 25/01/13]

Department of Health (DoH) (2012) New start date and more funding announced for local HealthWatch bodies. Press release, 3 January, http://www.dh.gov.uk/health/12/01/local-healthwatch/ [accessed 10/12/12]

Development GAP (1999) Statement of the Development GAP on the proposed multilateral and G7 debt-reduction plan, http://www.developmentgap.org/debtstatement.html [accessed 22/09/03]

DFID (2005) Partnerships for Poverty reduction: rethinking conditionality. UK Policy Paper, http://www.dfid.gov.uk/pubs/files/conditionality.pdf [accessed 15/11/06]

Diderichson F (1995) Market reforms in health care and sustainability of the welfare state: lessons from Sweden. *Health Policy* 32: 141–53

Dixon A, Mossialos E (eds) (2002a) *Health care systems in eight countries: trends and challenges*. European Observatory on Health Care Systems and London School of Economics, London

Dixon A, Mossialos E (eds) (2002b) Not much to write home about? *Health Service Journal*, 24 January

Dixon J, Smith P, Gravelle H, Martin S, Bardsley M, Rice N, Georghiou T, Dusheiko M, Billings J, DeLorenzo M, Sanderson C (2011) A person based formula for allocating commissioning funds to general practices in England: development of a statistical model. *British Medical Journal* 343 (22 November), d6608, doi: 10.1136/BMJ.d6608

Dixon J, Welch H (1991) Priority setting: lessons from Oregon. *Lancet* 337: 891–4 (13 April)

Docteur E, Oxley H (2003) Health Care Systems: Lessons from reform experience. 5 December, OECD, Paris

Dodd R, Hinshelwood E, Harvey C (2004) *PSRPs: their significance of health. Second synthesis report.* WHO, Geneva

Doherty J (2011) Expansion of the private health sector in east and South Africa. Equinet, http://www.equinetafrica.org/bibl/docs/EQ%20Diss%2087%20Private%20HS.pdf [accessed 25/01/13]

Donnelly J (2002) Briton to head global fund on diseases. *Boston Globe*, 25 April, http://www.healthgap.org/press_releases/a02/042502_BG_FUND_ED.html [NOT found]

Dorman T (1999) Managed Care – A Review. *Medical Sentinel* 4(1) (January–February)

Downer A (1998) *Health in Australia's Aid Program.* Australian Agency for International Development, http://www.ausaid.gov.au [accessed 15/11/06]

Doyal L (1979) *The Political Economy of Health.* Pluto Press, London

Drache D, Sullivan T (eds) (1999) *Health Reform: public success, private failure.* Routledge, London & New York

Drechsler D, Jütting JP (2007) Scope, limitations and policy responses. Chapter 7 in Preker et al. 2007

Drinkard J (2005) Drugmakers go furthest to sway Congress. USATODAY.com, 25 April, http://usatoday30.usatoday.com/money/industries/health/drugs/2005-04-25-drug-lobby-cover_x.htm [accessed 14/01/13]

Drucker P (2012) HCA: the unsustainable private equity bubble in US health care. Forbes, 15 August, http://www.forbes.com/sites/stevedenning/12/08/15/private-equity-wont-fix-health-care-either/ [accessed 26/08/12]

Duffin C (2011) Referral management centres across London under review. *Pulse*, 25 October, http://www.pulsetoday.co.uk/newsarticle-content/-/article_display_list/12941966/referral-management-centres-across-london-under-review [accessed 25/01/13]

Dunlop DW, Martins JM (eds) (1996) *An International Assessment of Health Care Financing: Lessons for Developing Countries.* World Bank, Washington

Dyer G (2003) How do you price AIDS treatment? *Financial Times*, 25 March

Dyer G, Anderlini J, Sender H (2011) China's lending hits new heights. *Financial Times*, 17 January, http://www.ft.com/cms/s/0/488c60f4-2281-11e0-b6a2-00144feab49a.html [accessed 02/03/13]

Eaton J, McCay L, Semrau M, Chatterjee S, Baingana F, Araya R, Btulo C, Thornicoft G, Saxena S (2011) Scaling up of services for mental health in low-income and middle income countries. *Lancet* 378: 1,592–603 (17 October), DOI:10.1016/S0140-6736(11)60891-X

ECB (European Central Bank) (2003) The need for comprehensive reforms to cope with population ageing. *ECB Economic Policy Committee Monthly Bulletin*, ECB Frankfurt, http://www.ecb.int/pub/pdf/mobu/mb200304en.pdf [accessed 14/01/13]

ECB Bulletin (2003) 'The need for comprehensive reforms to cope with population ageing'. April, http://www.ecb.int/pub/pdf/mobu/mb200304en.pdf [accessed 25/01/13]

Economist (2006) The birth of philanthrocapitalsim. February, http://www.economist.com/node/5517656?story_id=5517656 [accessed 25/01/13]

Economist (2007) Of markets and medicines. Big donors are betting on Africa's private sector to improve health. December, http://www.economist.com/node/10339384 [accessed 23/03/13]

Economist (2008) Operating profit. Why put up with expensive, run-of-the-mill care at home when you can be treated just as well abroad? August, http://www.economist.com/node/119 19622?Story_id= 11919622 [accessed 29/01/12]

Economist (2011a) Charity begins abroad. August, http://www.economist.com/node/21525836 [accessed 25/01/13]

Economist (2011b) Aid 2.0. 13 August, http://www.economist.com/node/21525899 [accessed 25/01/13]

Economist (2012) New cradles to graves. 8 September, http://www.economist.com/node/21562210 [accessed 23/03/13]

Economist Intelligence Unit (2011a) Hungary pharma. Yet more cuts. Views Wire, June, http://viewswire.eiu.com/index.asp?layout=ib3Article&article_id=1537865538&country_id=&pubtypeid=1152462500&industry_id=&catcgory_id=&fs=true [accessed 28/07/12]

Economist Intelligence Unit (2011b) Spain pharma: The pain in Spain. Views Wire, September, http://viewswire.eiu.com/index.asp?layout=ib3Article&article_id=100818 8885&pubtypeid=]152462500&country_id= 1420000142&fs=true&fs=true [accessed 28/07/12]

Economist Intelligence Unit (2011c) Greece pharma: Roche in a hard place. Views Wire, September, http://www.eiu.com/index.asp?layout=ib3Article&article_id=1948471379&pubtypeid=1152462500&country_id=1370000137&fs=true&rf=0 [accessed 10/04/12]

Economist Intelligence Unit (2011d) Portugal healthcare: Hospitals for sale. Views Wire, September, http://vic\vswire.eiu.com/indcx.asp?layout=ib3Article&article_id=138843392 3&pubtypeid=1152462500&country_id=1740000174&fs=true [accessed 28/07/12]

Economist Intelligence Unit (2011e) Western Europe: Healthcare outlook. Views Wire, November, http://viewswire.eiu.com/index.asp?layout=ib3Article&article_id=238582408 &pubtypeid=1152462500&country_id=1030000303&fs=true [accessed 28/07/12]

Edwards N, Hensher M (1998) Managing demand for secondary care services: the changing context. *British Medical Journal* 317: 135–8 (11 July)

Edwards N, Hensher M, Wernecke U (2000) Changing Hospital Systems. In Saltman et al. 2000

Edwards S (2010) Abolishing User Fees: Making it work in Sierra Leone and beyond. Health Poverty Action, March, http://www.healthpovertyaction.org/wp-content/uploads/downloads/2011/01/AbolishingUserfeesMarch20101/pdf [accessed 25/01/13]

Eggleston K, Ling L, Meng Q, Lindelow M, Wagstaff A (2006) Health Service Delivery in China: a Literature Review. *World Bank Policy Research Working Paper* 3,978, August

Egyptian Initiative for Personal Rights (EIPR) (2009) Preliminary analysis of the New Health Insurance Bill. Committee for the Defense of the Right to Health, 21 October, http://li293-174/members.linode.com/sites/default/files/reports/pdf/Preliminary_ Analysis_of__the_New_Health_Insurance_Bill_EIPR_EN.pdf [accessed 15/01/13]

Egyptian Initiative for Personal Rights (EIPR) (2010) EIPR Welcomes Withdrawal of Flawed Health Insurance Bill, and Asks Minister of Health to Submit a New Bill to the Public to Remedy the Failure of the Latest Bill, 24 March, http://eipr.org/en/ pressrelease/2010/03/24/705 [accessed 02/03/13]

EHMA (European Health Management Association) (2000) *The impact of market forces on health systems*. Dublin

Elliott L (2003a) NHS is being railroaded. *Guardian*, 5 May

Elliott L (2003b) Third-way addicts need a fix. *Guardian*, 14 July

Elliott L (2006) Britain issues World Bank £50m ultimatum. *Guardian*, 14 September

Emmett B (2006) *In the public Interest*. Oxfam

England R (2004) Market forces can help fight AIDS. *Financial Times*, 11 July

England S, Kaddar M, Nigam A, Pinto M (2001) *Practice and policies on user fees for immunization in developing countries*. Department of vaccines and biologicals, World Health Organization, Geneva

Enthoven AC (1985) National Health Service: some reforms that might be politically feasible. *Economist*, 22 June, p. 19

Enthoven AC (1988) *Theory and practice of managed competition in healthcare finance*. Elsevier, New York

Enthoven AC (1997) Market-based reform of US health care financing and delivery: managed care and managed competition. In Schieber 1997

Enthoven AC (2003) Employment-based health insurance is failing: now what? *Health Affairs* web exclusive, 28 May, http://www.healthaffairs.org/WebExclusives/Enthoven_ Web_Excl_052803.htm [accessed 19/06/03]

Equinet (2000) Equity in health in Southern Africa: Turning values into practice. Paper for the Regional Conference 'Building Alliances for Equity in Health', Equinet, Harare

Esping-Andersen G (1990) *The Three Worlds of Welfare Capitalism*. Polity Press

Europa (2004) The State of Mental Health in the European Union. European Commission, Luxembourg, http://ec.europa.eu/health/archive/ph_projects/2001/monitoring/fp_ monitoring_2001_frep_06_en.pdf [accessed 02/03/13]

Europa (2008) Commission adopts proposal for directive on patients' rights in cross-border healthcare. Europa press releases, 2 July, Brussels, http://europa.eu/rapid/press-release_ IP-08-1080_en.htm [accessed 18/01/13]

European Community (2012) *The 2012 Ageing Report: Economic and budgetary projections for the 27 EU Member States (2010–2060)*. European Economy, 2 May, Brussels, http://ec.europa.eu/economy_finance/publications/ european_economy/2012/2012-ageing-report_en.htm

European Health Management Association – see EHMA

European Public Health Association (2006) EPHA's briefing on the European Commission Green Paper on Mental Health. EPHA, January, http://www.epha.org/IMG/pdf/mental_ health_briefing_20060111final.pdf [accessed 14/01/13]

European Union (2004) The state of mental health in the European Union. Health & Consumer Protection Directorate General, http://ec.europa.eu/health/archive/ph_ projects/2001/monitoring/fp_monitoring_2001_frep_06_en.pdf [accessed 14/01/13]

Eurotreaties (2003) Text of the Treaty Establishing a Constitution for Europe. http://www.
eurotreaties.com/constitutiontext.html [accessed 02/03/13]

Evans RG (1997) Going for the gold: the redistributive agenda behind market-based health
care reform. *Journal of Health Politics, Policy and Law* 22(2): 427–65 (April)

Evans RG, Barer ML, Stoddart GL, Bhatia V (1993) Who are the zombie masters, and
what do they want? Vancouver: Centre for Health Services and Policy Research,
University of British Columbia, http://www.chspr.ubc.ca/files/publications/1993/
hpru93-13D.pdf [accessed 31/08/10]

Families USA (2003) Tax free savings accounts for medical expenses: a tax cut
masquerading as help for the uninsured. *Issue Brief*, 22 July, Washington DC, http://
www.familiesusa.org

Fan V (2012a) What indicators reveal about interest in global health: the World
Health Statistics Report. International Health Partnerships Plus, http://www.
internationalhealthpartnership.net/.eveal-about-interest-in-global-health-the-world-
health-statistics-report-323641 [accessed 10/12/12]

Fan V (2012b) Is the Global Fund getting better? IHP plus, 25 April, http://www.
internationalhealthpartnership.net/en/news-events/article/is-the-global-fund-getting-
better-327/ [accessed 10/12/12]

Farrant W (1991) Addressing the contradictions: Health promotion and community health
action in the United Kingdom. *International Journal of Health Services* 21(3): 423–39

Feachem R, Preker A (1997) Presentation of the new strategy of the World Bank on Health,
Nutrition and Population, 9 July. In WHO 1997, https://extranet.who.int/iris/restricted/
bitstream/10665/63719/1/PPE_PAC_97.7.pdf [accessed 02/03/13]

Feachem R (1999) A new role for the Bulletin. *Bulletin of the World Health Organization*
77(1): 2

Feachem RA (2001) Globalisation is good for your health, mostly. *British Medical Journal*
323: 504–6 (1 September)

Ferge Z (2001) Welfare and 'Ill-Fare' systems in Central-Eastern Europe. In Sykes et al.
2001

Figueras J, Saltman RB, Sakellarides C (1998) Introduction to Saltman et al. 2000

Finkel E (2012) The Continuing Struggle: Helping Individuals and Families in the Criminal
Justice System. National Alliance on Mental Health, http://www.nami.org/Template.
cfm?Section=CIT&Template=/ContentManagement/ContentDisplay.cfm&ContentID=1
44470&MicrositeID=0 [accessed 15/09/12]

Fitzpatrick M (2012) The Colorado Tragedy: mental health system concerns. NAMI blog,
1 August, http://blog.nami.org/12/08/the-colorado-tragedy-mental-health.html [accessed
15/01/13]

Flood CM (2000) *International Health Care Reform*. Routledge, London

Flood CM (2011) It pays to drive a hard bargain. *The Mark News*, 14 June, http://www.
themarknews.com/articles/5536-it-pays-to-drive-a-hard-bargain/ [accessed 14/01/13]

Flores W (2006) Equity and health sector reform in Latin America and the Carribbean
from 1995 to 2005: Approaches and Limitations. Report Commissioned by the
International Society for Equity in Health – Chapter of the Americas

Fontana A (2005) *'In Limbo': current status of some HIPC decision point countries*. EURODAD
European Network on Debt and Development, 26 July, http://www.eldis.org/static/
DOC19218.htm [accessed 24/08/06]

Ford N, Mills E, Calmy A (2009) Rationing antiretroviral therapy in Africa – treating too few, too late. *New England Journal of Medicine* 360(18): 1,808–10 (30 April)

Forget EL, Deber R, Roos LL (2002) Medical Savings accounts: will they reduce costs? *CMAJ* 167(2): 143–7 (23 July)

Forsberg BC, Montagu D, Sundewall J (2011) Moving towards in-depth knowledge on the private sector in low- and middle-income countries. *Health Policy and Planning*, 13 June, 26: i1–i3, doi: 10.1093/heapol/czr050

Fotaki M, Boyd A (2005) From Plan to Market: a comparison of health and old age care policies in the UK and Sweden. *Public Money and Management* Vol. 25, pp. 237–43, August

Fouquet H, Cimino A (2012) French parliament passes transaction tax in Hollande's budget. Bloomberg, 1 August, http://www.bloomberg.com/news/12-07-31/french-lawmakers-pass-budget-bill-including-transaction-tax.html [accessed 29/09/12]

Fox M (2009) Healthcare system wastes up to $800 billion a year. Reuters, 26 October, http://www.reuters.com/article/2009/10/26/us-usa-healthcare-waste-idUSTRE59P0L320091026 [accessed 25/01/13]

Foy H (2012) India to give free generic drugs to hundreds of millions. Reuters, 5 July, http://www.reuters.com/article/12/07/05/us-india-drugs-idUSBRE8630PW20120705 [accessed 10/12/12]

France Diplomatie (2012) UNITAID: the International solidarity levy on air tickets. France Diplomatie, 4 June, http://www.diplomatie.gouv.fr/en/global-issues/development-and-humanitarian/institutions-and-issues-of/innovative-ways-to-fund/unitaid-the-international/ [accessed 29/09/12]

Francis R (2013) The Mid Staffordshire NHS Foundation Trust Public Inquiry. February, http://www.midstaffspublicinquiry.com/report [accessed 17/02/13]

Francome C, Marks S (1996) *Improving the Health of the Nation*. Middlesex University Press

Frankel, Ebrahim and Davey Smith (2000) The limits to demand for health care. *British Medical Journal* 321: 42–5 (1 July)

Frayer L (2012) Portugal's sick economy triggers health crisis. *Los Angeles Times*, 13 May, http://articles.latimes.com/print/12/may/13/world/la-fg-portugal-health-20120513 [accessed 21/09/12]

Freeman CW, Boynton XL (eds) (2011) *China's Emerging Global Health and Foreign Aid Engagement in Africa*. Center for Strategic and International Studies, Washington DC, http://csis.org/files/publication/111122_Freeman_ChinaEmergingGlobalHealth_Web.pdf [accessed 25/01/13]

Freeman R (2000) *The Politics of Health in Europe*. Manchester University Press, Manchester

Freidson E (1999) Professionalism and institutional ethics. In Baker et al. 1999

Frenk J (2006) Bridging the divide: global lessons from evidence-based health policy in Mexico. *Lancet* 368: 954–61 (9 September)

Frenk J, de Ferranti D (2012) Universal health coverage: the third global health transition? *Lancet* 380: 862–4 (8 September), doi:10.1016/S0140-6736(12)61341-5 http://www.thelancet.com/journals/lancet/article/PIIS0140-6736(12)61341-5/fulltext#article_upsell [accessed 10/12/12]

Frum D (2011) Arizona's mental health budget crunch. 13 January, http://www.frumforum.com/arizonas-mental-health-budget-crunch [accessed 25/01/13]

Fryatt R, Mills A, Nordstrom A (2010) Financing of health systems to achieve Millennium Development Goals in low-income countries. *Lancet* 375: 419–26 (30 January)

Funk M, Drew N, Saraceno B (2007) Global perspective on mental health policy and service development issues: the WHO angle. Chapter 18 in Knapp et al. 2007

Garrett L (2012) The US promotes universal health care, but only in other countries. *Atlantic*, 29 June, http://www.theatlantic.com/international/archive/12/06/the-us-promotes-universal-health-care-but-only-in-other-countries/259160/ [accessed 21/09/12]

Gates B (2011) Innovation with Impact, Financing 21st Century Development. A report by Bill Gates to G20 leaders, Cannes Summit, November, http://www.thegatesnotes.com/~/media/Images/GatesNotes/G20/G20-Documents/g20-report-english.pdf [accessed 14/01/13]

Gates B (2012) Bill Gates Celebrates Philanthropy In China. *Inquisitor*, 17 January, http://www.inquisitr.com/18236//bill-gates-celebrates-philanthropy-in-china/#hYqzP4jQsvyfyaIP.99 [accessed 10/12/12]

Gates Foundation (2012a) Private and Public Partners Unite to Combat 10 Neglected Tropical Diseases by 2020. Gates Foundation press release, http://www.gatesfoundation.org/press-releases/Pages/combating-10-neglected-tropical-diseases-120130.aspx [accessed 10/12/12]

Gates Foundation (2012b) Brazil's Ministry of Health and Bill & Melinda Gates Foundation Announce Strategic Alliance to Advance Innovation in Global Health. Gates Foundation press release, April, http://www.gatesfoundation.org/press-releases/Pages/brazil-ministry-of-health-global-health-innovation-120416/aspx [accessed 10/12/12]

Gates Foundation (2012c) Bill Gates Outlines Stark Choice: Invest in Innovations for Poorest or Let Millions Starve. Gates Foundation press release, http://www.gatesfoundation.org/press-releases/Pages/fourth-annual-letter-120124/aspx [accessed 10/12/12]

Gaynor M (2012) Reform, Competition, and Policy in Hospital Markets. In OECD 2012c, pp. 333–58

George S (1999) A short history of neo-liberalism. Conference on Economic Sovereignty in a Globalising World, http://www.globalexchange.org/economy/econ101/neoliberalism.html [accessed 20/01/01]

George V and Wilding P (2002) *Globalization and Human Welfare*. Palgrave Macmillan, Basingstoke

Gershman J, Irwin A (2000) Getting a Grip on the Global Economy. In Kim et al. 2000, pp. 11–43

Gibson R, Singh JP (2012) *The Battle over Health Care: What Obama's Reform Means for America's Future*. Rowman & Littlefield Publishers, Inc. 2012

Giles C (2006) UK healthcare's reliance on public funding rises. *Financial Times*, 27 June

Gillam S (2008) Is the declaration of Alma Ata still relevant to primary health care? *British Medical Journal* 336: 536, http://www.BMJ.com/cgi/content/full/336/7643/536 [accessed 25/01/13]

Gilmore A, Fooks G, McKee M (2009) The International Monetary Fund and Tobacco: a product like any other? *International Journal of Health Services* 39(4): 789–93, doi:10.2190/HS.39/4/1

Gilson L, Erasmus E, Mathews P, Ngulube TJ, Scott V (2006) Applying Policy Analysis in Tackling Health-equity Related Implementation Gaps. Equinet Discussion Paper No. 28

Gilson L, McIntyre D (2005) Removing user fees for primary care in Africa: the need to care for action. *British Medical Journal* 331: 762–5, http://www.BMJ.com/cgi/content/extract/331/7519/762 [accessed 25/01/13]

Girach M, Irwin R (2012) How patients could benefit from top-up payments. *Health Service Journal*, 12 July, http://www.hsj.co.uk/resource-centre/best-practice/finance-and-efficiency-resources/how-patients-could-benefit-from-top-up-payments/5046147/article [accessed 10/12/12]

Glassman A, Duran D (2012) Global Health Initiative 2.0: effective priority setting in a time of austerity. Centre for Global Development, 30 January, http://www.cgdev.org/content/publications/detail/1425913 [accessed 14/01/13]

Glennerster H, Midgley J (eds) (1991) *The Radical Right and the welfare state: an international assessment*. Harvester Wheatsheaf, Hemel Hempstead

Glinos IA (2011) Cross border collaboration. Chapter 7 in Wismar et al. 2011

Global Action on Aging (2001) The Ageing of the World's Population. http://www.globalaging.org/waa2/documents/theagingoftheworld.htm [accessed 25/01/13]

Global Fund (2011) Annual Report 2011. http://www.theglobalfund.org/en/library/publications/annualreports/ [accessed 25/01/13]

Global Fund (2012) Donor Governments. http://www.theglobalfund.org/en/donors/?lang=en, [accessed 14/07/12]

Global Insight (2006a) Africa's health insurance initiatives gain momentum. http://www.globalinsight.com/SDA/SDADetails 6281/htm [accessed 29/08/06]

Global Insight (2006b) Belgium to Pilot Toned-Down Version of 'Kiwi Model' for Drug Reimbursement in 2007. http://www.ihs.com/products/global-insight/industry-economic-report.aspx?id=106599255 [accessed 25/01/13]

Goddard M, Mannion R (2006) Decentralising the NHS: rhetoric, reality and paradox. *Journal of Health Organisation and Management* 20: 67–73, http://dx.doi.org/10.1108/14777260610656561 [accessed 25/01/13]

Godlee F (1996) New hope for WHO? *British Medical Journal* 312: 1,376, http://dx.doi.org/10.1136/bmj.312.7043.1376 (1 June)

Godlee F (1998) Change at last at WHO. *British Medical Journal* 317: 296 (1 August)

Godlee F (1994a) The World Health Organization (series). *British Medical Journal* 309: 1,424–8 (26 November)

Godlee F (1994b) WHO in retreat: is it losing its influence? *British Medical Journal* 309: 1,491–5 (3 December)

Godlee F (1994c) WHO at country level – a little impact, no strategy. *British Medical Journal* 309: 1,636–9 (17 December)

Goldberg M (2012) Healthy Dose: World Leaders Meet on polio at the UN. *Healthy Dose*, 28 September, https://groups.google.com/forum/?hl=en&fromgroups#!topic/TheHealthyDose/WcJwQZ34hM0 [accessed 30/09/12]

Gonzalez-Block MA (2004) Health policy and systems research agendas in developing countries. *Health Policy and Systems* August 2: 6

Gottret P, Schieber GJ (2006) *Health Financing Revisited: A Practitioner's Guide*. World Bank, Washington DC

Gottret P, Schieber GJ, Waters HR (eds) (2008) *Good Practices in Health Financing*. World Bank, Washington DC

Gough I (2000) Globalisation and regional welfare regimes: the East Asian case. International Social Security Association, International Research Conference, Helsinki, http://www.issa.int/pdf/helsinki2000/topic1/2gough.pdf [accessed 25/01/13]

Govindaraj R, Obuobi AAD, Enyimayew NKA, Antwi P, Ofusu-Amaah S (1996) Hospital autonomy in Ghana: the experience of Korle Bu and Komfo Anyoke teaching hospitals. August, Data for Decision Making, Harvard

GPOBA (2007) Project Information Document (PID) 38677, Concept Stage, 2 February, http://goo.gl/bgtZ9 [NOT found]

GPOBA (2008) Yemen Queen of Sheba Safe Motherhood Project Operations Manual. Global Partnership on Output-Based Aid, August, http://www.gpoba.org/gpoba/sites/gpoba.org/files/OperationsManual/Operations%20Manual%20-%20Yemen%20Health.pdf [accessed 25/01/13]

GPOBA (2010) Lesotho: New public–private partnership set to boost access to health care for the poor. 15 June, http://www.gpoba.org/gpoba/node/472 [accessed 25/01/13]

Grant J (2003) GM pumps $3 bn into employee health fund. *Financial Times*, 11 August

Gratzer D (2002) It's time to consider Medical Savings Accounts. *CMAJ* 167(2) 151–2, 23 July

Graul AI, Cruces F. (2011) The year's new drugs & biologics, 2010. *Drugs of Today* (Barcelona) 47(1): 27–51 (January), http://www.ncbi.nlm.nih.gov/pubmed/21373648 [accessed 25/01/13]

Greer S (2009) Cross-border trade in health services: lessons from the European laboratory. University of Michigan, http://sitemaker.umich.edu/scottlgreer/files/crossborder_trade_in_health_services_revised.pdf [accessed 18/01/13]

Greku E (2009) The added value of the Euro Health Consumer Index to existing mechanisms of national health care systems evaluation provided by the OECD and WHO. University of Twente School of Management and Governance, http://essay.utwente.nl/58997/1/scriptie_E_Greku.pdf [accessed 25/01/13]

Gryta T (2011) What is a 'Pharmacy Benefit Manager?' *Wall Street Journal*, 21 July, http://online.wsj.com/article/SB10001424053111903554904576460322664055328.html [accessed 25/01/13]

Guardian Development Network (2011) Lesotho's ailing public health system. http://www.guardian.co.uk/global-development/2011/oct/07/lesotho-ailing-public-health-system [accessed 25/01/13]

Guha K (2006) Reform of IMF 'is less pressing than tackling global economic imbalances'. *Financial Times*, 11 September

Guha K, Condon C (2006) IMF questions Hungary's fiscal rescue plan. *Financial Times*, 22 June

Guha K, Giles C, McGregor R (2006) IMF heads for wrangle on voting power. *Financial Times*, 15 September

Guilloux A, Moon S (2002) Hidden Price Tags: Disease Specific Drug Donations: Costs and Alternatives. Drugs for neglected diseases working group, New York, http://www.deolhonaspatentes.org.br/media/file/Publicacoes/hidden_price_tags.pdf [accessed 25/01/13]

Gupta AS (2008) Medical tourism in India: winners and losers. *Indian Journal of Medical Ethics* V(1) (January–March)

Gupta S, Clements B, Coady D (2012) The challenge of health care reform in advanced and emerging economies. In Clements et al. 2012

Gupta S, Clements B, Guin-Siu MT, Leruth L (2001) Debt relief and health spending in Heavily Indebted Poor Countries, reprinted in Health and Development (IMF December 2004). *Finance and Development*, September

Gupta MD, Rani M (2004) India's Public Health System: How Well Does It Function at the National Level? *World Bank Policy Research Working Paper* 3,447, November

Gwatkin DR, Guillot M (2000) The Burden of Disease among the Global Poor. Global Forum for Health Research, World Bank, Washington DC

HAI (Help Age International) (2002) State of the World's Older People 2002. Help Age International, London, http://www.helpage.org/resources/publications/?adv=0&ssearch=&filter=f.yeard&type=&region=&topic=&language=&page=34 [accessed 23/01/13]

HAI (Help Age International) (2011) Insights on Ageing: a survey report. Help Age International, London, http://goo.gl/nzay8 [accessed 23/01/13]

Hall D (2009) A Crisis for Public–private Partnerships (PPPs)? Crisis and public services note 2: Public Services International Research Unit, January, www.psiru.org/reports/2009-01-crisis-2.doc [accessed 15/03/13]

Hall MA, McCue MJ (2012) Estimating the impact of the Medical Loss Ratio Rule: a state-by-state analysis. The Commonwealth Fund, http://www.commonwealthfund.org/~/media/Files/Publications/Issue%20Brief/12/Mar/1587_Hall_medical_loss_ratio_ib.pdf [accessed 15/01/13]

Ham C (1997) Why rationing is inevitable in the NHS. In New 1997

Ham C (1998) Retracing the Oregon trail: the experience of rationing and the Oregon health plan. *British Medical Journal* 316: 1,965–9 (27 June)

Ham C (1999) Health Policy in Britain (4th Ed). Macmillan, London

Ham C and Honigsbaum F (1998) Priority setting and rationing health services. In Saltman et al. 2000

Hamid H, Abanilla K, Bauta B, Huang K-K (2008) Evaluating the WHO assessment instrument for mental health systems by comparing mental health policies in four countries. *Bulletin of the WHO* 2008, 86: 467–73

Hancock J (2012) The new normal in health insurance: high deductibles. *Kaiser Health News*, 3 June, http://www.kaiserhealthnews.org/Stories/12/June/04/high-deductible-health-insurance.aspx [accessed 20/09/12]

Handal S (2012) Tories plan to sell off NHS blood supplier. Liberal Conspiracy blog, 15 July, http://liberalconspiracy.org/2012/07/15/tories-plan-to-sell-off-nhs-blood-supplier/ [accessed 02/03/13]

Hanefield J (2008) How have global health initiatives impacted on health equity? *Global Health Promotion* 15(1): 19–23, DOI 10. 1177/1025382307088094

Hann A (ed.) (2000) *Analysing Health Policy.* Ashgate, Aldershot

Hansard (House of Commons debates) (1996) Ministerial answer on Health Care Reforms. Hansard, 1 July, Column 338, http://www.publications.parliament.uk/pa/cm199596/cmhansrd/vo960701/text/60701w17/htm [accessed 25/01/13]

Hanson K, Gilson L, Goodman C, Mills A, Smith R, Feachem R, Feachem NS, Koehlmoos TP, Kimlaw H (2008) Is private healthcare the answer to the health problems of the world's poor? *PloS Medicine* 5(11): 1,528–31, e233/ Doi:10.1371/journal/pmed.0050233

Hanvoravongchai P (2002) Medical Savings Accounts: lessons learned from international experience. EIP/HFS/PHF Discussion Paper No. 52, World Health Organization, 15 October, http://www.who.int/healthinfo/paper52/pdf [accessed 20/01/13]

Hardon A (2000) Vaccination Policy and the Public–Private Mix. *Report on the Health Action International Europe/BUKO Pharma-Kampagne Seminar*, 3 November, HAI Europe, http://www.haiweb.org/campaign/PPI/seminar200011.html#item5 [accessed 12/06/04]

Harper RW (2004) New Health System for Australia. http://www.pc.gov.au/inquiry/ncp/subs/subdr142/rtf [NOT found]

Hart, J Tudor (1971) The Inverse Care Law. *Lancet* 1: 405–12 (27 February)

Hart, J Tudor (1994) *Feasible Socialism: The National Health Service past present and future*. Socialist Health Association, London

Hart, J Tudor (2003) Health care or health trade? A historic moment of choice. Paper presented at European Social Forum anti-summit conference on globalisation, Thessaloniki, 18 June, *International Journal of Health Services* 34(2): 245–54

Hart, J Tudor (2010) *The Political Economy of Health Care* (2nd Edition). The Policy Press, Bristol

Harvey T (2001) Do the performance tables measure up? *British Journal of Health Care Management* 7(12): 497–8

Haugh D (2011) Analysing FairCare, Fine Gael's proposal for mandatory universal health insurance. 18 February, http://www.macliam.org/Health/AnalysisFineGaelFaircare.pdf [accessed 18/01/13]

Hazarika I (2010) Medical tourism: its potential impact on the health workforce and health systems in India. *Health Policy and Planning*, 25: 248–51, DOI: 10.1093/heapol/czp050

Health and Social Care Information Centre (2012) NHS Workforce: Summary of staff in the NHS: Results from September 2011 Census. March, http://www.ic.nhs.uk/webfiles/publications/010_Workforce/NHS%20STAFF%20ANNUAL%202001-11/NHS_Workforce_Census_Bulletin_2001_2011/pdf [accessed 10/12/12]

Health for North East London (2009) Pre-consultation business case. December, http://www.healthfornel.nhs.uk/resources/publications/?entryid49=25452 [accessed 02/03/13]

Health Policy Consensus Group (2001) Why we need market-based health care reform (two parts). Part 1, 1 March; Part 2, 1 April; Heartland Institute, 9 January, http://www.heartland org

Health Poverty Action (2012) International Health Partnership. http://www.healthpovertyaction.org/policy-and-resource/aid-financing-and-debt/international-health-partnership [accessed 04/07/12]

Health Systems 20/20 (USAID) (2012) Data. http://www.healthsystems2020.org/

Healthcare Europa (2011) Stockholm outsources psychiatric care. http://www.healthcareeuropa.com/articles/20081121_2/print [accessed 04/04/11]

Healthcare Europa (2012) Payment by results saves Stockholm 17%. Healthcare Europa, http://www.HealthcareEuropa.com, June

Healthcare for London (2010) Delivering Healthcare for London: An Integrated Strategic Plan 2010–2015. NHS London, http://www.london.nhs.uk/webfiles/Corporate/HFL_First%20Stage%20Report_V2.1.pdf [accessed 02/03/13]

Heaton A (2001) Joint public–private initiatives: meeting children's right to health? Save the Children Fund UK, May

Heighway-Bury R (2007) Knowledge Bankrupted: Evaluation says key World Bank research was 'not remotely reliable'. Bretton Woods Project, 31 January, http://www.brettonwoodsproject.org/art-549070 [accessed 14/01/13]

Heldrup J (2007) Health development – a global perspective. *Danish Medical Bulletin* 54(1): 37–8

Hennessy P (1995) Social Protection for dependent elderly people: perspectives from a review of OECD countries. Labour Market and Social Policy Occasional Paper No. 16, OECD, Paris, http://dx.doi.org/10.1787/271344236402 [accessed 14/01/13]

Henry JS (2012) The price of offshore revisited. Tax Justice Network, July, http://www.tjn-usa.org/storage/documents/The_Price_of_Offshore_Revisited_-_22-07-2012/pdf [accessed 15/01/13]

Hensher M, Edwards N, Stokes R (1999) International trends in the provision and utilisation of hospital care. *British Medical Journal* 319: 845–8 (25 September)

Hercot D, Meessen B, Ridde V, Gilson L (2011) Removing user fees for health services in low income countries: a multi-country review framework for assessing the process of policy change. *Health Policy and Planning* 26: ii5–ii15, doi:10.1093/czr063

Hernández-Quevedo C, Olejaz M, Nielsen AJ, Rudkjøbing A, Birk HO, Krasnik A (2012) Do Danes enjoy a high-performing chronic care system? *Eurohealth* 18(1): 26–9

Herper M (2012) The global drug market will swell to $1.2 trillion while big Pharma treads water. Forbes, 12 July, http://www.forbes.com/sites/matthewherper/12/07/12/the-global-drug-market-will-swell-to-1-2-trillion-while-big-pharma-treads-water/ [accessed 10/12/12]

Hickel J (2011) Fallacy of 'freedom': USAID and neoliberal policy in Egypt. The Africa Report, 14 March, http://eprints.lse.ac.uk/41295/ [accessed 25/01/13]

Hilary J (2005) DFID, UK and services privatisation: time for change. *Global Social Policy* 5(2): 134–6, http://peer.ccsd.cnrs.fr/docs/00/57/17/73/PDF/PEER_stage2_10.1177%252F146801810500500202/pdf [accessed 13/07/12]

Hillstrom S (2000) Charitable donations of drugs by corporations. Tax driven practices and consequences. http://www.drugdonations.org/eng/charitable_drug_donations_by_c.html, [accessed 12/02/11]

Hindle D, McAuley I (2004) The effects of increased private health insurance: a review of the evidence. *Australian Health Review* 28(1): 119–38 (September)

Hitipieuw J (2012) Indonesia's government planning health insurance for all poor people. Kompas.com, 24 February, http://english.kompas.com/read/12/02/24/09103884/Indonesias.Govt.Planning.Health.Insurance.for.All.Poor.People [accessed 08/09/12]

HM Treasury (1997) An introduction to the private finance initiative. London, HM Treasury

HM Treasury (2012) PFI signed projects list. March, http://www.hm-treasury.gov.uk/ppp_pfi_stats.htm

Hoggett P (1994) The politics of the modernisation of the UK welfare state. In Burrows and Loader 1994

Holland W (2000) Extra Money for the United Kingdom National Health Service. *Euro Observer: Newsletter for the European Observatory on Health Care Systems* Winter 00/01, Vol. 2, No. 4, WHO Europe, Copenhagen

Hollande F (2012) 'The Globalization of Solidarity': France praises UNITAID for setting example. UNITAID, http://www.unitaid.eu/component/content/article?id=1001 [accessed 08/09/12]

Holst J (2010) Patient cost sharing: reforms without evidence. Discussion Paper SP I 2010-303, November, Wissenscahtszentrum Berlin für Sozialforschung (WZB), https://www.econstor.eu/dspace/bitstream/10419/56932/1/689987234.pdf [accessed 25/01/13]

Holt E (2012) Romania redrafts health-care law after violent protests. *Lancet* 379(9,815): 505 (11 February), doi:10.1016/S0140-6736(12)60214-1 http://www.theLancet.com/journals/Lancet/article/PIIS0140-6736(12)60214-1/fulltext [accessed 14/01/13]

Homedes N, Ugalde A (2005a) Human resources: the Cinderella of health reform in Latin America. *Human Resources for Health* 3(1), January

Homedes N, Ugalde A (2005b) Why neoliberal health reforms have failed in Latin America. *Health Policy* 71: 83–96

Hood C (1991) A public Management for all seasons. *Public Administration* 69 (Spring): 3–19

Hood M (2011) Global Fund faces billion-dollar gap. AFP, 19 May, http://www.google.com/hostednews/afp/article/ALeqM5h6Ih8CYz1SqAKYjI-SiowJgu8BSA?docId=CNG.07d4a47a8ce76f0e07e322726bdf65a2/6f1 [accessed 25/01/13]

HOPE (European Hospital, Healthcare Federation) (2009) Hospitals in the 27 member states of the European Union. Dexia Editions, January, European Hospitals and Healthcare Federation, http://www.hope.be/03activities/1_0-facts_and_figures.html [accessed 20/01/13]

HOPE (European Hospital, Healthcare Federation) (2011) The Crisis, Hospitals and Healthcare. http://www.hope.be/05eventsandpublications/docpublications/86_crisis/86_HOPE-The_Crisis_Hospitals_Healthcare_April_2011/pdf [accessed 25/01/13]

Horn JS (1969) *Away with All Pests: An English Surgeon in People's China.* Paul Hamlyn, London

Hovhannisyan K (2012) Campaign averts savage cuts to health budget in Armenia but out-of-pocket payments still dangerously high. Oxfam, *Global Health Check*, 19 June, http://www.globalhealthcheck.org [accessed 10/12/12]

Hrobon P, Machácek T, Julínek T (2005) Healthcare Reform for the Czech Republic in 21st Century Europe. http://www.healthrcform.cz/content/files/en/Reform/1_Publications/EN_publikace.pdf [accessed 25/01/13]

Hsiao W, Heller PS (2007) What should Macroeconomists know about healthcare policy? IMF working paper WP/07/13, International monetary fund, Washington DC, http://www.imf.org/external/pubs/ft/wp/2007/wp0713/pdf [accessed 18/01/13]

HSJ Local (2012) Formal grievance lodged over outsourcing plans. *Health Service Journal*, 28 May, http://www.hsj.co.uk/hsj-local/formal-grievance-lodged-over-outsourcing-plans/5045306/article [accessed 25/09/12]

Hsu J (2010a) The relative efficiency of public and private service delivery. World Health Report, Background Paper No. 39, WHO Geneva

Hsu J (2010b) Medical savings accounts: what is at risk? WHO World Health Report, Background Paper No. 17, http://www.who.int/healthsystems/topics/financing/healthreport/MSAsNo17FINAL.pdf [accessed 20/01/13]

Huang Y (2011) Domestic factors and China's health programs in Africa. In Freeman and Boynton 2011, http://csis.org/files/

publication/111122_Freeman_ChinaEmergingGlobalHealth_Web.pdf [accessed 25/01/13]

Huber M, Rodrigues R, Hoffmann F, Marin B (2009) Facts and figures on long☒term care for older people: Europe and North America. European Centre for Social Welfare Policy and Research, http://www.euro.centre.org/data/1253897823_70974/pdf [accessed 25/01/13]

Hujer M, Reiermann C (2012) 'Emerging Nations Vie for Power at IMF', *Spiegel Online*, 18 April, http://spiegel.de/international/business/0,1518,druck-827790,00.html

Human Rights Watch (2006) A high price to pay: Detention of poor patients in Burundian Hospitals. New York, Human Rights Watch, http://www.hrw.org/reports/2006/ burundi0906/.

Hundal S (2012) Tories plan to sell off NHS blood supplier. Liberal Conspiracy, 15 July, http://liberalconspiracy.org/12/07/15/tories-plan-to-sell-off-nhs-blood-supplier/ [accessed 20/01/13]

Hunter D (1998) Public Private mix in *health care restructuring. ILO/PSI workshop on employment and labour practices in health care in Central and Eastern Europe*, Part 5, ILO Geneva

Hunter DJ (2008) *The Health Debate.* The Policy Press, Bristol

Hunter N (2010) End state subsidies for private care. irishhealth.com, 2 October, http:// www.irishhealth.com/article.html?id=17968 [accessed 06/09/12]

Hurst J, Jee-Hughes M (2001) Performance measurement and performance management in OECD health systems. *Labour Market and Social Policy Occasional Papers* No. 47, OECD, Paris

Hutchinson P, LaFond AK (2004) Monitoring and evaluation of decentralization reforms in developing country health sectors. Partners for Health Reformplus, Abt Assiciates Inc, Bethesda MD

Hutton G (2004) Charting the path to the World Bank's 'No blanket policy on user fees'. DFID Health Systems Research Centre, May, http://hdrc.dfid.gov.uk/wp-content/ uploads/2012/10/Charting-the-path-to-the-World-Banks-policy.pdf [accessed 25/01/13]

Hygeia Group (2012) Hygeia HMO. http://www.hygeiagroup.com/hmo/index.php?category_ id=124 [accessed 14/05/12]

IDB (2012) Public Health. Inter-American development Bank, http://www.iadb.org/en/ about-us/public-health,6222/html [accessed 13/07/12]

IFC (2002) Topical Briefing on health and investing in private healthcare: strategic directions for IFC. 'Official use only', restricted circulation, 22 February, International Finance Corporation, Washington DC

IFC (2007a) Factsheet: Investment Boom for Health Care in Middle East and North Africa, Says IFC. International Finance Corporation, Washington DC, http:// www1/ifc.org/wps/wcm/connect/86d09a804970bfb89919db336b93d75f/Factsheet_ InvestmentBoomHealthCareinMENA.pdf?MOD=AJPERES [accessed 23/09/12]

IFC (2007b) The Business of Health in Africa. International Finance Corporation, Washington DC, http://www.unido.org/fileadmin/user_media/Services/PSD/BEP/IFC_ HealthinAfrica_Final.pdf [accessed 23/09/12]

IFC (2008) Landmark public–private partnership (PPP) healthcare agreement signed. Press release, 27 October, http://www.netcare.co.za/live/content.php?cookie=k&Item_ID=4784

IFC (2009a) Success Stories – Lesotho: National Referral Hospital. June, International Finance Corporation, Washington DC, http://www.ifc.org/ifcext/psa.nsf/AttachmentsByTitle/PPPseries_Lesotho/$FILE/SuccessStories_LesothoWEB.pdf [link does not go to this article]

IFC (2009b) Breaking new ground: Lesotho Hospital Public Private Partnership – a model for integrated health services delivery. Smartlessons, International Finance Corporation, Washington DC, http://www.ifc.org/ifcext/psa.nsf/AttachmentsByTitle/Smartlesson_LesothoHospital/$FILE/LesothoHospital_Smartlesson.pdf [link does not go to this article]

IFC (2009c) Summary of Proposed Investment. International Finance Corporation, Washington DC, http://www.ifc.org/ifcext/spiwebsite1/nsf/DocsByUNIDForPrint/BAD8195B71440864852576BA000E2DE3?opendocument [accessed 25/01/13]

IFC (2009d) Lesotho National Referral Hospital Public Private Partnership. 11 September, p. 2, http://www.mofep.gov.gh/documents/pfa_ppp_presentation_2009_10.pdf

IFC (2009e) Leasing in Development. Guidelines for Emerging Economies. International Finance Corporation, Washington DC, http://rru.worldbank.org/Documents/Toolkits/Leasing/IFC-Leasing-Guide-2009-2nd-ed.pdf

IFC (2010) IFC's $93 Million Investment in South African Provider, Life Healthcare to Expand Emerging Market Health Coverage, IFC, Washington DC, http://www1.ifc.org/wps/wcm/connect/industry_ext_content/ifc_external_corporate_site/industries/health+and+education/news/features_health_southafrica_061010 [accessed 02/03/13]

IFC (2011) Integrated Health systems, Lesotho's pioneering model. Handshake, Issue 3, International Finance Corporation, Washington DC, http://viewer.zmags.com/publication/6c527326#/6c527326/1 [accessed 25/01/13]

IFC (no date) Frequently asked questions. http://www1.ifc.org/wps/wcm/connect/CORP_EXT_Content/IFC_External_Corporate_Site/IFC+Projects+Database/Projects/AIP+Policy+in+Detail/ProjectFAQs [accessed 04/03/13]

Ilie L (2012) Romania withdraws controversial healthcare bill. Reuters, 13 January, http://www.reuters.com/article/12/01/13/us-romania-healthcare-idUSTRE80C28720120113 [accessed 15/01/13]

IMA (2011a) Executive Summary. Israeli Medical Association, http://www.ima.org.il/ENG/ViewCategory.aspx?CategoryId=6153 [accessed 20/09/12]

IMA (2011b) Background – The Crisis in the Healthcare System. Israeli Medical Association, http://www.ima.org.il/ENG/ViewCategory.aspx?CategoryId=6156 [accessed 20/09/12]

IMF (2012) Global financial stability report. World Economic and Financial Surveys, International Monetary Fund, Washington DC, April, http://www.imf.org/external/pubs/ft/gfsr/12/01/ [accessed 14/01/13]

IMF and World Bank (2005) Review of the Poverty Reduction Strategy Approach: Balancing Accountabilities and Scaling Up Results. IMF and World Bank, 19 August, International Monetary Fund, Washington DC, http://siteresources.worldbank.org/INTPRS1/Resources/PRSP-Review/2005_Review_Final.pdf [accessed 14/01/13]

IMF External Affairs (2012) Poverty reduction Strategy Papers (PRSP). Factsheet, April, International Monetary Fund, Washington DC, http://www.imf.org/external/np/exr/facts/prsp.htm [accessed 10/12/12]

Indianstocksnews.com (2009) Apollo hospitals buy stock to keep portfolio health good. http://www.indianstocksnews.com/2009/01/apollo-hospitals-buy-stock-to-keep.html [accessed 25/01/13]

InPharm (2012) Europe's pharma sector: living through the crisis. 14 March, http://www. pharmafile.com/news/171773/europe-s-pharma-sector-living-through-crisis [accessed 15/01/13]

Insurance News Net (2010) Private Equity Taps Health Sector Growth. 26 April, http:// insurancenewsnet.com/print.aspx?id=183449&type=newswires [accessed 25/01/13]

International Finance Corporation (IFC) (2010) IFC's $93 Million Investment in South African Provider, Life Healthcare to Expand Emerging Market Health Coverage. IFC press release, Washington DC, http://www1/ifc.org/wps/wcm/connect/industry_ ext_content/ifc_external_corporate_site/industries/health+and+education/news/ features_health_southafrica_061010 [accessed 25/01/13]

IRIN (2006) Lesotho: Lack of healthcare workers a drain on new HIV/AIDS plan, 27 April, http://www.irinnews.org/PrintReport.aspx?Reportid=58858

Irwin A, Scali E (2005) Action on the Social Determinants of Health: Learning From Previous Experiences, A Background Paper. WHO Commission on Social Determinants of Health, March, http://www.who.int/social_determinants/resources/action_sd.pdf [accessed 25/01/13]

Jaffe DJ (2012) Closing New York State Psychiatric Hospitals is Dangerous. *Huffington Post*, 19 March, http://www.huffingtonpost.com/dj-jaffe/kingsboro-psychiatric-center-closing_b_1342887/html [accessed 15/01/13]

Jakarta Post (2011) Govt kicks off pilot project for universal health care in W. Java. 1 March, http://uhcforward.org/headline/govt-kicks-pilot-project-universal-health-care-w-java [accessed 02/03/13]

Jakarta Post (2012a) Universal health insurance by 2019. 4 September, UHC Forward, http://uhcforward.org/headline/universal-health-insurance-2019 [accessed 02/03/13]

Jakarta Post (2012b) Indonesia's National Health Scheme Untapped. 13 May, http:// uhcforward.org/headline/indonesias-national-health-scheme-untapped [accessed 02/03/13]

Jarman B (1993) Is London overbedded? *British Medical Journal* 306: 979–82 (10 April)

Jeffs E, Baeten R (2011) Simulation on the EU cross-border care directive. Final report Brussels, 24 November, European health Management Association, http://www.uems. net/uploads/media/CrossBorderHealthcareSimulation_FinalRep_09052012/pdf [accessed 18/01/13]

Jenkins PL (2012) The Mental Health Cuts Being Made Behind Closed Doors. *Huffington Post*, 23 May, http://www.huffingtonpost.co.uk/paul-i-jenkins/mental-health-cuts-the-mental-health-cuts-be_b_1537453/html [accessed 10/12/12]

Jessop B (2003) From Thatcherism to New Labour: neo-liberalism, workfarism and labour market regulation. In Overbeek 2003, pp. 137–53

Jha P, de Beyer J, Heller PS (1999) Death and taxes: the economics of tobacco control. IMF, Washington DC, *Finance & Development* 36(4) (December), http://www.imf.org/ external/pubs/ft/fandd/1999/12/jha.htm [accessed 14/01/13]

Johnston T, Stout S (1999) *Investing in Health. Development effectiveness in the Health Nutrition and Population Sector.* Operations Evaluation Department, World Bank, Washington DC

Joumard I, André C, Nicq C (2010) Health care systems: efficiency and institutions. OECD Economics Department Working Papers No. 769, OECD Publishing, Paris, http://dx.doi.org/10.1787/5kmfp51f5f9t-en [accessed 25/01/13]

Kahenya G, Lake S (1994) User Fees and their Impact on Utilization of Key Health Services. UNICEF, Lusaka

Kahn CN (2006) Intolerable risk, irreparable harm: the legacy of physician-owned specialty hospitals. *Health Affairs* 25(1): 130–3, DOI: 10.1377/hlthaff.25/1/130

Kaiser Family Foundation (KFF) (2012) Health care costs: a primer Key information on health care costs and their impact. KFF, May, http://www.kff.org/insurance/upload/7670-03/pdf [accessed 10/12/12]

Kanzler L, Ng A (2012) The future of public and private health care insurance in Asia. In Clements et al. 2012

Kar D, Curcio K (2011) Illicit Financial Flows from Developing Countries 2000–2009. Ford Foundation, January, http://www.gfintegrity.org/storage/gfip/documents/reports/IFF2010/gfi_iff_update_report-web.pdf [accessed 14/01/13]

Kastrup MC, Ramos AB (2007) Global mental health. *Danish Medical Bulletin* 54: 42–3 (February)

Kaufman J (2005) China: the intersections between Poverty, Health Inequity, Reproductive health and HIV/AIDS. Palgrave Macmillan Ltd

Kay JA, Thompson DJ (1986) Privatisation: a policy in search of a rationale. *Economic Journal* 96(381): 18–32 (March), http://www.jstor.org/stable/2233423 [accessed 01/01/13]

Kelley A, McGarry K, Fahle S, Marshall S, Du Q, Skinner J (2012) Out-of-Pocket Spending in the Last Five Years of Life. *Journal of General Internal Medicine*, http://dx.doi.org/10.1007/s11606-012-2199-x [accessed 10/12/12]

Kelley R (2009) Where can $700 billion in waste be cut annually from the U.S. Healthcare system? Thomson Reuters, http://www.ncrponline.org/PDFs/2009/Thomson_Reuters_White_Paper_on_Healthcare_Waste.pdf [accessed 25/01/13]

Kelly J, Malone S (eds) (2006) *Ecosocialism or Barbarism*. Socialist Resistance, London

Kelsey J (1995) *Economic fundamentalism*. Pluto Press, London

Kemkes J, van der Meer J, Mooren H, de Wildt G (1997) Economic adjustment in developing countries is too painful for health care: Time for a signal from the medical profession. *Bulletin medicus mundi*, April, http://www.medicusmundi.cj/bulletin/bulletin641.html [accessed 29/06/02]

Kerrison SH, Pollock AM (2001) Caring for older people in the private sector in England. *British Medical Journal* 323: 566–9 (8 September)

Kessler T (2003) Assessing the Risks in the Private Provision of Essential Services. Discussion paper for G-24 Technical Group Geneva, Switzerland. Citizens' Network on Essential Services, http://unctad.org/en/Docs/gdsmdpbg2420047_en.pdf [accessed 25/01/13].

Khalegian P (2001) Immunization financing and sustainability: a review of the literature. GAVI, http://www.gaviftf.info/docs_activities/background_docs.html#planning [accessed 15/11/03]

Kickbusch I (2006) Gender – a critical determinant of health in a global world. *International Journal of Public Health* 51: 1–2, DOI 10.1007/s00038-006-6076-4

Kim JY, Millen JV, Irwin A, Gershman J (eds) (2000) *Dying for Growth: Global Inequality and the Health of the Poor*. Maine: Common Courage Press

Kippenberg J (2006) A High Price to Pay Detention of Poor Patients in Burundian Hospitals. *Human Rights Watch* 18(8a) (September)

Kirigia J, Emrouznejad A, Sambo LG (2002) Measurement of technical efficiency of public hospitals in Kenya: using data envelopment analysis. *Journal of Medical Systems* 26: 1, 39–45 (February)

Kirigia JM, Nganda BM, Mwikisa CN, Cardoso B (2011) Effects of global financial crisis on funding for health development in nineteen countries of the WHO African Region. *BMC International Health and Human Rights* 11: 4, doi:10.1186/1472-698X-11-4, http://www.biomedcentral.com/1472-698X/11/4 [accessed 15/01/13]

Klein N (2008) Free market ideology is far from finished. *Guardian*, 19 September, http://www.guardian.co.uk/commentisfree/2008/sep/19/marketturmoil.usa [accessed 16/01/13]

Klein R (2000) *The New Politics of the NHS* (4th Edition). Longman, London

Klein R (2004) The first wave of NHS foundation trusts. Editorial, *British Medical Journal* 328: 1,332 (5 June)

Kleinke JD (2001a) *Oxymorons: the myth of a US health care system.* Jossey-Bass, San Francisco

Kleinke JD (2001b) The price of progress: prescription drugs in the health care market. Editorial, *Health Affairs* 20(5) 43–59 (September–October)

Klugman J, Schieber G (1996) A survey of health reform in Central Asia. World Bank Technical Paper No. 344, Washington DC

Kmietowicz Z (2003) Some operating theatres are used only eight hours a week. *British Medical Journal* 326: 1,349 (21 June)

Knapp M, McDaid D (2007) Financing and funding mental health services. Chapter 4 in Knapp et al. 2007

Knapp M, McDaid D, Mossialos E, Thornicroft G (2007) *Mental Health Policy and Practice Across Europe.* European Health Observatory, Open University Press, McGraw Hill, Maidenhead

Knobler S, Mahmoud A, Lemon S, Mack A, Sivitz L, Oberholtzer K (eds) (2004) *Learning from SARS. Preparing for the next disease outbreak.* Institute of Medicine Workshop Summary, National Academies Press, Washington DC, http://www.nap.edu/catalog/10915/html [accessed 25/01/13]

Knowles JC, Leighton C, Stinson W (1997) Measuring results of health sector reform for system performance: a handbook of indicators. Partnerships for Health Reform, Bethesda MD, September

Kocher B (2007) Global provider trends. McKinsey & Company Presentation at IFC Conference for Private Health Care in Emerging Markets, April, IFC: Washington DC, http://www.ifc.org/ifcext/che.nsf/AttachmentsByTitle/Healthpres_2007_BobKocher/$FILE/Healthpres_2007_Bob+Kocher.pdf [NOT found]

Koivusalo M (2003) Health systems solidarity and European Community policies. In Sen 2003

Kroger T (2001) Comparative research on social care: the state of the art. European Commission 5th Framework Programme, Brussels, February, http://cordis.europa.eu/documents/documentlibrary/90834291EN6/pdf [accessed 12/09/12]

Kronfol NM (1999) Perspectives on the health care system of the United Arab Emirates. *Eastern Mediterranean Health Journal* 5(1): 149–67

Kruk ME, Goldman E, Galea S (2009) Borrowing and selling to pay for health care in low and middle income countries. *Health Affairs*, July–August, doi 10.1377/hlthaff.28/4/1056

KTN Prime (Standard Digital media) (2012) (Video) Nairobi Women's Hospital Fiasco. 8 August, http://www.standardmedia.co.ke/index.php?videoID=2000059555&video_ title=nairobi-womens-hospital-fiasco [accessed 10/12/12]

Küçükel B (2009) Transforming the Turkish Healthcare System. Aspects of Health Reform in Turkey. *Hospital* 11(2): 36–9, http://myhospital.eu/

Kurian B, Bharadwaj S, Mukherjee R (2011) PE biggies chase healthcare deals. *Times of India*, 7 February, http://articles.timesofindia.indiatimes.com/2011-02-07/india-business/28360741_1_private-equity-healthcare-industry-growth-capital [accessed 26/08/12]

Kutzin J (2008) Health financing policy: a guide for decision-makers. Health Financing Policy Paper, Division of Country Health Systems, WHO Europe, Barcelona

Kyobutungi C, Ezeh AC, Zulu E, Falkingham J (2009) HIV/AIDS and the health of older people in the slums of Nairobi, Kenya: results from a cross sectional survey. BMC Public Health, 27 May, http://www.biomedcentral.com/1471-2458/9/153 [accessed 25/01/13]

Labonté R, Blouin C, Chopra M, Lee K, Packer C, Rowson M, Schrecker T, Woodward D (2007) Towards Health-Equitable Globalisation: Rights, Regulation and Redistribution Final Report to the Commission on Social Determinants of Health. WHO, http://www.who.int/social_determinants/resources/gkn_final_report_042008.pdf [accessed 02/03/13]

Labonté R, Schrecker T, Packer C, Runnels V (eds) (2009) *Globalization and Health*. Routledge, New York & London

Labonté R, Schrecker T, Sanders D, Meeus W (2004) Fatal Indifference: The G8, Africa and Global Health. University of Cape Town Press, International Development Research Centre

Lagarde M, Palmer N (2008) The impact of user fees on health service utilization in low- and middle-income countries: how strong is the evidence? *Bulletin of the World Health Organization* 86 (11) 839–48 (November)

Lagomarsino G, Garabrant A, Adyas A, Muga R, Otoo N (2012) Moving towards universal health coverage: health insurance reforms in nine developing countries in Africa and Asia. *Lancet* 380(9,845): 933–43 (8 September), DOI: 10.1016/S0140-6736(12)61147-7 http://www.theLancet.com/journals/Lancet/article/PIIS0140-6736(12)61147-7/fulltext#article_upsell [accessed 10/12/12]

Laing & Buisson (2012a) Health and care providers are safe in the hands of private equity. Laing & Buisson press release, 17 July, http://www.laingbuisson.co.uk/MediaCentre/PressReleases/Healthandcareprovidersaresafe.aspx [accessed 03/09/12]

Laing & Buisson (2012b) Private medical cover – better, but still suffering the woes of a weak economy. Laing & Buisson press release, 28 August, http://www.laingbuisson.co.uk/Portals/1/PressReleases/HealthCover_12_PR.pdf [accessed 10/12/12]

Lakhani N (2011) Cuts are pushing mental health services to the edge, says study. *Independent*, 21 November, http://www.independent.co.uk/life-style/health-and-families/health-news/cuts-are-pushing-mental-health-services-to-the-edge-says-study-6265387/html [accessed 18/09/12]

Lamberti A (2011) African Medical Investments Upbeat on Prospects. 24 August, http://
www.proactiveinvestors.co.uk/companies/news/32318/african-medical-investments-
upbeat-on-prospects--32318/html [accessed 14/05/12]

Langer A, Catino J (2006) A gendered look at Mexico's health-sector reform. *Lancet*
368(9,549): 1,753–5, PMID 17113408 DOI: 10.1016/S0140-6736(06)69527-5

Lanjouw JO (2002) Intellectual Property and the Availability of Pharmaceuticals in Poor
Countries. Centre for Global Development Working Paper No. 5, April

Laterveer L, Niessen LW, Yazbeck AS (2003) Pro-poor health policies in poverty reduction
strategies. *Health Policy And Planning* 18(2): 138–45, doi: 10.1093/heapol/czg018

Laurell AC, Arellano OL (1996) Market commodities and poor relief: the World Bank
proposal for health. *International Journal of Health Services* 26(1): 1–18

Lawrence F (2012) Serco out-of-hours GP service failures create spike in Cornwall A&E
use. *Guardian*, 31 August, http://www.guardian.co.uk/uk/12/aug/31/serco-gp-service-
cornwall [accessed 20/01/13]

Le Grand J (2007) *The Other Invisible Hand*. Princeton University Press, New Jersey and
London

Leach-Kemon K, Chou DP, Schnneider MT, Tardiff A, Dieleman JL, Brooks BPC, Hanlon
M, Murray CJL (2012) The global financial crisis has led to a slowdown in growth of
funding to improve health in many developing countries. *Health Affairs* 31(1): 228–35,
Doi: 10.1377/hlthaff.2011/1154 [accessed 09/01/12]

Lee C (2008) Physician-owned hospitals faulted on emergency care. *Washington Post*,
10 January, http://www.washingtonpost.com/wp-dyn/content/article/2008/01/09/
AR2008010903140.html [accessed 18/01/13]

Lee K, Buse K, Fustukian S (eds) (2002) *Health Policy in a Globalising World*. Cambridge
University Press

Lee K, Goodman H (2002) Global health networks: the propagation of health care
financing reforms since the 1980s In Lee et al. 2002

Lee K, Koivusalo M, Ollila E, Labonté R, Schuftan C, Woodward D (2009) Global
Governance for Health. In Labonté et al. 2009, Chapter 12

Leighton C (1995) 22 Policy questions about health care financing in Africa. HFS Project,
Abt Associates Inc, Bethesda MD

Leighton C, Wouters A (1995) Strategies for achieving health financing reform in Africa.
World Development Also in HFS 24(9): 1,511–25, Policy Paper 10, Abt Associates,
Bethesda MD

Lenaghan J (1997) *Hard Choices in Health Care. BMJ* Publishing Group, London

Lenin VI (1917) Imperialism the Highest Stage of Capitalism. Chapter 1, full text, http://
www.marxists.org/archive/lenin/works/1916/imp-hsc/ch01/htm [accessed 25/01/13]

Leon DA, Walt G (eds) (2001) *Poverty, Inequality and Health*. Oxford University Press

Leon DA, Walt G, Gilson L (2001) International perspectives on health inequalities and
policy. *British Medical Journal* 322: 591–4 (10 March)

Lesotho MHSW (Ministry of Health and Social Welfare) (2008) Annual Joint Review
Report 2007/08FY, p. 21, http://www.ted-biogas.org/assets/download/HEALTH_AJR_
Report_February_2008%20.pdf [accessed 25/01/13]

Lesotho Times (2011) Hospital turns away pregnant woman. *Lesotho Times*, 12 October,
http://www.lestimes.com/?p=7361 [accessed 25/01/13]

Lesotho–Boston Health Alliance on behalf of Boston University (2009) Queen Elizabeth II and the New PPP Hospital: Baseline Study, Vol. 1, Draft Final Report, 12 March, p. 72; cited by Matthew Smith in Case Study 3: Financing a New Referral Hospital Lesotho, CABRI Dialogue: Ensuring Value for Money in Infrastructure Projects (p. 6 footnote), December, http://cabri-sbo.org/images/documents/6thAnnualSeminar/session_4_group_a_lesotho_mathundsane_mohapi_english.pdf [accessed 25/01/13]

Lethbridge J (2002a) International Finance Corporate (IFC) health care policy briefing. *Global Social Policy* 2(3) 349–54

Lethbridge J (2002b) Forces and reactions in healthcare: a report on worldwide trends for the PSI health services taskforce. December, Public Services International Research Unit, Greenwich, UK

Lethbridge J (2011) Care services for older people in Europe – challenges for labour. EPSU, February, http://www.epsu.org/a/7431 [accessed 14/01/13]

Lethbridge J (2012) Empty promises. The impact of outsourcing on the delivery of NHS services. PSIRU, published by UNISON, London, http://www.unison.org.uk/acrobat/20682/pdf [accessed 20/01/13]

Lewis M (2006) Governance and Corruption in Public Health Care Systems. Center for Global Development, Working Paper No. 78, January

Lewis M (2008) Contracting out health services. Broadening coverage, raising quality, lowering cost. ID 21 insights health, DFID, May, http://www.eldis.org/assets/Docs/47671/html [accessed 20/01/13]

Leys C (2001) *Market Driven Politics*. Verso, London

Leys C, Player S (2011) *The Plot Against the NHS*. Merlin Press, London

Library of Congress (2006) Iraq country profile. Federal Research Division, August, http://lcweb2.loc.gov/frd/cs/profiles/Iraq.pdf

Lieberman T (2011) Turning 65: Finding a Medigap Policy. Prepared Patient Forum, 12 May, http://blog.preparedpatientforum.org/blog/2011/05/turning-65-finding-a-medigap-policy/ [accessed 25/01/13]

Lien L (2003) Financial and organisational reforms in the health sector: implications for the financing and management of mental health care services. *Health Policy* 63(1): 73–80 (January)

Light D (1997) The real ethics of rationing. *British Medical Journal* 315: 112–15 (12 July)

Light D (2003) Choice bites in Boca Raton. *HSJ*, 25 September, pp. 18–19

Ling T (2000) Unpacking partnership: health care. In Clarke et al. 2000

Lintern S (2012) Private MH hospitals facing tighter margins. *Health Service Journal*, 5 July, http://www.hsj.co.uk/news/private-mh-hospitals-facing-tighter-margins/5046612/article?referrer=RSS [accessed 18/09/12]

Lisac M, Reimers L, Henke K-D, Schlette S (2009) Access and choice – competition under the roof of solidarity in German health care: an analysis of health policy reforms since 2004. *Health Economics, Policy and Law* (2010), 5: 31–52, http://journals.cambridge.org/action/displayAbstract;jsessionid=4C6E141A639777722D3E0F0B0DA02FF0.journals?fromPage=online&aid=6851252 [accessed 25/01/13]

Lister G (2002) Hopes and fears for the future of health: scenario for health and care for 2022. Nuffield Trust, http://www.ukglobalhealth.org/content/Text/Nuffut.doc [accessed 26/05/03]

Lister J (1998a) Taking Liberties, a response to the North Essex Health Authority consultation document 'Taking the Initiative'. January, UNISON Eastern Region, Chelmsford

Lister J (1998b) Into the Wilderness: a response of West Hertfordshire Health Authority's document 'Choosing the Right Direction'. September, UNISON Eastern Region, http://www.healthemergency.org.uk [accessed 01/11/03]

Lister J (1999) The Care Gap. UNISON, London, 27 May

Lister J (2001) PFI in the NHS: a dossier. GMB, London, http://www.gmb.org.uk/docs/pdfs/PFIDossier.pdf [accessed 12/06/04]

Lister J (2003a) SW London Hospitals under Pressure. Battersea & Wandsworth TUC, London

Lister J (2003b) The PFI Experience, Voices from the frontline. UNISON, London

Lister J (2005) *Health Policy reform: Driving the Wrong Way?* Middlesex University Press, London

Lister J (2007) Globalization and Health Systems Change, http://www.globalhealthequity.ca/electronic%20library/Globalization%20and%20Health%20Systems%20Change%20Lister.pdf

Lister J (2008a) *The NHS After 60, for Patients or Profits?* Middlesex University Press, London

Lister J (2008b) Hinchingbrooke Hospital Up for Grabs? UNISON Eastern Region, Chelmsford

Lister J (2011a) Lesotho hospital public private partnership: new model or false start? *Global Health Check*, 16 December, http://www.globalhealthcheck.org/?p=481 [accessed 25/01/13]

Lister J (ed.) (2011b) *Europe's Health for Sale: The Heavy Cost of Privatisation*. Libri Publishing, Faringdon

Lister J (2012a) In Defiance of the Evidence: Conservatives threaten to 'reform' away England's National Health Service. *International Journal of Health Services* 42(1): 137–55

Lister J (2012b) Will Liberal Democrats take the chance to kill the Health Bill? *Lancet* 379(9,819): 869–70

Lister J (2012c) Eastern Eye, newspaper of UNISON Eastern Region Health Services Committee, UNISON, Chelmsford

Lister J (2012d) SYRIZA: building the movement and ready for government (Interview with Alexis Benos). *Socialist Resistance* 70: 17–19 (September–October)

Lister J (2013) Private sector runs Circle round Hinchingbrooke: How NHS East of England asked the wrong question, and wound up with the wrong answer. UNISON Eastern Region, January, http://www.healthemergency.org.uk/pdf/PrivatesectorrunsCircleroundHinchingbrooke.pdf

Lister J, Labonté R (2009) Globalization and Health Systems Change. In Labonté et al. 2009

Little AD (2001) Public Finance Balance of Smoking in the Czech Republic. Philip Morris CR, http://hspm.sph.sc.edu/courses/Econ/Classes/cbacea/czechsmokingcost.html [accessed 29/09/12]

Liu X, Hotchkiss DR, Bose S (2007) The effectiveness of contracting-out primary healthcare services in developing countries: a review of the evidence. *Health Policy and Planning* 2008, 23: 1–13, doi: 10.1093/heapol/czm042

Liu Y (2000) Understanding and setting up the process for health equity. *Bulletin of the World Health Organization* 78(1): 82–3

Lloyd-Sherlock P (2002) Ageing and health policy: global perspectives. In Lee et al. 2002

Lloyd-Sherlock P, Redondo N (2009) Institutional care for older people in developing countries: the case of Buenos Aires, Argentina. *Population Ageing* 2: 41–56, DOI: 10.1007/s12062-010-9017-1

Lockwood DNJ (2002) Leprosy elimination – a virtual phenomenon or a reality? *British Medical Journal* 324: 1,516–8 (22 June)

Loevinsohn B (2008) Performance-based contracting for health services in developing countries: A toolkit. World Bank Institute, Washington DC, http://siteresources. worldbank.org/INTHSD/Resources/topics/415176-1216235459918/ContractingEbook. pdf [accessed 20/01/13]

Loevinsohn B, Harding A (2004) Contracting for the delivery of Community Health Services: a review of global experience. Health, Nutrition and Population (HNP) Discussion Paper, World Bank, September

Loevinsohn B, Harding A (2005) Buying results? Contracting for health service delivery in developing countries. *Lancet* 366: 676–81 (20 August)

Lovelace JC (2003) Foreword, in Preker and Harding 2003

Löwy M (2006) What is Ecosocialism? In Kelly and Malone 2006

Maarse H (2006) The privatisation of health care in Europe: an eight country analysis. *J Health Polit Policy Law* 31(5): 981–1,014 (October), DOI: 10.1215/0361 6878-2006-014

Maarse H (2009a) Health care reform – more evaluation results. Health Policy Monitor, http://hpm.org/en/Surveys/BEOZ_Maastricht_-_Netherlands/13/Health_care_reform_-_ more_evaluation_results.html [accessed 05/09/12]

Maarse H (2009b) Private Health Insurance in the Netherlands. Maastrict University, http://www.cef-see.org/health/healthfiles/materials/report_Private_Health_Insurance_in_ the_Netherlands.pdf [accessed 25/01/13]

Maarse H (2012) The reform of long-term care in the Netherlands. *Eurohealth* 18(2): 33–5

Macalister T (2012) Pharma overtakes arms industry to top the league of misbehaviour. *Guardian*, 8 July, http://www.guardian.co.uk/business/12/jul/08/pharma-misbehaviour- gsk-fine [accessed 14/01/13]

Maceira D (1998) Provider payment mechanisms in health care: incentives, outcomes and organisational impact in developing countries. *Major Applied Research No. 2, Working Paper 2*, PHR, Abt Associates, Bethesda MD

Macinko JA, Starfield B (2002) Annotated Bibliography on Equity in Health, 1980–2001. *Int J for Equity in Health* 1:1, 1–20, May

Maciocco G (2008) From Alma Alta to the Global Fund: the history of international health policy. *Social Medicine* 3(1) (January)

Mackintosh J (2003) Healthcare keeps GM care cheap. *Financial Times*, 20 August

Mackintosh M (2001) Do health care systems contribute to inequalities? In Leon and Walt 2001

Madarasz N (2003) A trap for Lula. *News from Brazil*, http://www.brazil-brasil.com/2003/ html/news/articles/jul03/p118jul03.htm [accessed 28/07/03]

Magnussen J, Vrangbaek K, Saltman RB (eds) (2009) *Nordic Health Care Systems*. Open University Press, McGraw Hill Education

Mahler H (1981) The meaning of health for all by the year 2000. *World Health Forum* 2 (1) 5–22

Makinen M, Sealy S, Bitrán RA, Adjei S, Muñoz R (2011) Private Health Sector Assessment in Ghana. World Bank Working Paper No. 210, World Bank, Washington DC, http://www.oneworldtrust.org/climategovernance/sites/default/files/publications/ ebaines/Private%20health%20sector%20assessment%20in%20Ghana.pdf [accessed 25/01/13]

Maldonado C (2012) New Orleans' mental health crisis. Gambit, 13 March, http://www. bestofneworleans.com/gambit/new-orleans-mental-health-crisis/Content?oid=1972425 [accessed 15/09/12]

Malin N, Wilmot S, Manthorpe J (2002) Key concepts and debates in health and social policy. Open University Press, Buckingham

Management Sciences for Health (MSH) (2001) Conference: Innovations in Health Care Financing: Experiences from Kenya, May, http://www.msh.org/features/conferences/ AFS/publications.html

Manning N (2000) The new public management and its legacy. Administrative and civil service reform, World Bank, http://www1.worldbank.org/publicsector/covilservice/debate. htm [accessed 15/02/03]

Mannion R, Marini G, Street A (2008) Implementing payment by results in the English NHS. *Journal of Health Organisation and Management* 22(1): 79–88, http://www. emeraldinsight.com/1477-7266/htm [accessed 25/01/13]

Marmor TR (1998) The procompetitive movement in American medical politics. In Ranade 1998

Marmor TR (1999) The rage for reform: sense and nonsense in health policy. In Drache and Sullivan 1999

Marmor TR (2001) Comparing Global health systems. Lessons and caveats. In Wieners 2001

Marmor TR (2002) Policy and political fads: the rhetoric and reality of managerialism. *British Journal of Health Care Management* 8(1): 16–23 (January)

Marmot M (2001) Future links between socio-economic status and health. Proceedings of a conference, Health Trends Review, Barbican Centre London

Marriott A (2009a) Your Money or Your Life. Will leaders act now to save lives and make health care free in poor countries? Oxfam, 14 September, http://policy-practice.oxfam. org.uk/publications/your-money-or-your-life-will-leaders-act-now-to-save-lives-and-make-healthcare-115075 [accessed 25/01/13]

Marriott A (2009b) Blind optimism. Challenging the myths about private health care in poor countries. Oxfam Briefing Paper, February, http://www.oxfam.org/policy/bp125-blind-optimism [accessed 20/01/13]

Marriott A (2011) Direct health care by government best option says World Bank Health Economist. *Global Health Check*, 22 July, http://www.globalhealthcheck.org/?m=201107 [accessed 10/07/12]

Marriott A (2012a) Partners in Health call for action against user fees in health care. *Global Health Check*, 1 May, http://www.globalhealthcheck.org [accessed 10/12/12]

Marriott A (2012b) World Bank champions free health care! *Global Health Check*, 9 September, http://globalhealthcheck.org/?m=201109 [accessed 10/07/12]

Martin C (2011) Four months later: the legacy of the Tucson shooting. *Time* online, 9 May, http://www.time.com/time/printout/0,8816,2069848,00.html [accessed 07/07/11]

Martinez E, Garcia A (1997) What is 'neo-liberalism'? A brief definition for activists. *Corporate Watch*, http://www.corpwatch.org/trac/corner/glob/neolib.html [accessed 20/01/01]

Martinussem PE, Magnussen J (2009) Health care reform: the Nordic experience. In Magnussen et al. 2009

Marx K (1852) The Eighteenth Brumaire of Louis Bonaparte. In Marx and Engels 1970a

Marx K (1867) *Capital*. Volume 1, available https://www.marxists.org/archive/marx/works/1867-c1/commodity.htm [accessed 10/07/12]

Marx K, Engels F (1970a) *Selected Works in One Volume*. Lawrence & Wishart, London

Marx K, Engels F (1970b) *The German Ideology*. Lawrence & Wishart, London

Masson R (2012) $270 million in cuts threatens services for the mentally ill and disabled. fox8live.com, New Orleans local news, 29 May, http://www.fox8live.com/story/18427586/health-cuts [accessed 15/09/12]

Mathiason N (2012) Five steps to end global tax evasion. *Guardian*, 24 January, http://www.guardian.co.uk/commentisfree/12/jan/24/five-steps-global-tax-evasion [accessed 22/09/12]

Maynard A, Bloor K (2000) Payment and regulation of providers. Flagship course on Health Sector Reform, World Bank Institute, November

Maynard A, Dixon A (2002) Private health insurance and medical savings accounts: theory and experience. In Mossialos et al. 2002

Maynard A, Sheldon T (2001) Rationing is needed in a national health service. *British Medical Journal* 322: 734

Mays N (2011) Is there evidence that competition in health care is a good thing? No. *British Medical Journal* 343, d4205, doi: 10.1136/BMJ.d4205

McCoy D, Chand S, Sridhar D (2009) Global health funding: how much, where it comes from and where it goes. *Health Policy and Planning* 24: 407–17

McGregor D (2003a) Democrats commit themselves to healthcare reforms, in all but name. *Financial Times*, 22 May

McGregor D (2003b) Senate votes to allow Canada drug purchases. *Financial Times*, 21–2 June

McIntyre D (2007) Learning from Experience: health care financing in low- and middle-income countries. Global Forum for Health Research, Geneva, http://whqlibdoc.who.int/publications/2007/2940286531_eng.pdf [accessed 14/01/13]

McIntyre D, Whitehead M, Gilson L, Dahlgren G, Tang S (2007) Equity impacts of neoliberal reforms: what should the policy responses be? *International Journal of Health Services* 37(4): 693–709

McKee M (2001) The World Health Report 2000: advancing the debate. WHO Denmark, http://www.who.int/health-systems-performance/regional_consultations/euro_mckee_background.pdf [accessed 02/03/13]

McKee M, Karanikolos M, Belcher P, Stuckler D (2012) Austerity: a failed experiment on the people of Europe. *Clinical Medicine* 12(4): 346–50, http://www.rcplondon.ac.uk/sites/default/files/documents/clinmed-124-p346-350-mckee.pdf [accessed 15/01/13]

McKee M, Stuckler D (2011) The assault on universalism: how to destroy the welfare state. *British Medical Journal* 343doi, http://dx.doi.org/10.1136/BMJ.d7973 [accessed 25/01/13]

McKinsey (2009) Achieving World Class Productivity in the NHS 2009/10–2013/14: Detailing the Size of the Opportunity. Department of Health, London, March, http://www.dh.gov.uk/prod_consum_dh/groups/dh_digitalassets/documents/digitalasset/dh_116521/pdf [accessed 25/01/13]

McLeod D (2007) Monitoring MDG 1 poverty reduction in middle income countries. Final report to UNDP-BDP Poverty Group, New York

McPake B, Brikci N, Cometto G, Schmidt A, Araujo E (2011) Removing user fees: learning from international experience to support the process. *Health Policy and Planning* 26: ii104–ii117, doi:10.1093/heapol/czr21064

McSmith A (2004) Letwin: 'NHS will not exist under Tories'. *Independent*, 6 June, http://www.independent.co.uk/life-style/health-and-families/health-news/letwin-nhs-will-not-exist-under-tories-6168295/html [accessed 25/01/13]

Mechanic RE, Altman SH (2009) Payment reform options: episode payment is a good place to start. *Health Affairs* 28(2): w262–71, http://content.healthaffairs.org/content/28/2/w262/full.html [accessed 18/01/13]

Meessen B, Hercot D, Noirhomme M, Ridde V, Tibouti A, Bicaba A, Tashobaya C, Gilson L (2009) Removing user fees in the health sector: a multi-country review. UNICEF, New York, http://www.itg.be/itg/Uploads/Volksgezondheid/unicef/UNICEF_Multi-Country_review.pdf [accessed 25/01/13]

Mehra N (2005) Flawed, failed, abandoned: 100 P3s. Canadian and international evidence. Ontario Health Coalition, March, http://cupe.ca/privatization/Flawed_failed_abando [accessed 16/01/13]

Mental Health Foundation (2012) The Mental Health Strategy, system reforms and spending pressures: what do we know so far? Mental Health Foundation, January, http://www.mentalhealth.org.uk/publications/mental-health-strategy/ [accessed 14/01/13]

Mental Health Network (2011) Personal health budgets: countdown to roll-out. NHS Confederation Briefing 222, October, http://www.nhsconfed.org/Publications/Documents/Personal_health_budgets_061011/pdf [accessed 25/01/13]

mhGAP (2008) Scaling up care for mental, neurological and substance abuse disorders. Mental Health Gap Action Programme, WHO Geneva, http://www.who.int/mental_health/mhgap_final_english.pdf [accessed 15/01/13]

Michaud C (2003) Development Assistance For Health (DAH): recent trends and resource allocation. Paper prepared for the Second Consultation Commission on Macroeconomics and Health, World Health Organization, Geneva, October, http://www.who.int/macrohealth/events/health_for_poor/en/dah_trends_nov10.pdf [accessed 02/03/13]

Mills A, Bennett S, Russell S (2001) *The challenge of health sector reform: What must governments do.* Palgrave, Basingstoke UK

MIND (2011) Listening to experience: an independent inquiry into acute and crisis mental healthcare. November, http://www.mind.org.uk/assets/0001/5921/Listening_to_experience_web.pdf [accessed 25/01/13]

Minvielle E (2006) New Public Management à la Française: The Case of Regional Hospital Agencies. *Public Administration Review*, September–October, pp. 753–63

Mladovsky P, Srivastava D, Cylus J, Karanikolos M, Evetovits T, Thomson S, McKee M (2012) Health policy responses to the financial crisis in Europe. WHO Europe, http://www.euro.who.int/__data/assets/pdf_file/0009/170865/e96643/pdf [accessed 10/12/12]

Moberly T (2012a) 90% of PCTs are now rationing care. GP online, 19 June, http://www.gponline.com/News/article/1136671/Exclusive-90-PCTs-rationing-care/ [accessed 10/12/12]

Moberly T (2012b) Labour demands 'immediate' review of NHS rationing. GP online, 3 July, http://www.gponline.com/News/article/1139246/labour-demands-immediate-review-nhs-rationing/ [accessed 10/12/12]

Mohan J (1995) *A National Health Service? The restructuring of health care in Britain since 1979.* Macmillan, Basingstoke

Mohapi (2011) PPPs and Social Infrastructure. SADC PPP Forum and Network Launch, 15–17 February, South Africa, http://www.sadc-dfrc.org/assets/files/Ms%20Zondy%20Mohapi.pdf

Mokoro Ltd (2005) *DFID conditionality in developing assistance to partner governments.* Final Report, 12 August, DFID, http://www.dfid.gov.uk/pubs/files/conditionality-mokoro-report.pdf, [accessed 15/11/06]

Molina N, Pereira J (2008) Critical conditions: The IMF maintains its grip on low-income governments. Eurodad, April, http://eurodad.org/uploadedfiles/whats_new/reports/critical_conditions.pdf [accessed 14/01/13]

Monbiot G (2004) At the edge of Lunacy. 6 January, http://www.monbiot.com/2004/01/06/on-the-edge-of-lunacy [accessed 25/01/13]

Monbiot G (2008) Labour's perverse polyclinic scheme is the next step in privatising the NHS. *Guardian*, 29 April, http://www.guardian.co.uk/commentisfree/2008/apr/29/nhs.health [accessed 25/01/13]

Montagu D, Prata N, Campbell MM, Walsh J, Orero S (2005) Kenya: reaching the poor through the private sector – a network model for expanding access to reproductive health services. Health, Nutrition and Population (HNP) Discussion Paper, May

Mooney G (2012) *The Health of Nations: Towards a New Political Economy.* Zed Books, London & New York

Moran M (1999) *Governing the health care state: a comparative study of the United Kingdom, the United States and Germany.* Manchester University Press

Moreno Torres M, Anderson M (2004) Fragile States: Defining Difficult Environments for Poverty Reduction. PRDE Working Paper 1, Poverty Reduction in Difficult Environments Team Policy Division, UK Department for International Development, August

Morestin F, Ridde V (2009) The abolition of user fees for health services in Africa: Lessons from the literature. University of Montreal, July, http://www.medsp.umontreal.ca/vesa-tc/pdf/publications/abolition_en.pdf [accessed 14/01/13]

Mossialos E, Dixon A, Figueras J, Kutzin J (eds) (2002) *Funding Health Care: Options for Europe.* Open University Press, Buckingham & Philadelphia

Mossialos E, Mrazek M (2002) Entrepreneurial behaviour in pharmaceutical markets and the effects of regulation. In Saltman et al. 2002, pp. 146–62

Mountjoy S (2012) Unions angry at health consortium's ideas for South West. BBC News, 23 August, http://www.bbc.co.uk/news/uk-england-cornwall-19353569 [accessed 02/03/13]

MSI Healthcare (2000) MSI healthcare: Germany. October, MSI, Devon, UK

Muchhala B (2009) The IMF's Financial Crisis Loans: no change in conditionalities. Third World Network, 11 March, http://goo.gl/saMVa 925/01/13]

Mudyarabikwa O (2000) *An Examination of Public Sector Subsidies to the Private Health Sector: A Zimbabwe Case Study.* Equinet Policy Series No. 8, Regional Network for Equity in Health in Southern Africa (EQUINET) with University of Zimbabwe Medical School

Munishi GK (1995) Private sector delivery of health care in Tanzania. Major Applied Research Paper No. 14, HFS, Abt Associates, Bethesda MD

Muntaner C, Salazar RMG, Benach J, Armada F (2006) Bucking the neoliberal trend: the Venezuelan Health Care reform initiative. *International Journal of Health Services* 36(4): 803–11

Muraskin W (2004) The Global Alliance for Vaccines and Immunization: is it a new model for effective public–private cooperation in international public health? *American Journal of Public Health* 94(11): 1,922–5

Murphy R (2012) Why are they increasing the tax gap? PCS (Public & Commercial Services Union), http://www.pcs.org.uk/en/campaigns/tax-justice/why-are-they-increasing-the-tax-gap.cfm [accessed 10/12/12]

Murray CJL, Frenk J (2000) A framework for assessing the performance of health systems. *Bulletin of the World Health Organization* 78(6): 717–31

Murray CJL, Lopez AD (1996) The global burden of disease: a comprehensive assessment of mortality and disability. Harvard School of Public Health, for World Bank, Cambridge MA

Murray CJL, Lopez AD, Wibulpolprasert S (2004) Monitoring global health: time for new solutions. *British Medical Journal* 329: 1,096–100 (6 November)

Murray Brown J, Timmins N, Wise P (2004) Brussels acts to exclude private finance for public works from stability pact rules. *Financial Times,* 7 February, International News

Musau SN (1999) Community-based health insurance: experiences and lessons learned from East and Southern Africa. *Technical Report 34,* August, Partnerships for Health Reform, Bethesda MD

Mwabu G, Mwanzia J, Laimbila W (1995) User Charges in Government Health Facilities in Kenya. *Health Policy and Planning* 10(2): 164–70

Mwase T, Kariisa E, Doherty J, Hoohlo-Khotle N, Kiwanuka-Mukiibi P, Williamson T (2010) Lesotho Health Systems Assessment 2010. June, Bethesda MD, Health Systems 20/20, Abt Associates Inc, http://www.healthsystems2020.org/files/2833_file_Lesotho_HSA_2010.pdf [accessed 25/01/13]

Naidoo Y (2007) Hospitals can expect further drastic cuts. *Cape Argus,* 2 September, http://www.iol.co.za/news/south-africa/hospitals-can-expect-further-drastic-cuts-1/369008 [accessed 25/01/13]

NAMI (2011) State mental health cuts: the continuing crisis. National Alliance on Mental Health, November, http://www.nami.org/ContentManagement/ContentDisplay.cfm?ContentFileID=147763 [accessed 14/01/13]

Nanda P (2002) Gender dimensions of user fees: implications for women's utilisation of health care. *Reproductive Health Matters* 10(20): 127–34

Nash E (2003) The Spanish prototype: efficient, but controversial. *Independent,* 15 May: 4

National Academies (2006) Medication errors injure 1.5 million people and cost billions of dollars annually. Press release, 20 July, Office of News and Public Information, New York, http://www/nationalacademies.org/onpinews/newsitem.aspx?RecordID=11623 [accessed 03/09/12]

National Coalition on Health Care (2004) Building a Better Health Care System: Specifications for Reform. NCHC, Washington DC

National Drug Intelligence Center (2011) The Economic Impact of Illicit Drug Use on American Society. US Department of Justice, April, http://www.justice.gov/archive/ndic/pubs44/44731/44731p.pdf [accessed 15/01/13]

Navarro V (2000) Assessment of the World Health Report 2000. *Lancet* 356: 1,598–601 (4 November)

Navarro V, Muntaner C (eds) (2004) *Political and economic determinants of population health and well-being.* Baywood Publishing, Amityville, New York

Ncayiyana DJ (2002) Africa can solve its own health problems. *British Medical Journal*, 324: 688–9 (23 March)

Nebehay S, Lewis B (2011) WHO slashes budget, jobs in new era of Austerity. Reuters, 19 May, http://www.reuters.com/article/2011/05/19/us-who-idUSTRE74I5I320110519 [accessed 25/01/13]

New B (1996) The rationing agenda in the NHS. *British Medical Journal* 312: 1,593–601 (22 June)

New B (ed.) (1997) *Rationing: Talk and action in health care. BMJ* Publishing Group, King's Fund, London

New B (1999) *A Good Enough Service: Values, Trade-offs and the NHS.* IPPR, London

Newbrander W, Collins D, Gilson L (2000) *Ensuring equal access to health services: User fee systems and the poor.* Management Sciences for Health, Boston

Newman J (2000) Beyond the New Public Management? Modernising public services. In Clarke et al. 2000

Newman S, Lawler J (2009) Managing healthcare and the New Public Management. A Sisyphean challenge for nurses. *Journal of Sociology* 4(4): 419–32, doi: 10.1177/1440783309346477

NHS London (2010) Integrated Strategic Plan 2010-2015. First State Report, Healthcare for London, NHS London, January, http://www.london.nhs.uk/webfiles/Corporate/First%20Stage%20Report.pdf [accessed 27/07/12]

Nicolás AL, Vera Hernández M (2004) Are tax subsidies for private medical insurance self financing? Evidence from a microsimulation model. *Journal of Health Economics* 27: 1,285–98

Nikolic IA, Maikisch H (2006) Public–Private Partnerships and collaboration in the health sector: an overview with case studies from recent European experience. World Bank HNP Discussion Paper, http://siteresources.worldbank.org/INTECAREGTOPHEANUT/Resources/HNPDiscussionSeriesPPPPaper.pdf [accessed 16/01/13]

Nishtar S (2010) The mixed health systems syndrome. *Bulletin of the World Health Organization* 84: 74–5

Nys H, Goffin T (2011) Mapping national practices and strategies relating to patients' rights. In Wismar et al. 2011

O'Grady P (2012) Economic Crisis: Austerity and Privatisation in Healthcare in Ireland. *Irish Marxist Review* (2): 24–36, June, http://www.scribd.com/doc/96798763/Irish-Marxist-Review-2 [accessed 10/12/12]

OECD (1992) OECD Health Systems Facts and Trends 1960–1991. *Health Policy Studies* 1(3), OECD, Paris

OECD (1995a) New Directions in Health Care Policy. *Health Policy Studies*, No. 7, OECD, Paris

OECD (1995b) Social protection for dependent elderly people: perspectives from a review of OECD countries. *Labour market and Social Policy Occasional Paper*, No. 16, OECD, Paris

OECD (1998a) *Maintaining Prosperity in an Ageing Society*. OECD, Paris

OECD (1998b) Press Release: The New Social Policy Agenda A Caring World. OECD, Paris, 24 June

OECD (2001a) *Health at a Glance*. OECD, Paris

OECD (2001b) *OECD Health Project*. OECD, Paris, May

OECD (2001c) Measuring Up: Improving Health Systems Performance in OECD countries. Media Information for Ottawa conference, 5–7 November, OECD, Paris

OECD (2004) *Towards High-performing Health Care Systems: Policy Studies*. OECD Health Project, Paris, http://www.amcp.org/WorkArea/DownloadAsset.aspx?id=13176 [accessed 25/01/13]

OECD (2008) Recent Health Reforms in Turkey. OECD/World Bank Review of the Turkish Health System, http://go.worldbank.org/TRKAQ6NWS0 [accessed 25/01/13]

OECD (2009) Achieving Better Value for Money in Health Care. *Health Policy Studies*, OECD Publishing, doi: 10.1787/9789264074231-en

OECD (2011) Can We Get Better Value for Money in Long-term Care? In Colombo et al., *Help Wanted?: Providing and Paying for Long-Term Care*. OECD Publishing, doi: 10.1787/9789264097759-15-en, http://www.oecd.org/els/healthpoliciesanddata/47885662/pdf [accessed 25/01/13]

OECD (2012a) OECD Health Data 2012. OECD, Paris, June, http://www.oecd.org/document/60/0,3746,en_2649_33929_2085200_1_1_1_1,00.html [accessed 10/12/12]

OECD (2012b) Growth in health spending grinds to a halt. OECD, Paris, http://www.oecd.org/document/39/0,3746,en_21571361_44315115_50655591_1_1_1_1,00.html [accessed 10/12/12]

OECD (2012c) *Competition in Hospital Services*. OECD, Competition Committee, DAF/COMP(2012)9 OECD, Paris, June, http://www.oecd.org/daf/competition/50527122/pdf [accessed 15/01/13]

OECD Health Data (2012) http://www.oecd.org/els/health-systems/oecdhealthdata2012-frequentlyrequesteddata.htm [accessed 02/03/13]

Ollila E (2005) Global health priorities – priorities of the wealthy? *Globalization and Health* 1:6 (22 April), doi: 10.1186/1744-8603-1-6

Ollila E, Koivusalo M (2002) The World Health Report 2000: WHO health policy steering off course – changed values, poor evidence and lack of accountability. *International Journal of Health Services* 32(3): 503–14

Ooms G (2006) Health Development versus Medical Relief: The Illusion versus the Irrelevance of Sustainability. *PLoS Med* 3(8): e345/ DOI: 10.1371/ journal. pmed.0030345

Opensecrets (2010) Federal Lobbying Climbs in 2009 as Lawmakers Execute Aggressive Congressional Agenda. 10 February, http://www.opensecrets.org/news/2010/02/federal-lobbying-soars-in-2009/html [accessed 25/01/13]

Ortiz I, Cummins M (2011) Global Inequality: Beyond the Bottom Billion: A Rapid Review of Income Distribution in 141 Countries. UNICEF Social and Economic Policy Working Paper, April

Osborne D, Gaebler T (1992) *Reinventing government: how the entrepreneurial spirit is transforming the public sector.* Addison-Wesley, New York

Osborne D, Plastrik P (1997) *Banishing bureaucracy: The five strategies for reinventing government.* Addison-Wesley, Reading MA

Osborne D, Plastrik P (1998) *Banishing Bureaucracy: The Five Strategies for Reinventing Government.* Plume, reprint edition, 1 April

Ostlin P (2005) What evidence is there about the effects of health care reforms on gender equity, particularly on health? Health Evidence Network report, WHO, Copenhagen, http://www.euro.who.int/Document/E87674.pdf [accessed 24/08/06]

Over M (2009) AIDS treatment in South Asia. Equity and efficiency. Center for Global Development, Working Paper No. 161, February, http://www.cgdev.org/files/1421119_file_Over_Fiscal_Burden.pdf [accessed 15/01/13]

Overbeek H (ed.) (2003) *The Political economy of European Unemployment: European Integration and the Transnationalisation of the Employment Question.* Routledge, London

Owino W, Korir J (1997) Public health sector efficiency: estimation and policy implications. December, Institute of Policy Analysis and Research, Nairobi

Oxfam (2006) Zambia uses G8 debt cancellation to make health care free for the poor. Oxfam press release, 31 March

Oxfam (2008) Health insurance in low-income countries. Where is the evidence that it works? Joint NGO Briefing Paper, 7 May, http://policy-practice.oxfam.org.uk/publications/health-insurance-in-low-income-countries-where-is-the-evidence-that-it-works-123910 [accessed 25/01/13]

Oxley H (2009) Policies for Healthy Ageing: An Overview. *OECD Health Working Papers* No. 42, http://search.oecd.org/officialdocuments/displaydocumentpdf/?doclanguage=en&cote=DELSA/HEA/WD/HWP(2009)1 [accessed 25/01/13]

PA consulting (2008) Study of Unscheduled Care in 6 Primary Care Trusts Central Report. Healthcare for London, http://www.londonhp.nhs.uk/wp-content/uploads/2011/03/Study-unscheduled-care-in-6-PCTs.pdf [accessed 25/01/13]

Packer C, Labonté R, Runnels V (2009) Globalization and Cross Border Flow of Health Workers. In Labonté et al. 2009

Pafford B (2009) The third wave – medical tourism in the 21st-century. *Southern Medical Journal* 102(8): 810–13, http://journals.lww.com/smajournalonline/Abstract/2009/08000/The_Third_Wave_Medical_Tourism_in_the_21st_Century.9/aspx [accessed 18/01/13]

PAHO (Pan American Health Organisation) (2001a) Evaluating the impact of health reforms on gender equity: a PAHO guide. 23 April, PAHO, Washington

PAHO (Pan American Health Organisation) (2001b) Regional Consultation on Health Systems Performance Assessment. May, PAHO, Washington

PAHO (Pan American Health Organisation) (2001c) Regional Consultation on Health Systems Performance Assessment (Final Report). May, PAHO, Washington

PAHO (Pan American Health Organisation) (2008) Declaration of Alma Ata. Pan American Health Organization, http://www.paho.org/english/dd/pin/alma-ata_declaration.htm [accessed 16/01/13]

PAHO, WHO, International Development Research Centre (2001) Research on health sector reforms in Latin America and the Caribbean: contribution to policymaking. Paper for pre-summit of the Americas Forum, Montreal, March, http://www.idrc.ca/lacro/docs/conferencias/paho_idrc.html [accessed 17/09/03]

Palier B, Sykes R (2001) Challenges and change: Issues and perspectives in the analysis of globalisation and the European welfare states. In Sykes et al. 2001

Palmer N (2000) The use of private sector contracts for primary health care: theory, evidence and lessons for low-income and middle-income countries. *Bulletin of the World Health Organization* 78(6): 821–9

Palmer S, Torgerson DJ (1999) Definitions of efficiency. *British Medical Journal* 318: 1,136

Park E, Lav IJ (2003) Proposed expansion of medical savings accounts could drive up insurance costs and increase the number of uninsured. 30 April, Center on Budget and Policy Priorities, Washington

Parussini G, Horobin W (2012) French Budget Hits Rich and Businesses with Tax Boost. wsj.com, 28 September, http://online.wsj.com/article/SB10000872396390443843904578024593559854134.html

Patel K, Rushefsky ME (1999) Health care politics and policy in America. ME Sharpe Inc, New York

Patel N (2011) India to create central foreign aid agency. *Guardian*, 26 July, http://www.guardian.co.uk/global-development/2011/jul/26/india-foreign-aid-agency [accessed 25/01/13]

Paton C (2000) New Labour, New Health Policy? In Hann 2000

Pauly M (2000) Foreword to Feldman RD (ed.), *American Health Care*. Transaction Publishers, New Brunswick (US) and London

Payne D (2001) German company offers 'package deal ops' to Ireland. *British Medical Journal* 323: 471 (1 September)

Pearlstein S (2005) Free-market philosophy doesn't always work for healthcare. *Washington Post*, 8 June, http://www.washingtonpost.com/wp-dyn/content/article/2005/06/07/AR2005060702014/html [accessed 18/01/13]

Pearson M (2004) Economic and financial aspects of the Global Health Partnerships. GHP Study Paper 2, DFID Health Systems Research Centre

Pein C (2011) For every 1,000 seriously mentally ill people in Arizona 1 mental hospital and 253 gun shops. War Is Business, 8 February, http://warisbusiness.com/3226/news/arizona-has-1564-gun-dealers-but-only-396-mental-hospitals [accessed 25/01/13]

People's Health Movement (PHM) (2005) Global Health Watch. PHM, http://reliefweb.int/sites/reliefweb.int/files/resources/AF558D1E144DAD0BC1257130005C9B60-medico.pdf [accessed 02/03/13]

People's Health Movement (PHM) (2007) Against the privatization of health insurance in Egypt. PHM 17 June, http://www.phmovement.org/en/node/375 [accessed 15/01/13]

People's Health Movement (PHM) (2008) Declaration from the National Egyptian Committee on the Right to Health. PHM, http://www.phmovement.org/en/node/806 [accessed 15/01/13]

People's Health Movement (PHM) (2011) *Global Health Watch 3: An Alternative World Health Report*. People's Health Movement, Zed Books, London, http://www.ghwatch.org/sites/www.ghwatch.org/files/global%20health%20watch%203/pdf [accessed 25/01/13]

PEPFAR (2012a) Using science to save lives: latest PEPFAR funding. US President's Emergency plan for AIDS Relief. Washington DC, http://www.pepfar.gov/documents/organization/189671.pdf [accessed 10/12/12]

PEPFAR (2012b) Examples of PEPFAR Platforms Strengthening the Effectiveness and Sustainability of Country Efforts on Health. US President's Emergency plan for AIDS Relief, Washington DC, http://www.pepfar.gov/documents/organization/176785.pdf [accessed 10/12/12]

Peston R (2008) *Who Runs Britain?* Hodder & Stoughton, London

Petchesky RP (2003) *Global Prescriptions: Gendering Health and Human Rights.* Zed Books, London

Petrella R (1996) Globalisation and internationalisation: the dynamics of the emerging world order. In Boyer and Drache 1996

Pfeiffer J (2004) International NGOs in the Mozambique health sector: the 'velvet glove' of privatisation. In Castro and Singer 2004

Pharmiweb.com (2012) IMS Study Forecasts Rebound in Global Spending on Medicines, Reaching Nearly $1.2 Trillion by 2016. Press release, 12 July, http://www.pharmiweb.com/PressReleases/pressrel.asp?ROW_ID=61152 [accessed 10/12/12]

PHR (2000) Health Insurance models becoming more popular in Africa. *Healthwatch* (Abt Associates newsletter), Fall 2000

Phumaphi J (2009) The Affordable Medicines Facility – Malaria. Information Paper 47,428, World Bank Health Nutrition and Population Department, Washington DC, 2 February, http://apps.who.int/medicinedocs/documents/s17513en/s17513en.pdf [accessed 25/01/13]

Physicians for a National Health Program (PNHP) (2003a) (Unpublished) Proposal of the Physicians' Working Group for Single-Payer National Health Insurance, http://www.pnhp.org [password access; accessed 22/06/03]

Physicians for a National Health Program (PNHP) (2003b) 31% of health care spending is paperwork. Press release, 20 August, PNHP, Chicago, http://www.pnhp.org [accessed 20/08/03]

Physicians for a National Health Program (PNHP) (2012) Single-Payer National Health Insurance (resources). http://www.pnhp.org/facts/single-payer-resources [accessed 30/09/12]

Pickert K (2012) Fact check: Obamacare's Medicare Cuts. Time.com, 16 August, http://swampland.time.com/12/08/16/fact-check-obamacares-medicare-cuts/ [accessed 19/09/12]

Pierson C (1998) *Beyond the Welfare State: the new political economy of welfare.* Polity, Cambridge

Piller C, Sanders E, Dixon R (2007) Dark cloud over good works of Gates Foundation. *LA Times*, 7 January, http://www.latimes.com/news/la-na-gatesx07jan07,0,2533850.story [accessed 25/01/13]

Piller C, Smith D (2007) Unintended victims of Gates Foundation generosity. *LA Times*, 16 December, http://www.latimes.com/news/nationworld/nation/la-na-gates16dec16,0,3743924.story [accessed 25/01/13]

Pincus JR, Winters JA (2002) *Reinventing the World Bank.* Cornell University Press

Planning Commission of India (2011) *High Level Expert Group Report on Universal Health Coverage for India.* Planning Commission of India New Delhi, November 2011

Player S, Leys C (2008) Confuse and Conceal: the NHS and Independent Sector Treatment Centres. Merlin Press, Monmouth

Plumridge N, Kemp P (2004) New dawn for the NHS. *Public Finance*, 12–18 March, pp. 24–5

PNHP – see *Physicians for a National Health Program*

Pocock NS, Phua KH (2011) Medical tourism and policy implications their health systems: a conceptual framework from a comparative study of Thailand Singapore and Malaysia. *Globalization and Health* 7: 12, doi:10.1186/1744-8603-7-12 http://www. globalizationandhealth.com/content/7/1/12 [accessed 25/01/13]

Pollitt C (2000) Is the Emperor in his underwear? An analysis of the impacts of public management reform. *Public Management* 2(2): 181–99

Pollitt C (2003) *The Essential Public Manager*. Open University Press/McGraw Hill, Maidenhead

Pollock AM (2003) Foundation hospitals will kill the NHS. *Guardian*, 7 May

Pollock AM (2004) *NHS plc: The Privatisation of Our Health Care*. Verso, London

Pollock AM, Dunnigan MG (2000) Beds in the NHS: the National Beds Inquiry exposes contradictions in government policy. *British Medical Journal* 320: 461–2 (19 February)

Pollock AM, Dunnigan M, Gaffney D, Macfarlane A, Majeed FA (1997) What happens when the private sector plans hospital services for the NHS: three case studies under the private finance initiative. *British Medical Journal* 314: 1,266 (26 April)

Pollock AM, Macfarlane A, Greener I (2011a) Bad science concerning NHS competition is being used to support the controversial Health and Social Care Bill. LSE blog, http:// blogs.lse.ac.uk/politicsandpolicy/archives/21185 [accessed 02/03/13]

Pollock AM, Macfarlane A, Kirkwood GF, Majeed A, Greener I, Morelli, Boyle S, Mellett H, Godden S, Price D, Brhlikova P (2011b) No evidence that patient choice in the NHS saves lives. *Lancet* 378(9,809): 2,057–60 (17 December), DOI: 10.1016/ S0140-6736(11)61553-5

Pollock AM, Price D (2000) Rewriting the regulations: how the World Trade Organisation could accelerate privatisation in health care systems by undermining the voluntary basis of GATS. http://www.unison.org.uk/pfi/rewrite.htm [accessed 30/01/01]

Pollock AM, Price D (2003a) In Place of Bevan? Briefing on the Health and Social Care (Community health and standards) Bill 2003. September, Catalyst, London

Pollock AM, Price D (2003b) The BetterCare judgment – a challenge to health care. *British Medical Journal* 326: 236–7 (1 February)

Pollock AM, Price D (2011) How the secretary of state for health proposes to abolish the NHS in England. *British Medical Journal* 342:d1,695 (9 April)

Pope C (2011) Devil in the financial detail as cutbacks likely to have far-reaching consequences. *Irish Times*, 6 December, http://www.irishtimes.com/newspaper/ ireland/2011/1206/1224308620207/html [accessed 06/09/12]

Preker AS, Harding A (2000) The Economics of Public and Private Roles in Health Care: Insights from Institutional Economics and Organizational Theory. *Health Nutrition and Population*, June, World Bank, Washington DC

Preker AS, Harding A (eds) (2003) *Innovations in health service delivery: the corporatization of public hospitals*. Human development Network Health Nutrition and Population Series, World Bank, Washington DC

Preker AS, Scheffler RM, Bassett MC (eds) (2007) *Private voluntary health insurance in development*. World Bank, Washington DC

Preker AS, Zwiefel P, Schelekens OP (eds) (2010) *Global Marketplace for Private Health Insurance*. World Bank, Washington DC

PricewaterhouseCoopers (PWC) (2010) Build and beyond: the (r)evolution of health care PPPs. PricewaterhouseCoopers, December, http://www.pwc.com/us/en/health-industries/publications/build-and-beyond.jhtml [accessed 18/01/13]

PricewaterhouseCoopers (PWC) (2012) Build and Beyond: bridging the gap. PricewaterhouseCoopers, February, http://www.pwc.com/gx/en/healthcare/publications/bridging-the-gap-asia-healthcare-ppp.jhtml [accessed 20/01/13]

PricewaterhouseCoopers (PWC) Australia (2012) The growing role of PPPs in Australia's healthcare system. PricewaterhouseCoopers, February, http://www.pwc.com.au/media-centre/12/growing-role-of-PPPs-in-healthcare-feb12/htm [accessed 29/07/12]

Prince M, Bryce R, Ferri C (2011) World Alzheimer Report. The benefits of early diagnosis and intervention. Alzheimer's Disease International, September, http://www.alz.co.uk/worldreport2011 [accessed 25/01/13]

Private Equity Wire (2011) Aureos Africa Health Fund invests USD4.5m stake in Ghanaian hospital. 29 July, http://www.privateequitywire.co.uk/2011/07/29/126109/aureos-africa-health-fund-invests-usd45m-stake-ghanaian-hospital [accessed 02/03/13]

Provost C (2012) UK government cost-cutting could put aid programmes at risk. *Guardian*, 9 March, http://www.guardian.co.uk/global-development/12/mar/09/dfid-cost-cutting-puts-aid-at-risk [accessed 10/12/12]

PSP (Private Sector Partnership) (2006) PSP-One Policy. USAID, http://www.psp-one.com/section/technicalareas/policy [accessed 10/11/06]

Public Services International (PSI) (1999) Health and social services briefing notes. January, PSI, Paris

Publicprivatefinance.com (2003) Edinburgh hospital subject of investigations. 9 June, http://www.publicprivatefinance.com/pfi/news/ [accessed 13/06/03]

Publicprivatefinance.com (2004) Health FOCUS. PFP, London

Ramesh R (2010) MPs attack Labour inaction on inequality. *Guardian*, 2 November, http://www.guardian.co.uk/politics/2010/nov/02/health-inequality-labour-margaret-hodge [accessed 22/09/12]

Ramesh R (2012a) NHS will need extra £20bn a year by 2020, says thinktank. *Guardian*, 4 July, http://www.guardian.co.uk/society/12/jul/04/nhs-20-billion-pounds-2020?newsfeed=true [accessed 10/12/12]

Ramesh R (2012b) Mental health spending falls for first time in 10 years. *Guardian*, 7 August, http://www.guardian.co.uk/society/12/aug/07/mental-health-spending-falls [accessed 18/09/12]

Ramo JC (2001) The real price of fighting AIDS. *Time*, 9 July, http://www.time.com/time/magazine/printout/0,8816,1000261,00.html, [accessed 17/11/06]

Ranade W (ed.) (1998) *Markets and health care a comparative analysis*. Longman, London

Rannan-Eliya R, Somanathan A (2005a) Access of the very poor to health services in Asia: evidence on the role of health systems from Equitap. DFID Health Systems Resource Centre, London, Workshop Paper 10, February

Rannan-Eliya R, Somanathan A (2005b) Meeting the health related needs of the very poor. DFID Workshop, 14–15 February, Workshop Paper 10, DFID Health Systems Resource

Centre, London, http://www.eldis.org/fulltext/verypoor/10_rannan-eliya.pdf [accessed 14/01/13]

Rannan-Eliya R, van Zanten TV, Yazbeck A (1996) First year literature review for applied research agenda. Applied Research Paper 1, Partnerships for Health Reform, Abt Associates, Bethesda MD

Rathwell T (1992) Realities of health for all by the year 2000. *Social Science and Medicine* 35, 541–7

Ravindran TKS, de Pinho H (eds) (2005) *The Right Reforms? Health Sector Reform and sexual and reproductive health.* Women's Health Project, School of Public Health, University of the Witwatersrand

Ravishankar N, Gubbins P, Cooley R, Leach-Kemon K, Michaud CM, Jamison DT, Murray CJL (2009) Financing of global health: tracking development assistance for health from 1990 to 2007. *Lancet* 373(9,681): 2,113–24 (20 June)

RCS (Royal College of Surgeons) (1997) The provision of emergency surgical services. June, RCS, London

Rechel B, Doyle Y, Grundy E, McKee M (2009) How can health systems respond to population ageing? WHO Policy Brief 10 Health Systems and Policy Analysis, http://www.euro.who.int/__data/assets/pdf_file/0004/64966/E92560.pdf [accessed 25/01/13]

Regmi K, Naidoo J, Greer A, Pilkington P (2010) Understanding the effect of decentralisation on health services: The Nepalese experience. *Journal of Health Organization and Management* 24(4): 361–82, http://dx.doi.org/10.1108/14777261011064986 [accessed 15/08/12]

Relman AS (1980) The new medical-industrial complex. *New England Journal of Medicine* 303(17): 963–70 (23 October)

Relman AS (2002) For-profit health care: Expensive, Inefficient and Inequitable. PNHP, http://www.pnhp.org//Press/2002/Expensive_Inefficient_Inequitable4.21.02.htm [accessed 22/07/02]

Réthelyi JM, Miskovits E, Szócska MK (2002) Organizational Reform in the Hungarian Hospital Sector: Institutional Analysis of Hungarian Hospitals and the Possibilities of Corporatization. Health, Nutrition and Population (HNP) Discussion Paper, December

Reuters (2012) GlaxoSmithKline fined $3bn for healthcare fraud. guardian.co.uk, 2 July, http://www.guardian.co.uk/business/12/jul/02/glaxosmithkline-drug-fraud [accessed 10/12/12]

Revill J (2003) IVF free-for-all may cost £400m. 10 August

Richards T (1996) European health policy: must redefine its raison d'être. *British Medical Journal* 29 June, 312(7,047): 1,622–3

Ridde V (2011) Is the Bamako initiative still relevant for West African health systems? *International Journal of Health Services* 41(1): 175–84

Rivett G (1998) *From Cradle to Grave.* Kings Fund, London

Robbins CJ, Rudsenke T, Vaughan JS (2008) Private equity investment in health care services. *Health Affairs* 27(5): 1,389–98, http://content.healthaffairs.org/content/27/5/1389/full.html [accessed 25/01/13]

Robin C (2011) The War on Tax. *London Review of Books* 33(16): 8 (25 August)

Robinhoodtax.org (2012) Major new campaign for a Robin Hood tax on Wall Street launches in U.S. today with celebrities, economists and activists. Robinhoodtax.org media centre, http://robinhoodtax.org/content/

major-new-campaign-robin-hood-tax-wall-street-launches-us-today-celebrities-economists-and-a [accessed 10/12/12]

Robinson R (2002) Who's got the master card? *Health Service Journal*, 26 September, pp. 22–4

Rodin J, de Ferranti D (2012) Universal health coverage: the third global health transition? *Lancet* 380(9,845): 861–2 (8 September) DOI: 10.1016/S0140-6736(12)61340-3

Romanow R (2002b) The cost of health care: is it sustainable? Notes for a speech to the Weatherhead Center for International Affairs, Harvard University, 16 October, Council of Canadians, http://www.Canadians.org [accessed 14/11/03]

Romanow RJ (2002a) Building on values: the future of health care in Canada. November, Commission on the Future of Health Care in Canada, Ottawa

Roodman D (2012) The Health Aid Fungibility Debate: don't believe either side. International Health Partnerships Plus, http://www.internationalhealthpartnership.net/. vents/article/the-health-aid-fungibility-debate-dont-believe-either-side-323732 [accessed 10/12/12]

Rosenberg H, Peña R (2000) Dimensions of exclusion from social protection in health in Latin America and the Caribbean. International Social Security Association (ISSA) Research Programme

Rosenberg M (2012) Shocking revelations about the FDA exposed: rubberstamping drugs and dangerous medical equipment, spying on its own scientists. Truthout.org, 2 August, http://www.alternet.org/investigations/shocking-revelations-about-fda-exposed-rubberstamping-drugs-and-dangerous-medical [accessed 14/01/13]

Ruiters G, Scott B (2009) Commercialisation of health and capital flows in east and southern Africa: Issues and implications. EQUINET Discussion Paper 77, 2 August, Rhodes University Institute of Social and Economic Research, York University, Training and Research Support Centre, SEATINI, EQUINET, Harare

Rundell S (2010) Private healthcare Africa's latest boom. Insurance News Net, http://insurancenewsnet.com/article.aspx?id=213595&type=newswires [accessed 25/01/13]

Russell S, Gilson L (1997) User fee policies to promote health service access for the poor: a wolf in sheep's clothing? *International Journal of Health Services* 27(2): 359–79

S&P (2012) Mounting medical care spending could be harmful to the G20's credit. Standard & Poor's, 26 January, http://www.standardandpoors.com/ratings/articles/en/eu/?articleType=HTML&assetID=124538578642 [accessed 09/09/12]

Saadah F, Knowles J (2000) The World Bank Strategy for Health, Nutrition and Population in the Far East and Pacific Region. *Human Development Network*, June, World Bank, Washington DC

Saba DK, Levit KR, Elixhauser A (2008) Hospital stays related to mental health 2006. Healthcare Cost and Utilization Project (H-CUP), October, http://www.hcup-us.ahrq.gov/reports/statbriefs/sb62/jsp [accessed 14/01/13]

Sabado F (2009) Building the New Anti-capitalist Party. *International Socialism*, Issue 121 (2 January), http://www.isj.org.uk/?id=512 [accessed 25/01/13]

Saligram N (2012) Together, the US and India have what it takes to tackle NCDs. 15 June, http://www.smartglobalhealth.org/blog/entry/together-the-u.s.-and-india-have-what-it-takes-to-tackle-ncds [accessed 10/12/12]

Saltman RB (1996) The notion of planned markets and fixed budgets. In Schwartz et al. 1996, pp. 1–11

Saltman RB (2002) The Western European experience with health care reform. *European Observatory*, 4 April, http://www.observatory.dk [accessed 23/02/03]

Saltman RB (2008) Decentralisation, re-centralisation and future European health policy. *European Journal of Public Health* 18(2): 104–6, http://eurpub.oxfordjournals.org/content/18/2/104/full [accessed 20/01/13]

Saltman RB, Figueras J (eds) (1997) *European Health Care Reform, Analysis of Current Strategies.* European Observatory on Health Care Systems

Saltman RB, Von Otter C (1992) *Planned markets and public competition. Strategic Reform in Northern European Health Systems.* Open University Press, Buckingham

Saltman RB et al. (1998) 'Health reform in Sweden: the road beyond cost containment'. In Ranade 1998

Saltman RB, Figueras J, Sakellarides C (eds) (2000) *Critical Challenges for Health Care Reform in Europe.* Open University Press, Buckingham

Saltman RB, Busse R, Mossialos E (eds) (2002) *Regulating entrepreneurial behaviour in European health care systems.* Open University Press, Buckingham

SAMHSA (2011) Mental Health United States, 2010. Substance Abuse, Mental Health Services Administration, U.S. Department of Health and Human Services, http://www.samhsa.gov/data/2k12/MHUS2010/MHUS-2010.pdf [accessed 25/01/13]

Santa Cruz N, Powers A (2011) Mental health in Arizona: a case study. *LA Times*, 29 January, http://articles.latimes.com/2011/jan/19/nation/la-na-arizona-mental-health-20110120 [accessed 15/01/13]

Sapa-AFP (2004) Moms, babies can't leave hospital until they've paid. *Pretoria News*, 4 June, p. 4 (news report)

Save the Children (2005) User Fees: paying for health services at the point of use. Save the Children, London

Savedoff W (2003) How Much Should Countries Spend on Health? Discussion Paper No. 2, WHO Health System Financing, Expenditure and Resource Allocation Evidence and Information for Policy (EIP), Geneva

Savedoff W, de Ferranti D, Smith AL, Fan V (2012) Political and economic aspects of the transition to universal health coverage. *Lancet* 380(9,845): 924–32 (8 September), DOI: 10.1016/S0140-6736(12)61083-6, http://www.theLancet.com/journals/Lancet/article/PIIS0140-6736(12)61083-6/fulltext#article_upsell [accessed 10/12/12]

Scandlen G (2003) It's Up to Us. Heartland Institute, 1 February, http://www.heartland.org

Scheil-Adlung X, Bonan J (2012) Can the European elderly afford the financial burden of health and long-term care? Assessing impacts and policy implications. ESS Extension of Social Security Paper N° 31, Global Campaign on Social Security and Coverage for All, International Labour Office Social Security Department, Geneva, http://www.ilo.org/gimi/gess/RessShowRessource.do?ressourceId=30228 [accessed 14/01/13]

Schick A (1998) Why most developing countries should not try New Zealand reforms. *World Bank Research Observer* 13(1): 123–31 (February)

Schieber GJ, Maeda A (1997) A curmudgeon's guide to financing health care in developing countries. In Schieber 1997

Schieber GJ (ed.) (1997) Innovations in Health Care Financing. *World Bank Discussion Paper 365*, March, World Bank, Washington DC

Schrecker T (2011a) Social Determinants of Health: Resuscitating the Agenda in Rio. http://www.healthypolicies.com/2011/08/social-determinants-of-health-resuscitating-the-agenda-in-rio/ [accessed 25/01/13]

Schrecker T (2011b) Personal Communication: Comments on First Draft. World Conference on Social Determinants of Health

Schreuder B, Kostermans C (2001) Global health strategies versus local primary health care priorities – a case study of national immunisation days in Southern Africa. *South African Medical Journal* 91(3): 249–54 (March)

Schulz-Asche K (2000) A Case for Partnership? The German Government/Boehringer Ingelheim initiative on HIV/AIDS, Health Action International, http://www.haiweb.org/campaign/PPI/seminar200011.html#item4 [accessed 02/03/13]

Schwartz FW, Glennerster H, Saltman RB (eds) (1996) *Fixing Health Budgets: Experience from Europe and North America.* John Wiley & Sons, Chichester

Schwefel D, Vuckovic M, Korte R, Bichmann W, Brandrup-Lukanow A (2005) *Health Development and Globalisation.* GTZ, http://www.shi-conference.de/downl/geg_execsum.pdf [accessed 15/11/06].

ScienceDaily (2012) Health-Care Costs Hit the Elderly Hard, Diminish Financial Wellbeing. ScienceDaily, 4 September, http://www.sciencedaily.com/releases/12/09/120904162619/htm [accessed 09/09/12]

Scott C (2001) Public and private roles in health care systems. Open University Press, Buckingham

SCUK (2008) Freeing up health care: a guide to removing user fees. Save the children UK, London, http://www.savethechildren.org.uk/resources/online-library/freeing-healthcare-guide-removing-user-fees [accessed 25/01/13]

Sein T (2001) Health Sector Reform – Issues and Opportunities – Regional Health Forum. WHO website, http://w3.whosea.org/rh4/4a.htm [accessed 15/02/03]

Selvaraj S, Karan AK (2012) Why publicly-financed health insurance schemes are ineffective in providing financial risk protection. *Economic and Political Weekly* XLVII(11): 60–8 (17 March)

Sen K (ed.) (2003) *Restructuring Health Services: Changing Contexts and Comparative Perspectives.* Zed Books Ltd

Sen S (2010) Healthcare for all – a distant dream or a reality? *Express Healthcare*, March, http://www.expresshealthcare.in/201003/market16/shtml [accessed 23/09/12]

Shaffer ER, Waitzkin H, Brenner J, Jasso-Aguilar R (2005) Global trade and public health. *American Journal of Public Health* 95(1): 23–34 (January)

Shakow A (2006) Global Fund – World Bank HIV/AIDS Programs Comparative Advantage Study. Prepared for the Global Fund to Fight Aids, Tuberculosis & Malaria and the World Bank Global HIV/AIDS Program, 19 January, World Bank, Washington DC, http://goo.gl/CcaM7 [accessed 25/01/13]

Sharman D (2010) The global economic crisis and the need for World Bank reform. Global Research, 21 January, http://globalresearch.ca/index.php?context=va&aid=17114 [accessed 12/05/12]

Shaw RP (2002) World Health Report 2000 'Financial fairness indicator': useful compass or crystal ball? *International Journal of Health Services* 32(1): 195–203

Shaxson M (2011) *Treasure Islands: Tax Havens and the men who stole the world.* Bodley head, London

Sheldon T (2012) Dutch GP Association is fined €7.7 million for anti-competitive
    behaviour. *British Medical Journal* 344:e439, doi: 10.1136/BMJ.e439
Shetty P (2012) Grey matter: ageing in developing countries. *Lancet* 379: 1,285–7 (7 April)
Shipman T (2011) Sharks who made a killing out of 'care': how City predators destroyed
    firm caring for 31,000 old people. Mail Online, 2 June, http://www.dailymail.co.uk/
    news/article-1393294/Southern-Cross-Healthcare-destroyed-Stephen-Schwarzmans-
    private-equity-firm-Blackstone.html [accessed 14/01/13]
SHOPS (2012) Nigeria Holds Inaugural Private Health Sector
    Summit. http://www.shopsproject.org/about/announcements/
    nigeria-holds-inaugural-private-health-sector-summit
Shortt SED (2002) Medical Savings Accounts in publicly funded health care systems:
    enthusiasm versus evidence. *CMAJ* 167(2): 159–62 (23 July)
Shukrallah A (2009) Health and Human Rights – The Egyptian context. Health and
    Human Rights, Bahrain, May, http://www.upr.bh/projects/Health_and_human_
    rights_-_Dr[1]._Alaa.pps [NOT found]
Sibbald, McDonald, Roland (2007) Shifting care from hospitals to the community: a review
    of the evidence on quality and efficiency. *Journal of Health Services Research & Policy*
    12(2): 110–17
Silva C (2010) Physician-owned hospitals: Endangered Species Act? *AMANews*, 28 June,
    http://www.ama-assn.org/amednews/2010/06/28/gvsa0628/htm [accessed 02/09/12]
Simonet D (2008) The New Public Management theory and European health-care reforms.
    Canadian Public Administration 51(4): 617–35 (December)
Simonet D (2011) The New Public Management theory and the reform of European
    healthcare systems: an international comparative perspective. *International Journal of
    Public Administration* 34: 815 to 826, DOI: 10.1080/01900692/2011/603401/603401
Singer M (2007) Under the Influence. CBS News, 23 July, http://www.cbsnews.com/2102-
    18560_162-2625305/html?tag=contentMain;contentBody [accessed 25/01/13]
Siringi S, Nzioka P (2006) Revamped NHIF casts its net wide. *Nation* (Nairobi), 7
    November, http://allafrica.com/stories/printable/200611070174/html [accessed 21/11/06]
Skaar CM (1998) Extending coverage of priority health care services through collaboration
    with the private sector: selected experiences of USAID Cooperating Agencies. *Major
    Applied Research No. 4, Working Paper 1*, PHR, Abt Assiciates, Bethesda MD
Skolnik R, Jensen P, Johnson R (2010) Aid Without Impact: How the World Bank and
    Development Partners are Failing to Improve Health Through SWAps. ACTION
    Advocacy to Control TB Internationally, http://www.action.org/images/general/results_
    executive_summary_final_080910_highres.pdf [accessed 25/01/13]
Slack K, Savedoff WD (2001) Public purchaser-private contracting for health services.
    January, IADB, Washington DC
Smith M (2009) CASE STUDY: Financing a New Referral Hospital Lesotho, CABRI
    Dialogue: Ensuring Value for Money in Infrastructure Projects. December, http://
    cabri-sbo.org/images/documents/6thAnnualSeminar/session_4_group_a_lesotho_
    mathundsane_mohapi_english.pdf [accessed 25/01/13]
Smith P (2002) Stars in their eyes. *HSJ* 112(5,816): 10–12
Smith PC (ed.) (2000) *Reforming Markets in Health Care: an economic perspective*. Open
    University, Buckingham

Smith R (1996a) Being creative about rationing. *British Medical Journal* 312: 391–2 (17 February)

Smith R (1996b) Rationing health care: moving the debate forward. *British Medical Journal* 312: 1,553–4 (22 June)

Smith R (2002) A time for global health. *British Medical Journal* 325: 54–5 (13 July)

Smith R (2004) Foreign Direct Investment and Trade in Health Services: a review of the literature. *Social Science and Medicine* 59: 2313–23

Social Watch (2006) *Impossible Architecture: Social Watch Report 2006*. Instituto Del Tercer Mundo, Montevideo, Uruguay, http://www.socialwatch.org/en/informeImpreso/pdfs/SW-ENG-2006.pdf

Solomon L (2002) Rise of a 'zombie'. *National Post*, 31 July, Toronto

Sousa RM, Ferri CP, Acosta D, Albanese E, Guerra M, Huang Y, Jacob KS, Jotheeswaran AT, Rodriguez JJ, Pichardo GR, Rodriguez MC, Salas A, Sosa AL, Williams J, Zuniga T, Prince M (2009) Contribution of chronic diseases to disability in elderly people in countries with low and middle incomes: a 10/66 Dementia Research Group population-based survey. *Lancet* 374: 1,821–30, doi: 10.1016/S0140-6736(09)61829-8

Spinaci S, Currat L, Shetty P, Valerie Crowell V, Kehler J (2006) Tough choices: investing in health for development: experiences from national follow-up to the Commission on Macroeconomics and Health. WHO, Geneva

Sridhar D, Batniji R (2008) Misfinancing global health: a case for transparency in disbursements and decision making. *Lancet* 372: 1,185–91 (27 September)

Standard Digital (2008) When it costs Sh400,000 to give birth. Friday, 24 October, http://www.standardmedia.co.ke/?articleID=1143997756&pageNo=3 [accessed 25/01/13]

Stawicki E (2012) Minn. HMO profits keep rolling in. Minnesota Public Radio, 7 September, http://minnesota.publicradio.org/display/web/12/09/07/health/minnesota-health-plan-profits/ [accessed 10/12/12]

Steinhardt LC, Aman I, Pakzad I, Kumar B, Sigh LP, Peters DH (2011) Removing user fees for basic health services: a pilot study and national roll-out in Afghanistan. *Health Policy and Planning* 26: ii92–ii103, doi:10.1093/czr069

Stemmer E (2008) Contractual Structures and Risk Allocation and Mitigation in the Context of Public Private Partnerships in the Health Sector. Finance Economics & Urban Department Finance & Guarantees Group, February, pp. 10–11, http://siteresources.worldbank.org/INTGUARANTEES/Resources/RiskMitigationHealthSector_ERIC_STEMMER.pdf

Stevens S (2011) Is there evidence that competition in health care is a good thing? Yes. *British Medical Journal* 343: d4136, doi: 10.1136/BMJ.d4136

Stiglitz J (2002) *Globalisation and its discontents*. Penguin, London

Stoiciu V (2012) Austerity and structural reforms in Romania. Freidrich Ebert Stiftung, August, http://library.fes.de/pdf-files/id-moe/09310.pdf [accessed 14/01/13]

Stolt R, Winblad U (2009) Mechanisms behind privatisation: a case study of private growth in Swedish elderly care. *Social Science and Medicine* 68: 903–91, doi: 10.1016/j dots socscimed.2008/12/011

Stone D (2001) Think tanks, global lesson-drawing and networking social policy ideas. *Global Social Policy* 1(3): 338–60 (December)

Sturchio JL, Goel A (2012) The private sector role in public health. Reflections on the new global architecture in health. Center for Strategic and International Studies, Washington

DC, January, http://csis.org/publication/private-sector-role-public-health [accessed 10/12/12]

Sulku SN (2011) The impacts of health care reforms on the efficiency of the Turkish public hospitals: provincial markets. Munich Personal RePEx Archive, MPRA, 14 March, http://mpra.ub.uni-muenchen.de/29598 [accessed 25/01/13]

Sussex J (2001) *The economics of the private finance initiative in the NHS.* Office of Health Economics, London

Sykes et al. (eds) (2001) *Globalisation and European welfare states.* Palgrave, London

Tagaris K (2012) Greek health system crumbles under weight of crisis. Reuters Athens, 14 June, http://www.reuters.com/article/12/06/14/us-greece-health-idUSBRE85D1IO20120614 [accessed 15/01/13]

Tan C (2006) NGOs criticise outcome of IMF–World Bank meeting. Third World Network, press release, 20 September, http://www.twnside.org.sg/title2/finance/twninifofinance007.htm, [accessed 15/11/06].

Tangcharoensathien V, Patcharanarumol W, Ir P, Aljunid SM, Mukti AG, Akkhavong K, Banzon E, Huong DB, Thabrany H, Mills A (2011) Health-financing reforms in south-east Asia: challenges in achieving universal coverage, http://www.theLancet.com, published online 25 January, DOI:10.1016/S0140-6736(10)61890-9

Tanne JH (2007) US Health spending grew more slowly in 2005. *British Medical Journal* 334: 117 (20 January)

Taranto J (2012) Is he unelectable? *Wall Street Journal* Online, 31 January, http://online.wsj.com/article/SB10001424052970204740904577195172485772932/html#printMode [accessed 22/09/12]

Tarricone R, Tsouros AD (2008) The Solid facts: Home Care in Europe. WHO Europe, http://www.euro.who.int/__data/assets/pdf_file/0005/96467/E91884/pdf [accessed 25/01/13]

Tatar M, Kanavos P (2006) Health care reform in Turkey. *Eurohealth* 12(1): 20–2

Taylor J (2012) Achieving sustainability requires a great deal more energy. *Health Service Journal*, 27 September, pp. 18–21

Taylor M (2003) The reformulation of social policy in Chile 1973–2001: Questioning a Neoliberal Model. *Global Social Policy* 3(1): 21–44 (April)

Taylor R (2003) Singapore's innovative health financing system. *Flagship Online Journal*, May, World Bank, http://www.worldbank.org/wbi/healthandpopulation/oj.html [accessed 22/09/03]

Therborn G (1996) Critical Theory and the Legacy of Twentieth-century Marxism. In Turner 1996

Thiede M, Mutyambizi V (2010) South Africa. In Preker et al. 2010

Thiel V (2012) Social enterprises, big corporations and the NHS. The devil is in the details. *New Statesman*, 6 July, http://www.newstatesman.com/blogs/politics/12/07/social-enterprises-big-corporations-and-nhs [accessed 14/01/13]

Thomson S, Foubister T, Mossialos E (2009) Financing health care in the European Union. EU Health Observatory, *Observatory Studies* No. 17, http://www.euro.who.int/__data/assets/pdf_file/0009/98307/E92469/pdf [accessed 10/12/12]

Thomson S, Mossialos E (2009) Private health insurance in the European Union. Final report prepared for the European Commission Directorate General for Employment and

Social Affairs and Equal Opportunities, London School of economics health and social care, 24 June, http://eprints.lse.ac.uk/25511/ [accessed 25/01/13]

Tiemann O, Schreyögg J, Busse R (2011) Which type of hospital ownership has the best performance? Evidence and implications from Germany. *Eurohealth* 17(2–3): 31–3

Timmins N (1995) *The Five Giants: A Biography of the Welfare State*. Harper Collins, London

Timmins N (2002) Warning of spurious figures on value of PFI. *Financial Times*, 5 June

Tornaes U (2005) Strategy for Denmark's support to the International Fight against HIV/AIDS. Ministry of Foreign Affairs, Denmark, http://www.um.dk/en/menu/DevelopmentPolicy/DanishDevelopmentPolicy/HIVAIDSNewDanishPolicy/?wbc_purpose=Bas [accessed 15/11/06]

Torrey EF (1997) *Out of the Shadows: Confronting America's Mental Illness Crisis*. John Wiley, New York

Tran M (2012) Poorer countries must adapt to meet health needs of elderly, report says. *Guardian*, 4 April, http://www.guardian.co.uk/global-development/12/apr/04/poorer-countries-health-needs-ageing-population [accessed 13/09/12]

Triggle N (2012) South London Healthcare NHS Trust put into administration. BBC News, London, 12 July, http://www.bbc.co.uk/news/uk-england-londoin-18812193 [accessed 30/09/12]

True Cost (2012) How Much Will Insurance Cost Under Obamacare? 7 August, http://truecostblog.com/tag/health-care/ [accessed 02/03/13]

Tsolova T (2012) Bulgaria PM shuffles cabinet with eye on election. Reuters, 13 March, http://uk.reuters.com/article/12/03/16/bulgaria-politics-idUKL5E8EG18F20120316 [accessed 15/01/13]

Tuohy CH (1999) *Accidental Logics*. Oxford University Press, Oxford & New York

Turner BS (ed.) (1996) *The Blackwell Companion to Social Theory*. Blackwell, Oxford

Turner B (2009) Ireland. In Thomson and Mossialos 2009

Turshen M (1999) *Privatising Health Services in Africa*. Rutgers University Press, New Brunswick NJ

Twigg J (ed.) (2012) Russia's emerging global health leadership. Center for Strategic and International Studies, Washington DC, April, http://csis.org/publication/russias-emerging-global-health-leadership [accessed 10/12/12]

Tynan A, Draper DA (2008) Getting what we pay for: innovations lacking in provider payment reform to chronic disease care. Centre for studying Health System Change Research Brief No. 6, June, http://www.hschange.org/CONTENT/995/995/pdf [accessed 18/01/13]

Tyson J, Kashiwase K, Soto M, Clements B (2012) Containing public health spending: lessons from experiences of advanced economies. In Clements et al. 2012

Ulrich L, Jigidsuren A (2002) Report and Recommendations for Health Sector Public–Private Partnerships. Mongolia Second Health Sector Development Project, Asian Development Bank, May, http://www.infraproj.com/mongolian.pdf

UN (2002) Report on the Second World Assembly on Ageing. United Nations, New York, http://www.un.org/esa/socdev/ageing/waa/a-conf-197-9b.htm [accessed 08/01/03]

UN (2011a) Disability and the Millennium Development Goals. United Nations, New York, http://www.un.org/disabilities/documents/review_of_disability_and_the_mdgs.pdf [accessed 15/01/13]

UN (2011b) World Population Prospects: The 2010 Revision. Volume I: Comprehensive Tables. ST/ESA/SER.A/313 Department of Economic and Social Affairs, United Nations, New York, http://esa.un.org/unpd/wpp/Documentation/pdf/WPP2010_Volume-I_Comprehensive-Tables.pdf [accessed 14/01/13]

UN (2011c) World Population Prospects: The 2010 Revision. Highlights and Advance Tables. United Nations, http://esa.un.org/wpp/Documentation/pdf/WPP2010_Highlights.pdf [accessed 25/01/13]

UN Millennium Project (2005) Investing in Development: a practical plan to achieve the Millennium Development Goals. United Nations Development Programme, New York, http://www.unmillenniumproject.org/documents/MainReportComplete-lowres.pdf [accessed 15/01/13]

UN Office for the Coordination of Humanitarian Affairs (2005) Ghana: despite new health scheme, newborn babies detained in hospital pending payment. *IRINnews*, 16 September, http://www.irinnews.org/print.asp?ReportID=49114.

UN Office for the Coordination of Humanitarian Affairs (2006) Burundi: Nkurunziza announces free maternal healthcare, pay rise for workers. *IRINnews*, 1 May, http://www.irinnews.org/print.asp?ReportID=53075.

UNDESA (2011) The Global Social Crisis: Report on the World Social Situation. United Nations Department of Economic and Social Affairs New York, http://social.un.org/index/Publications/tabid/83/news/123/Default.aspx [accessed 25/01/13]

Unger JP, De Paepe P, Ghilbert P, Soors W, Green A (2006) Disintegrated care: the Achilles heel of international health policies in low- and middle-income countries. *International Journal of Integrated Care* Vol. 6 (18 September)

UNICEF (2008) India and China hold the key to world meeting MDGs, says UNICEF flagship report. Press release, New Delhi / Bangkok, 5 August, http://www.unicef.org/media/media_45009/html [accessed 23/09/12]

UNISON Scotland (2002) Sodexho booted out in South Glasgow. *Scottish Health Bulletin Autumn*: 7, http://www.healthemergency.org.uk/pdf/ScotlandNo1A4/pdf [accessed 29/09/12]

UNPFA and Help Age International (2011) Ageing in the Twenty-First Century: A Celebration and a Challenge. United Nations Population Fund, New York, and Help Aid International, London, http://www.helpage.org/resources/ageing-in-the-21st-century-a-celebration-and-a-challenge/ [accessed 02/03/13]

UNRISD (2000) Visible hands – taking responsibility for social development. Geneva, UNRISD

US Department of Health, Human Services (2012) Mental Health, United States, 2010. Substance Abuse and Mental Health Services Administration (SAMHSA), April, http://store.samhsa.gov/product/Mental-Health-United-States-2010/SMA12-4681 [accessed 14/01/13]

USAID (US Agency for International Development) (1999) Strategic Plan 1998–2003. January, Washington DC

USAID (US Agency for International Development) (2003a) Security, Democracy, Prosperity Strategic Plan, Fiscal Years 2004 –2009 Aligning Diplomacy and Development Assistance. USAID, Washington DC

USAID (US Agency for International Development) (2003b) USAID History. http://www.usaid.gov/about_usaid/usaidhist.html [accessed 31/12/03]

USAID (US Agency for International Development) (2003c) This is USAID. http://www.usaid.gov/about_usaid/ [accessed 31/12/03]

USAID (US Agency for International Development) (2007) Egypt's Health reform strengthened with Memorandum of Understanding signed by USAID, the Ministry of Health and Population and private pharmaceutical companies. Press release, 18 April

USAID (US Agency for International Development) (2011) Better Health for Development. Global Health Strategic Framework. http://apps.who.int/medicinedocs/documents/s19251en/s19251en.pdf [accessed 25/01/13]

Utomo B, Sucahya PK, Utami FR (2011) Priorities and realities: addressing the rich–poor gaps in health status and service access in Indonesia. *International Journal for Equity in Health* 10: 47, doi:10.1186/1475-9276-10-47, http://www.equityhealthj.com/content/10/1/47 [accessed 25/01/13]

Valentine W (1998) WHO spearheads multi-country study of decentralisation and health system change. *Bridge*, WHO, http://165.158.1.110/english/hsp/hspbb985.htm [accessed 15/02/03]

Valverde FD (2006) New strategies to extend health protection in the context of health reforms in Latin America and the Caribbean. International Social Security Association Regional Conference for the Americas, May

van de Ven WP, Schut FT (2008) Universal mandatory health insurance in the Netherlands: a model for the United States? *Health Affairs* 27(3): 771–81, doi:10.1377/hlthaff.27/3/771, http://content.healthaffairs.org/content/27/3/771/full.html [accessed 25/09/12]

van der Gaag J (1995) Private and public initiatives: Working together for health and education. In the Directions in Development Series, Washington DC, World Bank

van der Stuyft P, Unger JP (2000) Editorial: Improving the performance of health systems: the World Health Report as a go-between for scientific evidence and ideological discourse. *Tropical Medicine and International Health* 5(10): 675–7 (October)

van Mourik M, Cameron A, Ewen M, Laing RO (2010) Availability, price and affordability of cardiovascular medicines: a comparison across 36 countries using WHO/HAI data. *BMC Cardiovascular Disorders* 10: 25, http://www.biomedcentral.com/1471-2261/10/25 [accessed 25/01/13]

Varma S (2012) Unfair practices: Pharma companies fined $13bn in 4 years. *Times of India*, 16 July, http://timesofindia.indiatimes.com/business/international-business/Unfair-practices-Pharma-companies-fined-13bn-in-4-years/articleshow/14972186/cms [accessed 14/01/13]

Vaughan JP, Modegal S, Kruse S, Lee K, Walt G, de Wilde K (1996) Financing the World Health Organization: global importance of extrabudgetary funds. *Health Policy* 35(3): 229–45, March

Verheul E, Rowson M (2001) 'Poverty reduction strategy papers', *British Medical Journal* 323: 120–1

Vian T (2008) Review of corruption in the health sector: theory, methods and interventions. *Health Policy and Planning* 23: 83–94

Vidal J (2010) Why is the Gates foundation investing in GM giant Monsanto? http://www.guardian.co.uk/global-development/poverty-matters/2010/sep/29/gates-foundation-gm-monsanto [accessed 25/01/13]

Vienonen M, Jankauskiene D, Vask A (1999) Towards evidence-based health reform. *Bulletin of the WHO* 77(1): 44–7

Viroj Tangcharoensathien V, Patcharanarumol W, Ir P, Aljunid SM, Mukti AG, Akkhavong K, Banzon E, Huong DB, Thabrany H, Mills A (2011) Health-financing reforms in southeast Asia: challenges in achieving universal coverage. *Lancet* 377(9,768): 863–73 (5 March), DOI: 10.1016/S0140-6736(10)61890-9

Vladescu C, Radulescu S (2002) Improving primary care. Output based contracting in Romania. In Brook and Smith 2002

Vrangbæk K (2009) The political process of restructuring Nordic health care systems. In Magnussen et al. 2009

Vujicic M, Weber SE, Nikolic IA, Atun R, Kumar R (2011) Gavi, the Global Fund and the World Bank Support for human resources for health in developing countries. Health, Nutrition and Population (HNP) Discussion Paper, World Bank, http://goo.gl/CL0L7 [accessed 25/01/13]

Wagstaff A (2002) Reflections and alternatives to the WHO's fairness of financial contribution index. *Health Econ* 11(2): 103–15 (March)

Wagstaff A (2007) Social health insurance re-examined. *World Bank Policy Research Working Paper* 4, 111, January, World Bank

Waitzkin H (1994) The strange career of managed competition: from military failure to medical success? *Am J Public Health* March 84(3): 482–9, PMCID: PMC1614846

Waitzkin H (1997) Challenges of managed care: its role in health system reform in Latin America. *Informing and Reforming* No. 4, 2–4 ICHSRI (October–December)

Waitzkin H, Iriart C (2004) How the United States exports managed care to developing countries. In Navarro and Muntaner 2004

Waitzkin H, Jasso-Aguilar R, Iriart C (2007) Privatization of health services in less developed countries: an empirical response to the proposals of the World Bank and Wharton school. *International Journal of Health Services* 37(2): 205–27

Wall A, Owen B (2002) *Health Policy.* Gildredge Social Policy, Routledge

Wall M (2011) Subsidy for private treatment in public hospitals to be abolished. *Irish Times*, 26 November, http://www.irishtimes.com/newspaper/frontpage/2011/1126/1224308188759/html [accessed 06/09/12]

Wall Street Journal (2008) World Bank Disgrace. Editorial, 14 January, http://online.wsj.com/article/SB120026972002987225/html?mod=opinion_main_review_and_outlooks#printMode [accessed 25/01/13]

Wall Street Journal (2011) Arizona shootings shed light on mental health care for teens. *Wall Street Journal*, Juggle blog, 12 January, http://goo.gl/xOCfL [accessed 14/01/13]

Walt G (1994) Health Policy: an introduction to process and power. Witwatersrand University Press / Zed Books, London

Wang PS, Angermeyer M, Borges G, Bruffaerts R, Tat Chiu W, De Girolamo G, Fayyad J, Gureje O, Haro JM, Huang Y, Kessler RC, Kovess V, Levinson D, Nakane Y, Oakley Brown MA, Ormel JH, Posada-Villa J, Aguilar-Gaxiola S, Alonso J, Lee S, Heeringa S, Pennell BE, Chatterji S, Ustün TB (2007) Delay and failure in treatment seeking after first onset of mental disorders in the World Health Organization's World Mental Health Survey Initiative. *World Psychiatry* 6(3): 177–85 (October)

Wang'ombe JK (1997a) Health sector reform in Kenya. *Informing and Reforming* ICHSRI 1: 5–6 (January–March)

Wang'ombe JK (1997b) Cost Recovery Strategies in Sub-Saharan Africa. In Schieber 1997

Weich S, Lewis G (1998) Poverty, unemployment and common mental disorders: population based cohort study. *British Medical Journal* 317: 115–19 (11 July)

Weisbrot M (2001) *The 'Washington Consensus' and development economics*. UNRISD, http:// www.unrisd.org/unrisd/website/document.nsf/(httpPublications)/3AD5D5F2520B7436C 1256BC9004C3D2C?OpenDocument

Weisbrot M (2006) Latin America: The End of an Era. *International Journal of Health Services* 36(4), http://www.cepr.net/columns/weisbrot/2006_06_end_of_era.htm#article [NOT found]

Weissman R (2009) A new life for the IMF: Capitalizing on Crisis. *Multinational Monitor*, 30 June, http://www.multinationalmonitor.org/mm2009/032009/weissman.html [accessed 14/05/12]

Weiyuan C (2008) China's village doctors take great strides. *Bulletin of the World Health Organization* 86(12): 914–15, http://www.who.int/bulletin/volumes/86/12/08-021208/pdf [accessed 15/01/13]

Wellings R (2012) How to abolish the NHS. Institute of Economic Affairs, 23 January, http://www.iea.org.uk/blog/how-to-abolish-the-nhs [accessed 10/12/12]

Wells Fargo (2012) Invest in your health. Wells Fargo Bank, https://www.WellsFargo.com/ investing/hsa [accessed 07/09/12]

Wells Journal (2012) NHS cartel presses ahead with pay plans. 27 December, http://www. thisissomerset.co.uk/NHS-cartel-presses-ahead-pay-plans/story-17692840-detail/story. html#ixzz2Mr7UAb27 [accessed 02/03/13]

West E (2010) African Medical Investments opens new boutique hospital in Maputo, Mozambique. *Africa Medical & Healthcare News*, 10 May, http://www.expogr.com/ business_news/africa_medical_healthcare_business_news.htm#c [accessed 25/01/13]

Whelan D (2010) ObamaCare's first victim: physician-owned specialty hospitals. Forbes, 4 May, http://www.forbes.com/sites/sciencebiz/2010/04/05/obamacares-first-victim-physician-owned-specialty-hospitals/ [accessed 18/01/13]

Whitehead M (1992a) The concepts and principles of equity and health. *International Journal of Health Services* 22(3): 429–45

Whitehead M (1992b) *The Health Divide*. Penguin, London and New York

Whitehead M, Dahlgren G, Evans T (2001) Equity and health sector reforms: can low-income counties escape the medical poverty trap? *Lancet* 358: 833–6

Whitehead M, Dahlgren G, McIntyre D (2007) Putting equity centre stage: challenging evidence-free reforms. *International Journal of Health Services* 37(2): 353–61

WHO (1992) Basic documents (39th edition). WHO, Geneva

WHO (1995a) The World Health Report 1995 – Bridging the Gaps. http://www.who.int/ whr/1995/en/index.html

WHO (1995b) Report of the World Summit for Social Development. WHO, Copenhagen, http://www.un.org/documents/ga/conf166/aconf166-9/htm [accessed 25/01/13]

WHO (1996) The Ljubljana Charter on reforming health care. WHO, Europe, 18 June, http://www.euro.who.int/en/who-we-are/policy-documents/the-ljubljana-charter-on-reforming-health-care,-1996 [accessed 14/01/13]

WHO (1997) Key Issues in Health for All Renewal. WHO, Geneva, https://extranet.who.int/ iris/restricted/bitstream/10665/63719/1/PPE_PAC_97.7.pdf [accessed 02/03/13]

WHO (1998) Experiences of contracting: an overview of the literature. Macroeconomics, Health and Development Series, No. 33

WHO (1999) *Health 21: The health for all policy framework for the WHO European Region.* WHO, Copenhagen, http://www.euro.who.int/__data/assets/pdf_file/0010/98398/ wa540ga199heeng.pdf [accessed 02/03/13]

WHO (2000) *The World Health Report 2000 – Health Systems: Improving Performance.* WHO, Geneva

WHO (2001) Health in PRSPs. WHO Submission to World Bank/IMF Review of PRSPs. WHO, Department of Health and Development, Geneva

WHO (2002) Active Ageing a Policy Framework. A contribution of the World Health Organization to the Second United Nations World Assembly on Ageing, Madrid, Spain, April, http://whqlibdoc.who.int/hq/2002/who_nmh_nph_02/8/pdf [accessed 10/12/12]

WHO (2003) Climate Change and Human Health: risks and responses. Summary. WHO France, http://www.who.int/globalchange/publications/cchhsummary/en/ [accessed 14/01/13]

WHO (2004a) PRSPS: Their Significance for Health: Second Synthesis Report. WHO, Geneva

WHO (2004b) Disability, including prevention, management and rehabilitation. Resolution to 58th World Health Assembly, http://apps.who.int/gb/ebwha/pdf_files/WHA58/ WHA58_23-en.pdf [NOT found]

WHO (2005a) PRSPS: Their Significance for Health: Second Synthesis Report. WHO/ HDP/PRSP/04/1, MDGs, Health and Development Policy, Geneva, Switzerland

WHO (2005b) MDG: Health and the Millennium Development Goals. WHO, Geneva

WHO (2006a) *The World Health Report 2006 – Working together for health.* http://www.who. int/whr/2006/en/index.html [accessed 02/03/13]

WHO (2006b) Engaging for Health: 11th General Programme of Work, 2006– 2015, A Global Health Agenda. May, WHO, Geneva, http://whqlibdoc.who.int/ publications/2006/GPW_eng.pdf [accessed 02/03/13]

WHO (2007) Working for Health: an introduction to the World Health Organization. WHO, Geneva

WHO (2008a) Closing the gap in a generation: Health equity through action on the social determinants of health. WHO, Geneva, http://whqlibdoc.who.int/hq/2008/WHO_IER_ CSDH_08.1_eng.pdf [accessed 02/03/13]

WHO (2008b) The World Health Report 2008 – Primary Health Care (Now More Than Ever). WHO, Geneva, http://www.who.int/whr/2008/en/ [accessed 02/03/13]

WHO (2008c) Inequalities are killing people on a 'grand scale' reports WHO Commission. WHO press release, Geneva, 28 August, http://www.who.int/mediacentre/news/ releases/2008/pr29/en/print.html [accessed 09/09/08]

WHO (2008d) National Health Accounts: Ireland. WHO, http://www.who.int/nha/country/ irl/en/ [accessed 16/06/08]

WHO (2009) Mental health systems in selected low- and middle-income countries: a WHO-AIMS cross-national analysis. WHO, Geneva, http://www.who.int/mental_health/ evidence/who_aims_report_final.pdf [accessed 15/01/13]

WHO (2010) Proposed programme budget 2010–11: financial tables. Summary Table 2. Proposed programme budget by strategic objective, organizational level and source of financing, all levels, 2010–2011 (US$ million). WHO, Geneva, apps.who.int/gb/ebwha/ pdf_files/MTSP2009/PPB5-en.pdf [accessed 25/01/13]

WHO (2011) Implementation of the International Health Regulations 2005. Report by the Director-General A64/10, 5 May, WHO, Geneva, http://apps.who.int/gb/ebwha/pdf_files/WHA64/A64_10-en.pdf [accessed 16/01/13]

WHO (2012a) Outcome of the World Conference on Social Determinants of Health. WHO, Geneva, 26 May, http://www.who.int/sdhconference/background/A65_R8-en.pdf [accessed 10/12/12]

WHO (2012b) Good health adds life to years. Global brief for World Health Day, WHO, Geneva, http://www.who.int/mediacentre/news/releases/12/whd_20120403/en/index.html [accessed 14/01/13]

WHO (2012c) Global Health Observatory Data Repository, Health financing: Health expenditure per capita data by country. http://apps.who.int/gho/data/node.main.486 [accessed 02/03/13]

WHO and Alzheimer's Disease International (2012) Dementia: a public health priority. WHO, Geneva, http://whqlibdoc.who.int/publications/2012/9789241564458_eng.pdf [accessed 02/03/13]

WHO and World Bank (2011) World Report on Disability 2011. WHO, Geneva, http://whqlibdoc.who.int/publications/2011/9789240685215_eng.pdf [accessed 15/01/13]

WHO Eastern Mediterranean Regional Office (2012) Good practices in delivery of primary health care in urban settings. http://applications.emro.who.int/dsaf/EMPUB_2012_865.pdf

WHO Europe (1998) Health 21. An introduction to the health for all policy framework for the WHO European Region. European Health for All Series, No. 5, WHO Copenhagen, http://www.euro.who.int/en/what-we-publish/abstracts/health21-an-introduction-to-the-health-for-all-policy-framework-for-the-who-european-region [accessed 15/01/13]

WHO Europe (1999; document says 1996) The Ljubljana Charter on Reforming Health Care. Bulletin of the World Health Organization 77(1): 48–9, http://www.ncbi.nlm.nih.gov/pmc/articles/PMC2557573/pdf/10063661/pdf [accessed 25/01/13]

WHO Europe (2005) Mental health action plan for Europe. WHO, Helsinki, January, EUR/04/5047810/7, http://www.euro.who.int/__data/assets/pdf_file/0013/100822/edoc07/pdf [accessed 14/01/13]

WHO Global Forum (2011) Global noncommunicable disease network (NCDnet) Forum Report. WHO Global Forum, August, http://www.who.int/nmh/events/global_forum_ncd/forum_report.pdf [accessed 14/01/13]

Wieners W (ed.) (2001) Global Health Care Markets. Jossey Bass, San Francisco

Wiist B (2011) Philanthropic foundations and the public health agenda. Corporations and Health Watch, 3 August, http://www.corporationsandhealthwatch.org/news/202/62/Philanthropic-Foundations-and-the-Public-Health-Agenda/d,Article [accessed 25/09/11]

Williams M (1994) International Economic Organisations and the Third World. Harvester Wheatsheaf, London

Williamson J (1990) What Washington means by policy reform. In Williamson J (ed.), Latin American Adjustment: How much has happened? Institute for International Economics, Washington

Williamson J (2000) What should the World Bank think about the Washington Consensus? World Bank Research Observer

Wilson D (2010) Mistakes chronicled on Medicare patients. Nytimes.com, 15 November, http://www.nytimes.com/2010/11/16/business/16medicare.html?_r=0 [accessed 18/01/13]

Wismar M, Palm W, Figueras J, Ernst K, van Ginneken E (eds) (2011) *Cross-border healthcare in the European Union. Mapping and analysing practices and policies.* European Observatory on Health Systems and Policies, http://www.euro.who.int/en/ what-we-publish/abstracts/cross-border-health-care-in-the-european-union.-mapping-and-analysing-practices-and-policies [accessed 18/1/13]

Wohlforth T, Westoby A (1978) *Communists Against Revolution.* Folrose Books, London

Wolf (2006) Bad news for the IMF is good for its clients. *Financial Times,* 12 September

Wolfowitz P (2007) *Letter to Elizabeth Stuart, Oxfam.* 30 January, World Bank

Woodward D (2006) *The IMF and World Bank.* Research synthesis paper for Globalization Knowledge Network, WHO Commission on Social Determinants of Health

Woolf M (2006) Peerages of millionaire party donors are held up by new inquiry. *Independent,* 5 March, http://www.independent.co.uk/news/uk/politics/peerages-of-millionaire-party-donors-are-held-up-by-new-inquiry-468687/html [accessed 22/09/12]

Woolhandler S, Campbell T, Himmelstein DU (2003) Costs of Health Care Administration in the United States and Canada. *N Engl J Med* 2003, 768–75 (21 August)

Wootton I (2009) Privatisation in the healthcare industry. AEMH conference, Brussels, 7 May, PWC, http://www.aemh.org/pdf/PrivatisationinHealthcareIndustry_AEMH7/pdf [accessed 20/01/13]

World Bank (1987) Financing Health Services in developing Countries: An Agenda for Reform. Washington DC

World Bank (1993) *Investing in Health.* World Development Report, Washington DC

World Bank (1997) Health, Nutrition, Population (HNP) Sector Strategy. World Bank, Washington DC, http://go.worldbank.org/1BO4F9LL30

World Bank (2000) The role of the World Bank. Public and Private Initiatives, World Bank web site, http://www.worldbank.org/html/extdr/hnp/health/ppi/contents.htm [accessed 08/07/02]

World Bank (2001a) Mental health at a glance, http://www.worldbank.org/hnp [accessed 07/03/03]

World Bank (2001b) World Bank activities and position on aging. June, Washington DC, http://www.un.org/esa/socdev/ageing/worldbank200106.htm [accessed 22/02/03]

World Bank (2003a) World Bank seeks to ensure CAFTA helps reduce poverty. Press release, 9 January, Web.worldbank.org/WBSITE/EXTERNAL/NEWS [accessed 02/06/03]

World Bank (2003b) *World Development Report 2004.* 21 September, World Bank, Washington DC

World Bank (2007a) Detailed Implementation Review, India Health Sector. Vol. 2, World Bank, Washington DC, http://siteresources.worldbank.org/INTDOII/Resources/ WB250_Vol2_Web_011508/pdf

World Bank (2007b) Healthy Development. The World Bank Strategy for Health, Nutrition, and Population Results. 24 April, http://siteresources.worldbank.org/ HEALTHNUTRITIONANDPOPULATION/Resources/281627-1154048816360/ HNPStrategyFINALApril302007/pdf

World Bank (2009a) Improving Effectiveness and Outcomes for the Poor in Health, Nutrition, and Population. An Evaluation of World Bank Group Support Since 1997. IEG, World Bank, Washington DC

World Bank (2009b) Implementation of the World Bank's Strategy for Health, Nutrition, and Population (HNP) Results: Achievements, Challenges, and the Way Forward. World Bank, HNP Human Development, Washington DC, 19 March

World Bank (2009c) World Bank responds to new Oxfam health report. http://web.worldbank.org/WBSITE/EXTERNAL/TOPICS/EXTHEALTHNUTRITIONANDP OPULATION/0,,contentMDK:22068718~menuPK:282516~pagePK:64020865~piPK: 149114~theSitePK:282511,00.html [accessed 02/03/13]

World Bank (2010) 2010 Flagship Course on Health Sector Reform and Sustainable Financing (18 October to 5 November). Washington DC, http://wbi.worldbank.org/wbi/ news/2010/09/14/2010-flagship-course-health-sector-reform-and-sustainable-financing-october-18-novem [accessed 02/03/13]

World Bank (2012a) World Bank Program Budget. https://finances.worldbank.org/Budget/ World-Bank-Program-Budget/gprm-cvv7 [accessed 13/03/12]

World Bank (2012b) How we classify countries. World Bank, http://data.worldbank.org/ about/country-classifications [accessed 21/09/12]

World Bank Group (1997a) Sector Strategy, Health, Nutrition and Population. World Bank, Washington DC

Xu K, James C, Carrin G, Muchiri S (2006) An empirical model of access to health care, health care expenditure and impoverishment in Kenya: learning from past reforms and lessons for the future. Discussion Paper No. 3, WHO Health System Financing, Expenditure and Resource Allocation Evidence and Information for Policy (EIP), Geneva

Yach D, von Schirnding YE (1994) Towards a higher priority for health on the development agenda. *Public Health Review* 22(3–4): 339–74

Yeates N (2001) *Globalization and Social Policy.* Sage, London

Yip W, Mahal A (2008) The health care systems of China and India: performance and future challenges. *Health Affairs* 27(4): 921–32 (July–August)

Young S (2008) Outsourcing in public health: a case study of contract failure and its aftermath. *Journal of Health Organisation and Management* 22(5): 446–64

Yuwei Z (2010) More actions needed to sustain MDG progress. *China Daily,* 22 September, http://www.chinadaily.com.cn/cndy/2010-09/22/content_11336791/htm [accessed 25/01/13]

Zanon E (2011) Healthcare across borders: implications of the EU directive on cross-border healthcare for the English NHS. *Eurohealth* 17(2–3): 34–5

Index